Neurology Review for Psychiatrists

Neurology Review for Psychiatrists

Sean I. Savitz, MD
Co-Director, Stroke Program
Assistant Professor of Neurology
Department of Neurology
University of Texas Medical School at Houston
Houston, Texas

Michael Ronthal, MD
Professor of Neurology
Harvard Medical School
Beth Israel Deaconess Medical Center
Boston, Massachusetts

Wolters Kluwer | Lippincott Williams & Wilkins
Health
Philadelphia · Baltimore · New York · London
Buenos Aires · Hong Kong · Sydney · Tokyo

Acquisitions Editor: Charley Mitchell
Managing Editor: Sirkka Howes
Marketing Manager: Kimberly Schonberger
Designer: Teresa Mallon
Compositor: Maryland Composition/ASI

9 8 7 6 5 4 3 2 1

Library of Congress Cataloging-in-Publication Data

Neurology review for psychiatrists / [edited by] Sean I. Savitz, Michael Ronthal.
   p. ; cm.
   Includes bibliographical references and index.
   ISBN 978-0-7817-6666-1
   1. Neurology. 2. Nervous system—Diseases. 3. Psychiatrists. 4. Neuropsychiatry. I. Savitz, Sean I. II. Ronthal, Michael, 1938-
   [DNLM: 1. Nervous System Diseases—Problems and Exercises. 2. Neurobehavioral Manifestations—Problems and Exercises. 3. Neurologic Examination—methods—Problems and Exercises. WL 18.2 N4929 2009]
   RC346.N4558 2009
   616.80076—dc22
                      2008033490

DISCLAIMER

Care has been taken to confirm the accuracy of the information present and to describe generally accepted practices. However, the authors, editors, and publisher are not responsible for errors or omissions or for any consequences from application of the information in this book and make no warranty, expressed or implied, with respect to the currency, completeness, or accuracy of the contents of the publication. Application of this information in a particular situation remains the professional responsibility of the practitioner; the clinical treatments described and recommended may not be considered absolute and universal recommendations.

The authors, editors, and publisher have exerted every effort to ensure that drug selection and dosage set forth in this text are in accordance with the current recommendations and practice at the time of publication. However, in view of ongoing research, changes in government regulations, and the constant flow of information relating to drug therapy and drug reactions, the reader is urged to check the package insert for each drug for any change in indications and dosage and for added warnings and precautions. This is particularly important when the recommended agent is a new or infrequently employed drug.

Some drugs and medical devices presented in this publication have Food and Drug Administration (FDA) clearance for limited use in restricted research settings. It is the responsibility of the health care provider to ascertain the FDA status of each drug or device planned for use in their clinical practice.

To purchase additional copies of this book, call our customer service department at (800) 638-3030 or fax orders to (301) 223-2320. International customers should call (301) 223-2300.

Visit Lippincott Williams & Wilkins on the Internet: http://www.lww.com. Lippincott Williams & Wilkins customer service representatives are available from 8:30 am to 6:00 pm, EST.

Contents

Preface

Aspiring psychiatrists have to be well versed in organic neurology because many patients who have psychiatric sounding symptoms have underlying organic neurological dysfunction. The American Board of Psychiatry and Neurology recognizes this need and requires neurological training in the psychiatric residency and also, for Board Certification, candidates have to pass an examination in Neurology on Part 1 of their Boards.

How do we teach neurology? Clearly a hands on experience and broad exposure is best, but the budding psychiatrist in training has only a limited time for rotation on the neurology wards.

This book attacks the problems of teaching neurology by presenting a wide review of neurological subjects in a way that makes the information accessible and pertinent not only for examination purposes but also for daily practice. The novel format of each chapter is designed to easily facilitate learning the key points of diagnosis, investigation and management of neurological patients, particularly those presenting to the psychiatrist.

We have carefully chosen subspecialist authors who are not only excellent clinicians, but also the best teachers in our schools.

Learning neurology should be relatively easy, stimulating and fun if the material is presented in an easily assimilable form! We trust that our objectives have been met in this book.

Sean Savitz
Michael Ronthal
Boston, 2008

Introduction

Psychiatrists and neurologists have much in common – their practice is rooted in the brain, and both disciplines practice the art of listening. The excellent physician listens carefully and, in neurology, a good history leads to the correct diagnosis in about 80% of consultations. Psychiatric diagnoses are made almost entirely by listening and psychiatrists are adept at this, but today medical practice has become rushed and all too often technology dominates: patients often complain that their physician spent the whole interview typing and hardly ever made eye contact! Because we take it for granted that psychiatrists are excellent listeners we have not belabored history taking in this book, but we have provided a framework for neurological evaluation not only of the psychiatric patient with neurological complaints, but also of common neurological complaints in the general patient population.

Neurology may be the last clinical discipline in which, after a lengthy and complete history, the diagnosis is confirmed or made based on the hands-on clinical examination. It's possible nowadays to be a cardiologist or pulmonologist and never even use the stethoscope, relying on ultrasound and imaging to make the diagnosis! Examining is a skill that can be acquired only by constant practice and just as neurology residents are required to spend time on the psychiatry ward so too do budding psychiatrists spend time on the neurology wards. That time should be utilized to examine as many patients as possible. The resident should take an active rather than a passive role.

We have adopted a symptom based approach to neurological diagnosis and the technique of examining a patient is described. The bedside examination should lead one to a diagnosis of the site of pathology and in some instances that clinical diagnosis stands on its own. In other cases further studies are required to elucidate the pathological process, but unless one has a pretty good idea of "where its sick", the imaging may be of the wrong site. Too often patients are seen in the neurology clinic clutching an array of MRI studies, all missing the diagnosis because the wrong site was studied. Prudently chosen investigations lead us to a diagnosis of "what's wrong"—the pathological diagnosis.

It is estimated that around 15% of the costs of medical care are generated by "wrong" tests. The trigger for these unnecessary and costly tests is partly ignorance and partly physician and patient anxiety. A good neurological evaluation based on a superb history and examination may be worth more than a couple of MRI examinations and is certainly a lot cheaper.

The major disease categories have been described in the various chapters and, nowadays, a book like this would be incomplete without a review and approach to the biochemistry and genetics of neurological and psychiatric physiology and pharmacology. Equally, with the approaching baby boom, cognitive dysfunction will be more prevalent as the population ages and significant space has been devoted to cognitive neurology.

We trust that this book will be a constant companion at the bedside, and in the clinic. After reading it, we hope the physician will be sensitized to so-called "red flags" denoting primary neurological causes for psychiatric symptomatology and have the tools to localize and evaluate the various clinical syndromes.

Contributors

Michael P. Alexander, MD
Professor of Neurology, Harvard Medical School, Boston, Massachusetts; Rehabilitation Neurology, Youville Hospital, Cambridge, Massachusetts

Alexandra Degenhardt, MD, MMSc
Director, Multiple Sclerosis Center, Department of Neurology and Rehabilitation, New York Methodist Hospital; Weill Medical College Affiliate, Cornell University Brooklyn, New York

Patricia E. Greenstein, MB, BCh
Assistant Professor of Neurology, Harvard Medical School; Staff Neurologist, Beth Israel Deaconess Medical Center, Boston, Massachusetts

Harpreet K. Grewal, MD
Resident in Neurology, University of Texas-Houston, Houston, Texas

Jai Grewal, MD
Department of Neuro-oncology, Neurological Surgery, P.C., Long Island, New York; Attending Physician, South Nassau Communities Hospital, Oceanside, New York

Sara J. Hoffschmidt, PhD
Instructor in Neurology, Harvard Medical School; Staff Neuropsychologist, Division of Behavioral Neurology, Beth Israel Deaconess Medical Center, Boston, Massachusetts

Santosh Kesari, MD, PhD
Assistant Professor of Neurology, Harvard Medical School; Department of Neurology, Brigham & Women's Hospital, Boston, Massachusetts

Nancy K. Madigan, PhD
Instructor in Neurology, Harvard Medical School; Staff Neuropsychologist, Division of Behavioral Neurology, Beth Israel Deaconess Medical Center, Boston, Massachusetts

Bushra Malik, MD
Fellow in Headache and Pain, Department of Neurology, Cleveland Clinic Foundation, Cleveland, Ohio

Jean K. Matheson, MD
Associate Professor of Neurology, Harvard Medical School; Neurologist, Beth Israel Deaconess Medical Center, Boston, Massachusetts

Laura C. Miller, MD
Adult Neurology and Epilepsy, Suiter Neuroscience Institute, Sacramento, California

Josef Parvizi, MD, PhD
Clinical Fellow in Neurology, University of California, Los Angeles, Los Angeles, California

Daniel Z. Press, MD
Assistant Professor of Neurology, Harvard Medical School; Staff Neurologist, Beth Israel Deaconess Medical Center, Boston, Massachusetts

David B. Robinson, MD
Research Fellow, Behavioral Neurology Unit, Harvard Medical School; Beth Israel Deaconess Medical Center, Boston, Massachusetts

Ludy C. Shih, MD
Clinical Fellow in Neurology, Harvard Medical School; Beth Israel Deaconess Medical Center, Boston, Massachusetts

Nicholas J. Silvestri, MD
Clinical Fellow in Neurology, Harvard Medical School; Resident in Neurology, Beth Israel Deaconess Medical Center, Boston, Massachusetts

Magdi M. Sobeih, MD
Instructor of Neurology, Harvard University Medical School; Assistant in Neurology, The Children's Hospital, Boston, Massachusetts

Mark Stillman, MD
Head, Section of Headache and Facial Pain, Cleveland Clinic Foundation, Cleveland, Ohio

Alan C. Swann, MD
Pat R. Rutherford, Jr. Chair, Professor and Vice-Chair for Research, Department of Psychiatry, University of Texas Medical School; Harris County Psychiatric Center, Houston, Texas

Daniel Tarsy, MD
Professor of Neurology, Harvard Medical School; Vice Chair, Department of Neurology, Beth Israel Deaconess Medical Center, Boston, Massachusetts

Andrew W. Tarulli, MD
Instructor of Neurology, Harvard Medical School; Neurologist, Beth Israel Deaconess Medical Center, Boston, Massachusetts

Stephen J. Traub, MD
Assistant Professor of Medicine, Division of Emergency Medicine, Harvard Medical School; Co-Director, Division of Toxicology, Department of Emergency Medicine, Beth Israel Deaconess Medical Center, Boston, Massachusetts

Neurology Review for Psychiatrists

Symptom-Oriented Neurological Problems

CHAPTER 1

Cranial Nerve Symptoms

Michael Ronthal • Sean I. Savitz

■ INTRODUCTION

This chapter covers common symptoms referable to dysfunction of the cranial nerves or their proximal or distal connections. For certain symptoms, such as dizziness, for example, the vestibular nerve may be the site of pathology or the upper neuron pathways within the brainstem/cerebellum controlling the vestibular system. For each symptom, an approach to the evaluation of the cranial nerves involved and the differential diagnosis are provided. Overall, the nuclei for cranial nerves II to XII can be found scattered throughout the brainstem (Fig. 1.1). Specific symptoms are caused by disorders of the upper brainstem (visual), middle brainstem (facial), and lower brainstem (dysphagia). Details of each symptom are described in the following sections.

■ DOUBLE VISION

The normal upper motor neuron (UMN) control of eye movements results in smooth conjugate gaze. Diplopia, or double vision, implies a defect in the yoking mechanism of the eyes, and that in turn implies a defect in the lower motor neuron (LMN) mechanism.

The LMN stretches from and includes the ocular motor nuclei; the third, fourth, and sixth cranial nerves; the neuromuscular junctions; and the external ocular muscles.

Each muscle has a specific direction of pull, and weakness secondary to a defect somewhere along the line results in misalignment of the eyeball with resultant diplopia when the patient looks in the direction of gaze controlled by that muscle. The lateral or external rectus is applied by the sixth nerve on each side. The superior oblique is supplied by the fourth, or trochlear, nerve. All other muscles are innervated by the third nerve, which also supplies the pupil and the levator of the eyelid.

Clinical Examination

Patients may clearly describe a symptom as double vision, or they may simply complain of blurriness. To sort this out, two key questions should be asked: "What do you see?" and "What happens if you close one eye?" Resolution of the blurriness if one or the other eye is closed suggests that the true symptom is diplopia.

The next step in analysis is to sort out monocular from binocular diplopia. If vision is normal when using one eye only yet blurred or doubled when using the alternate eye only, the diagnosis is monocular diplopia, which implies a local ophthalmological problem rather than a neurological one.

If the diplopia is truly binocular, the examination should sort out which eye is involved and which muscle is weak.

A test object, for example, a finger or light source, is held before the patient in the prime directions of gaze. Horizontally, it will be to left and right, but for vertical gaze, given the direc-

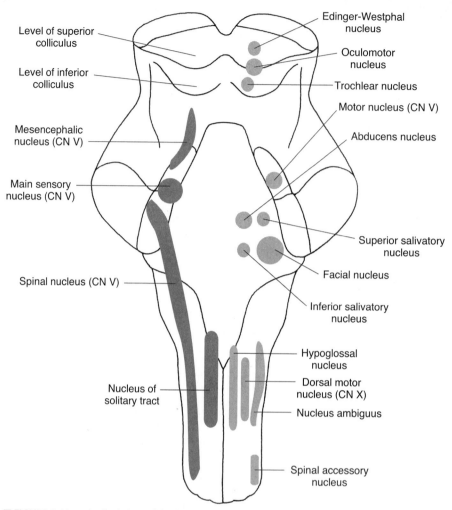

■ FIGURE 1.1 Longitudinal view of the brainstem depicting the position and arrangement of the sensory, motor, and autonomic cell groups that comprise first- and second-order neurons associated with cranial nerves. Motor nuclei of cranial nerves (CNs) III, IV, VI, and XII are located near the midline. Motor nuclei of CNs V, VII, IX, X (nucleus ambiguous for nerves IX and X), and XI are located slightly lateral to neurons associated with CNs III, IV, VI, and XII. Autonomic nuclei are derived from CNs III (Edinger-Westphal nucleus), VII (superior salivatory nucleus), IX (inferior salivatory nucleus), and X (dorsal motor nucleus) and are situated slightly more laterally. Sensory neurons lie lateral to motor neurons. Neurons for CNs IX and X innervate the general viscera. CNs I (not shown in this figure), VII, IX, and X include special visceral afferernt components (involving the nucleus of the solitary tract [solitary nucleus] for each of these nerves except CN I). The nerves innervating the somatic components of the head and face are found among CNs V (main sensory nucleus of SN V), IX, and X (spinal nucleus of CN V receives inputs from CNs IX and X). CNs II (optic) and VIII (auditory vestibular) are not shown in this illustration. (Reprinted from Siegel A, Sapru HN. *Essential Neuroscience.* Revised first edition. Philadelphia, Pa: Lippincott Williams & Wilkins; 2006:227, with permission.)

tion of pull of the muscles, as shown in Figure 1.2, the object is held not directly vertically but off to one side. Figure 1.3 shows the distribution of cranial nerves (CNs) VI, IV, and III.

The "false" object, that is, the object subtended by the weak eye, is always external to the "true" object. It remains to sort out which object is indeed "false." This can be ascertained by closing one eye and asking which image disappears, or, better still by using a red glass. The red glass is, by convention, held over the right eye. Objects seen with the right eye will be red, those

External Ocular Muscles

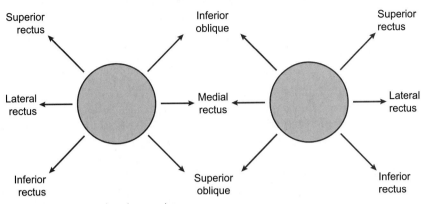

■ FIGURE 1.2 External ocular muscles.

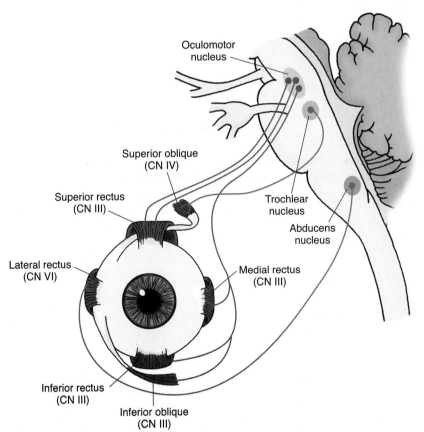

■ FIGURE 1.3 Origin and distribution of cranial nerves (CNs) VI, IV, and III, which innervate extraocular eye muscles. The focus of the *upper part* of this figure includes the abducens (CN VI) nerve of the oculomotor (CN III) nerve, which is essential for horizontal gaze. The *lower part* of this figure depicts the muscles of the eye and their relationship with CNs III, IV, and VI. (Reprinted from Siegel A, Sapru HN. *Essential Neuroscience.* Revised first edition. Philadelphia: Lippincott Williams & Wilkins; 2006:241, with permission.)

with the left eye normal in color. In the absence of diplopia the object will appear single and pink. Each direction of gaze is tested and the weak muscle diagnosed.

Once diplopia in a specific direction of gaze is established, the test object should be held in position for a minute or two to establish or deny a fatigue or myasthenic response. If the two perceived objects separate progressively, the diagnosis is ocular myasthenia.

Third Nerve Palsy

A third nerve lesion may be complete or partial. A partial deficit, that is, when only some of the muscles innervated by the nerve are weak, suggests that the lesion is in either the midbrain or retrobulbar area. The third nerve nucleus is large, and pathology such as tiny infarctions can affect only part of the nerve. From the nucleus itself, strands of nerve course ventrally through the brainstem; a partial lesion of these strands is termed a fascicular third nerve palsy.

From the ventral brainstem the nerve courses forward to the cavernous sinus and through it to the superior orbital fissure, where it divides into a superior division to levator palpebrae and superior rectus and an inferior division that then breaks up to supply the various extraocular muscles. Local pathological processes in the orbit should be excluded by imaging, and activity tests in the blood should be done to exclude an inflammatory cause such as arteritis.

A lesion along the course of the third nerve at the base of the brain usually results in a complete palsy with ptosis, sparing of lateral movement of the eyeball, and intorsion movement of the eyeball when looking downward past the horizontal meridian. The differential diagnosis includes a posterior communicating aneurysm compressing the nerve or a meningitic process. If the pupil is spared, the cause is likely diabetes with microvascular infarction ("pupil-sparing third"). Imaging, including angiography and a spinal tap, if there is no aneurysm, are indicated.

Fourth Nerve Palsy

Diplopia will be present when looking down and inward. If the head is tilted to one or the other side, it may be possible to see misalignment of the eyeballs.

The nerve is thin and has a tortuous course, emerging from the dorsal brainstem and coursing around it before passing anteriorly at the base in the direction of the orbit. Usually the cause of a fourth nerve lesion is obscure; it could be traumatic, infective, postinfective, or microvascular in origin.

Sixth Nerve Palsy

Diplopia is present on lateral gaze. The causes of a sixth nerve palsy are legion, and its presence, as with any of the previously described syndromes, triggers extensive imaging, blood studies, and a spinal fluid study.

Neuromuscular Junction

Myasthenia results in fluctuating diplopia and may or may not be associated with weakness of other somatic muscles. Reversal of an overt external ocular muscle palsy or just diplopia by an intravenous injection of edrophonium confirms the diagnosis. The drug should be administered with electrocardiographic control, and atropine should be at the bedside as a muscarinic antidote in case of severe bradycardia. The response for a positive test should be dramatic and not equivocal.

Botulism paralyzes the eye muscles and can also affect the pupil, a sign that is never seen in myasthenia. There is often a history of ingestion of imperfectly preserved food.

Ocular Muscles

Orbital myositis is an inflammatory myopathy affecting the extraocular muscles. Pain on eye movement is the clue, and imaging of the orbit may show swollen or edematous muscles. It responds to steroids.

■ VISUAL LOSS

As with the analysis of diplopia, loss of vision may be binocular, which implies a retrobulbar problem, or monocular, which implies a pathological condition locally in the eye or optic nerve. Retrobulbar problems affect the fields of vision of both eyes and have specific patterns.

Clinical Examination

If we are to evaluate visual loss, we must have reliable methods to measure vision. A reading card is used for near vision, and for distant vision a Snellen chart suffices. Refractive errors should be compensated for with appropriate spectacles; if these are not available, a pinhole eliminates refractive error. Subtle visual loss can be appreciated by testing color vision—a red object looks red with the normal eye or field and washed-out pink or black in the defective areas.

If there is a mild monocular visual loss, the swinging flashlight test may demonstrate it. The very bright flashlight is shone into one eye, which results in equal constriction of both the ipsilateral and contralateral pupils. The beam of the flashlight is then switched to the contralateral eye and trained on that eye for a short while. If the pupil dilates, that eye has a defect of the afferent loop of the reflex. If not, the test is repeated, starting on the side opposite to the initial trial.

The visual fields need to be evaluated. One can simply "wiggle" fingers in various parts of the fields, but this is relatively inaccurate; a more reliable test would be to use a small red object to test each eye separately. The test object is slowly moved from the periphery to the focal point around the compass. To test the accuracy of the examination, which requires patient cooperation, it is worthwhile to map the blind spot, which is subtended by the optic nerve head. It is on the horizontal meridian and lateral to the focal point.

The most accurate field analysis is done with a perimeter operated by a trained technician (Figs. 1.4 and 1.5).

Monocular Visual Loss

Sudden-onset monocular visual loss may be vascular or demyelinating in origin. Ischemic optic neuropathy is hypertension-linked and represents an infarct of the optic nerve. Fundoscopy may be normal, or with central retinal artery occlusion the retina becomes gray with a cherry red spot at the macula.

Retinal vein occlusion usually does not produce extremes of visual loss, such as with arteriolar pathology, but certainly affects vision, and fundoscopy reveals dilated veins and hemorrhagic lesion in the retina.

Demyelinating optic neuritis results in a large central scotoma or even blindness. The inflammatory process may cause swelling of the optic disc (papillitis), but if the demyelination is more posteriorly situated, the optic nerve looks normal. These patients frequently complain of pain on eyeball movement.

Ophthalmological causes such as macular edema will yield to retinoscopy for diagnosis.

Gradual-onset monocular visual loss could be due to progressive pathology such as a meningioma in the optic canal or growing from the sphenoid wing, but an ophthalmological cause such as glaucoma, which causes arcuate scotomas, simple cataract, or uveitis must be excluded by the ophthalmologist.

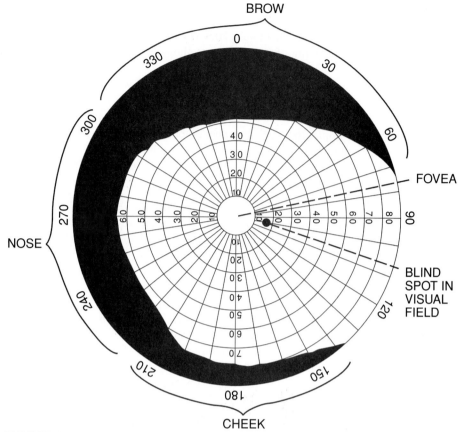

■ **FIGURE 1.4** Perimetric chart.

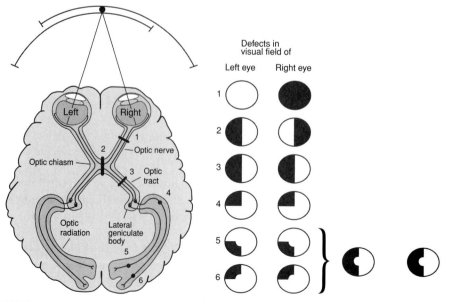

■ **FIGURE 1.5** Visual pathways.

Binocular Visual Loss

Bitemporal hemianopia is usually due to chiasmatic compression by a pituitary tumor, but other compressive lesions can do the same. These include schwannoma, meningioma, and occasionally a giant aneurysm.

Homonymous hemianopia is due to a lesion in the optic tract and is of varied etiology. If the defects are congruous, that is, almost identical, the lesion is likely posterior in the occipital lobe. If incongruous, the pathological condition will be found more anteriorly in the optic tract. The Meyer loop courses through the posterior temporal lobe and causes a homonymous upper quadrantic loss.

The pathology diagnosis will be suspected based on the tempo of the deficit (acute suggests a stroke of sorts), imaging, and, if necessary, spinal fluid examination.

■ FACIAL PAIN

Facial pain may be primarily neurogenic or arise from a pathological condition at the skull base, sinuses, teeth, or temporomandibular joint (Fig. 1.6).

Trigeminal neuralgia (tic douloureux) is seen usually in patients over the age of 50 and is a syndrome of symptoms without signs. Episodes of pain may last weeks to months, and the

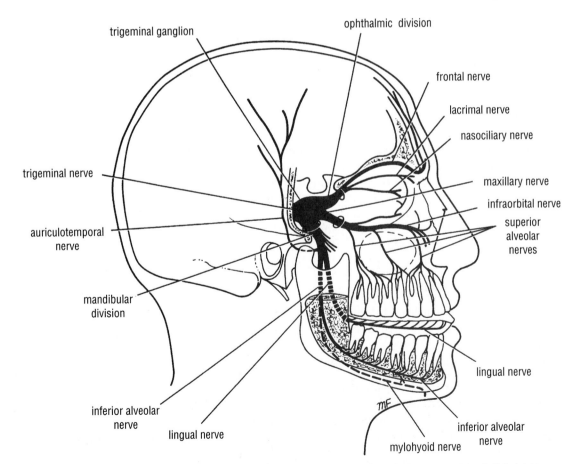

■ **FIGURE 1.6** Distribution of the trigeminal nerve. (Reprinted from Snell RS. *Clinical Anatomy.* 7th ed. Philadelphia: Lippincott Williams & Wilkins; 2003, with permission.)

pain-free intervals tend to shorten with the passage of time. The pain may be in the distribution of any of the three major divisions of the trigeminal nerve, very rarely affects more than one division, and is never bilateral. The pain is described as severe, lancinating, recurrent jabs occurring spontaneously or if a "trigger" area is stimulated. Even wind blowing on the face could be a trigger. The patient indicates the area involved not by touching or rubbing it, but by pointing. A response to carbamazepine, which usually works at least initially, is confirmatory. Imaging is negative apart from the occasional patient with an ectatic vessel syndrome when the vessels at the base of the brain may impinge on the nerve. If anticonvulsants fail to control the pain, injection therapy, high-frequency radiotherapy locally, or stereotactic radiotherapy may help.

In younger patients, trigeminal neuralgia may be a sign of demyelinating disease, such as multiple sclerosis.

If a neurological deficit is present, that is, a defect of sensation or motor function in the distribution of the trigeminal nerve, the diagnosis is "trigeminal neuropathy" rather than "trigeminal neuralgia." If neuropathy is diagnosed, the nerve should be imaged along its length for compressive or infiltrative lesions, blood should be checked for systemic disease, and a spinal tap should be considered to diagnose a possible meningitic process.

Temporomandibular joint dysfunction (Costens syndrome) may mimic trigeminal neuralgia in that the pain is sudden and lancinating and referred to the face. It may be triggered by jaw movement or chewing. One may feel a clicking sensation with jaw opening, and there is local tenderness. Referral to a dentist specializing in Costens syndrome is the preferred route of treatment.

Postherpetic neuralgia is a constant, often severe facial pain in the distribution of one of the branches of the trigeminal nerve. There is a history of shingles; small, often depigmented, round skin lesions are present, and each lesion is insensitive to pain despite the complaint. Pregabalin in gradually increasing doses is often effective.

Cluster headache is a recurrent episodic, time-locked syndrome of pain around the orbit associated with tearing of the eye, injection of the conjunctiva, ptosis, and a small pupil. It responds to triptan drugs, and calcium channel blockers, such as verapamil, are prophylactic.

Lower-half headache is a migraine variant with episodes of throbbing facial pain. It responds to triptan drugs.

If the clinical syndrome does not fit one of those described previously and investigation for putative trigeminal neuropathy is negative, the diagnosis becomes "atypical facial pain." Approximately 80% of these patients respond to an antidepressant; the cause might be, but is not necessarily, psychogenic. Patients are often tempted to undergo surgical procedures. If no pathological condition is found and the history is not that of trigeminal neuralgia, the patient should be counseled against surgery, which could result in a numb face with persistent pain (anesthesia dolorosum), a worse state than the original complaint.

■ FACIAL WEAKNESS

The key point in diagnosis is to decide if facial weakness is central, that is, UMN in origin, or peripheral, that is, LMN in origin. Figure 1.7 shows the distribution of the facial nerve.

Upper Motor Neuron Facial Weakness

Because there are two central paths that control facial movement—one for pure volitional activity and one for emotional activation of the facial muscles—and it is highly unlikely that both will be affected simultaneously, dissociation of volitional from emotional facial weakness makes the diagnosis of UMN pathology. Thus, if movement is normal when the patient smiles in response to a humorous stimulus, yet one side of the face is slower to react or reacts incompletely or not at all when the patient is asked to show the teeth, dissociation is present and the pathological condition is central.

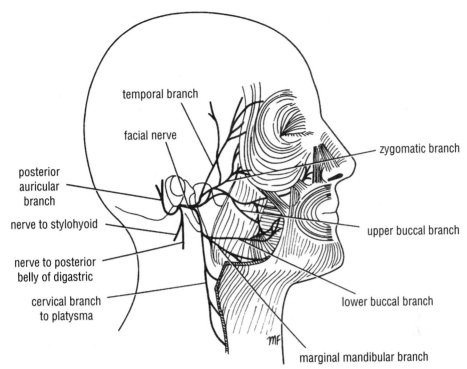

■ **FIGURE 1.7** Distribution of the facial nerve. (Reprinted from Snell RS. *Clinical Anatomy*. 7th ed. Philadelphia: Lippincott Williams & Wilkins; 2003, with permission.)

Bilateral UMN weakness, as in pseudobulbar palsy, is usually associated with a snout reflex—the lips are tapped with a reflex hammer and they pucker.

The upper part of the face (frontalis muscle) is innervated bilaterally, and sparing of the forehead may be suggestive of UMN dysfunction, but is not pathognomonic in that a partial or branch peripheral facial nerve lesion could spare the forehead.

Sudden onset of UMN facial weakness suggests stroke as the likely pathological condition, whereas a slowly progressive dysfunction is more in keeping with a slowly progressive pathological condition such as a tumor.

Lower Motor Neuron Facial Weakness

Weakness, whatever its degree, is present equally on both volition and emotional activation. Usually all divisions of the nerve are affected equally. Weakness of eye closure is tested by asking the patient to resist the examiner's attempts to pry open the eyelids with the fingers; if weakness is present, it usually has an LMN origin.

Hyperacusis from paralysis of the stapedius and loss of taste sensation on the ipsilateral tongue support a peripheral LMN localization. A contralateral hemiparesis suggests that the lesion is within the brainstem.

Bell's palsy is a rapidly progressive, idiopathic LMN facial weakness coming on over a day or two and sometimes associated with pain below and behind the earlobe. It may be infective in origin and is treated with an oral steroid and valacyclovir, based on the notion that herpes simplex is a likely pathogen. Serology for borreliosis should be checked, and inspection of the external auditory meatus will diagnose varicella or geniculate herpes by virtue of the finding of vesicles.

If the weakness does not improve after a month or so, imaging should be done to exclude a surgical cause.

Bilateral LMN facial weakness has a wide differential, but Lyme disease and sarcoidosis are at the top of the list.

■ DIZZINESS

The subjective complaint of dizziness is nonspecific, and one must be sure to decipher exactly what the patient means. It is convenient to separate the symptom into a sensation of spinning or movement, usually signifying a vestibular dysfunction, from nonspecific sensations such as light-headedness, which have many triggers.

Vertigo is, by definition, a sensation of movement in relationship to the environment. A spinning sensation almost always implicates the peripheral vestibular system or vestibular connections in the posterior fossa. Vestibular dysfunction is accompanied by nystagmus, a to-and-fro conjugate movement of the eyes in the horizontal or vertical plains or in a rotary fashion, and the character and direction of the nystagmus yields diagnostic clues. Nystagmus is named according to the quick or jerk phase, which is really the corrective movement and is a normal part of the eye movement. The slow phase or drift is due to vestibular imbalance.

Central Vertigo

The prime clue to a central pathological process is the presence of other central signs such as sensory loss, sudden headache, or other cranial neuropathies. Nystagmus beating to both right and left or with a spontaneous rotary component is highly suggestive of a central dysfunction in the brainstem or cerebellum. Upbeating or downbeating nystagmus is often due to a central disorder.

Sudden headache, ataxia, and nystagmus should always prompt urgent imaging to exclude a cerebellar hemorrhage or infarction, which are both treatable, and, if large, potentially life threatening.

Occasionally a focal seizure arising in one of the temporal lobes can present with a sensation of spinning.

If a central cause of vertigo is suspected, the brain should be imaged with computed tomography (CT), and, if hemorrhage is excluded, magnetic resonance imaging (MRI) is mandatory to assess for infarction or other structural abnormality. Acute vertigo that has a suspected central cause should immediately prompt an acute stroke evaluation. Misdiagnosis of cerebellar infarction can occur in patients with vertigo either in isolation or in conjunction with nonspecific symptoms, such as nausea or headache.

Peripheral Vertigo

Vestibular neuronopathy, or as it is sometimes called, labyrinthitis, is a self-limiting syndrome of rapid onset and characterized by a sense of spinning aggravated by movement and associated with sweating, pallor, and nausea and/or vomiting. Presumably it is a viral infection of sorts, but this has never been proved. Hearing is intact, and there is no tinnitus. If the symptoms persist for more than 2 weeks, imaging for other causes is indicated.

Ménière syndrome is characterized by repeated episodes of vertigo, nystagmus, pallor, and sweating associated with hearing loss, a feeling of fullness in the ears, and tinnitus. The diagnosis can be established by sophisticated hearing tests. The pathology is likened to hydrocephalus in the brain, referred to as hydrops.

Positional vertigo could be central in origin; however, if positional testing is positive, with a short latent period and fatigue of both the nystagmus and vertigo when the head is held 30 degrees below the horizontal and turned to one or the other side, the diagnosis is benign paroxysmal positional vertigo. The pathological process is thought to be migration of an otolith (canalith) from the saccule into a semicircular canal. The fleck of calcium may be repositioned by performing the Epley maneuver (http://www.aan.com/guidelines) or by referring for vestibular physical therapy.

Another form of postural vertigo for which no organic cause can be found, despite studies in a neuro-otological laboratory, has been labeled phobic postural vertigo and may respond to psychotherapy.

Chronic vestibulopathy is a label used for patients with vestibular dysfunction of unknown origin. They may have nystagmus or may veer to the side of the vestibulopathy when walking; this directional deviation can be tested by asking the patient to high step on a spot with the eyes closed—there is gradual turning toward the pathological side.

Vertebrobasilar disease is often invoked as a cause of vertigo, but transient posterior circulation ischemia is very rare. If the vertigo is associated with diplopia, or long tract signs or symptoms, the diagnosis could be viable.

A vestibular schwannoma is often considered in the differential diagnosis of vestibulopathy, but again this is a very unlikely diagnosis. Schwannomas present with deafness, and only if very large, such that they put pressure on the brainstem, do they trigger vertigo.

A neuro-otological laboratory can be used to test for hearing loss and to perform sophisticated vestibular studies.

There is no specific symptomatic treatment for vertigo. Mild sedatives help a bit, and meclizine is often prescribed because of its anticholinergic properties, but it is sedating and not tolerated by some patients. It usually is ineffective.

Nonspecific Dizziness

Dizziness that is not particularly a feeling of rotation can be caused by cardiorespiratory problems and could be the first symptom of, perhaps, syncope secondary to a cardiac arrhythmia. Hypoglycemia should be excluded. Postural hypotension should be excluded at the bedside.

In the office, if nothing specific is found, part of the examination is to attempt to reproduce the symptom by forced hyperventilation. If the provocative test is successful, a good symptomatic treatment is propranolol, which blocks somatic anxiety.

A vague feeling of imbalance may be triggered by spasm of the posterior cervical musculature, usually part of cervical spondylosis. This syndrome has been called cervical vertigo, but the sensation is never one of spinning or rotation. It responds to symptomatic treatment for spondylosis with local heat, massage, collar, and muscle relaxant drugs such as metaxalone.

■ DYSPHAGIA (FIG. 1.8)

Significant dysphagia is a major handicap. The "joy of eating" is lost. There may be weight loss from poor nutrition. There is the risk of aspiration.

Difficulty with swallowing may be neurogenic or have its cause in the gastrointestinal tract. The key question in the history is: "Where does the food stick?" Patients with esophageal problems are usually able to localize the site of dysfunction or obstruction with uncanny accuracy. If the patient points to the chest, further investigation should be performed by the gastrointestinal specialist.

If the patient points to the throat, the cause is likely to be neurogenic.

Swallowing has a voluntary phase when the food is chewed and the tongue propels it to the posterior pharynx. The larynx rises reflexively, the airway is closed by the epiglottis, the soft palate rises to block the nasal passage, and the food bypasses airways to the origin of the esophagus and is then propelled downward.

Problems with the voluntary phase suggest weakness of the muscles of mastication supplied by the mandibular branch of the trigeminal nerve or of the tongue supplied by the hypoglossal nerve. The muscles of mastication can be tested by palpation; the masseter in the cheek and temporalis in the temple region can be felt to be contracting on forced jaw closure. Weakness of the pterygoid causes deviation of the jaw to the side of the weak muscle on opening the mouth. In general, weakness of the muscles of mastication is almost certainly LMN in origin

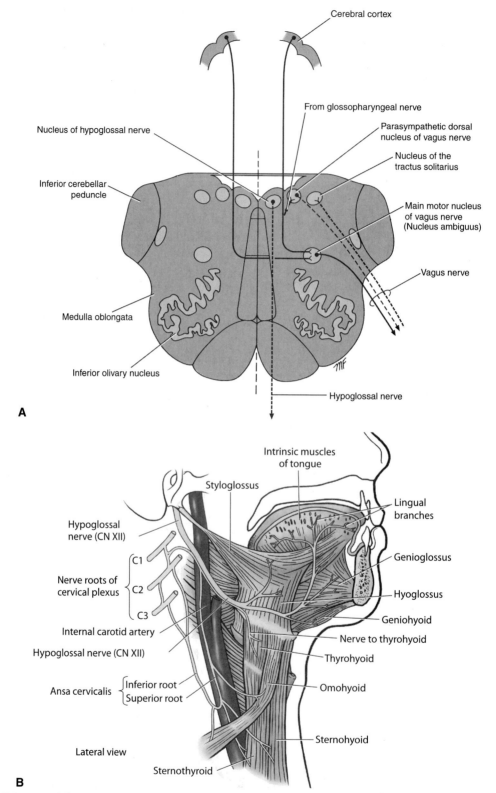

■ FIGURE 1.8 (A) Cranial nerves involved in swallowing have their inputs and outputs located in the medulla. These cranial nerves include CNs IX, X, and XII. Note that the gag reflex is mediated by CN IX (glossopharyngeal nerve) which provides sensory input from the throat to the parasympathetic dorsal nucleus of the vagus nerve. CN X controls movement of the pharynx and CN XII controls movement of the tongue. **(B)** The lower segments CN XII and the muscles it innervates are also shown. (**B** from Agur AMR, Dalley AF. *Grant's Atlas of Anatomy,* 11th ed. Baltimore: Lippincott Williams & Wilkins, 2004.)

and suggests a nuclear lesion in the pons, as in motor neuron disease; a lesion of the mandibular division of the trigeminal nerve whose cause must be sought by further investigation; or a problem at the neuromuscular junction, as in myasthenia. Rarely, a primary myopathy is the cause—oculopharyngeal dystrophy usually affects the pharyngeal muscles rather than the muscles of mastication.

LMN lesions of the 12th nerve caused by weakness of the tongue may be unilateral or bilateral. Unilateral weakness causes tongue deviation toward the side of the weakness. There may be atrophy, with wrinkling of the tongue mucosa because of loss of muscle bulk; fasciculations of the genioglossus may be present, but the tongue should be inspected in situ rather than protruded. Some normal individuals fasciculate with tongue protrusion. Spontaneous fasciculations and atrophy of the tongue suggest, again, a nuclear lesion or pathological condition along the course of the 12th nerve but are unlikely to be found in untreated myasthenia.

UMN lesions of the tongue must be bilateral to produce signs or symptoms. There is no atrophy or fasciculation, but the tongue lies in the floor of the mouth with little movement. In mild cases there is movement, but it is slow when the patient is asked to protrude the tongue and wiggle it from side to side. This is sometimes labeled poverty of tongue movement. Bilateral UMN weakness of the tongue is part of a pseudobulbar palsy. The signs will also include an increased jaw reflex, a snout reflex, and a delayed but vigorous gag reflex. There may be associated long tract motor signs in the limbs.

The swallowing reflex is medullary in origin. Much is made of an absent gag reflex. Many normal people do not gag, just as many normal people have a very brisk gag reflex. After a major hemisphere stroke the swallowing reflex may be inhibited and dysphagia is not uncommon, but whether or not the gag is present is of little relevance in regard to the function of swallowing and risk for aspiration. Swallowing should be tested by getting the patient to swallow—with or without videofluoroscopy. Dysphagia is common in lateral medullary strokes, but with the passage of time it usually improves.

If no obvious cause is found on examination, myasthenia gravis should be considered. The clue is that the complaint gets worse the more the muscles of swallowing are activated. Occasionally a myopathic process in cricopharyngeus is the cause. Ear, nose, and throat surgeons sometimes cut this muscle as a symptomatic treatment for dysphagia with no obvious cause; however, a snip of muscle should always be sent for histopathological examination.

Persistent and severe dysphagia indicates placement of a percutaneous gastric feeding tube for nutrition. A feeding tube of this sort does not prevent aspiration.

CHAPTER 2

Motor System: Weakness

Michael Ronthal

■ INTRODUCTION

The neurological examination begins with inspection.

Look for *abnormal movement, fasciculations, and atrophy*. Abnormal movements affecting whole limbs or parts thereof are discussed in the chapter on movement disorders. Fasciculations are spontaneous sudden, short-lived contractions of fiber groups that "flicker" under the skin. They are essentially nonspecific but are frequent in chronic degenerative diseases such as motor neuron disease. Fasciculations can be a normal phenomenon (benign fasciculation or cramp syndrome) or part of any peripheral neuropathic process.

Look for *atrophy*. The distribution of atrophy gives a clue to the site of pathology—it may be in the distribution of a root (myotome) or of a peripheral nerve.

■ TONE

Hypertonicity suggests central rather than peripheral disease.

Tone is tested by evaluating resistance of the muscles to passive movement. If the patient relaxes completely, the muscles are relatively flaccid and there is no resistance to passive joint movement by the examiner. In the lower limbs, with the patient supine and relaxed, rotate the leg from side to side—the foot should "flop" from side to side at the ankle. If the foot moves en bloc with the leg, there is hypertonia. Again, with the patient relaxed and supine, suddenly jerk the lower limb upward, tugging in the popliteal fossa. If the knee bends smoothly and the heel scrapes the bed, tone is normal; if there is a jerk of the leg upward before it relaxes, there is hypertonicity.

Extrapyramidal Hypertonicity

In the upper limbs a passive rotary movement of the hand on the wrist tests hypertonicity; the patient may be distracted by tapping the other hand on the knee, which will accentuate the hypertonicity or trigger it. The hypertonia of extrapyramidal disease is described as "plastic" or "lead pipe," meaning that the increase in tone is present throughout the range of movement. If a tremor is superimposed on the hypertonicity, the examiner records this as "cogwheeling." Plastic rigidity and cogwheeling are characteristic of Parkinson's disease.

Upper Motor Neuron Hypertonicity

Upper motor neuron (UMN) hypertonicity often shows a marked increase of tone at the beginning of the movement, followed by sudden release of tone. This has been likened to opening a clasp.

Hypotonicity is present in patients with peripheral paralysis and in those with cerebellar dysfunction.

■ WEAKNESS

Weakness as a *symptom* may or may not represent true motor dysfunction and should be confirmed by meticulous examination and documentation of the *signs*.

Although it is important to record the severity or grade of weakness, its *distribution* will usually guide one to the correct diagnosis.

By definition, any particular muscle is weak if the examiner can overcome its action by countering that action by applying pressure close to the joint that the muscle activates and using appropriate testing strength. If testing finger movement, one should use only the fingers to test that movement. If testing a more proximal and stronger muscle, one can use stronger opposing forces.

Grading Weakness

The severity of weakness is often recorded using a somewhat artificial grading system, as follows:

GRADING SYSTEM:
Grade 0 = Paralysis
Grade 1 = Only a flicker of voluntary movement
Grade 2 = Able to move the joint with gravity eliminated
Grade 3 = Able to move the joint against gravity
Grade 4 = "Weak"
Grade 5 = Normal strength

The grading system works reasonably well except for grade 4, which hides a multitude of sins. This is usually expanded in some way—simply the addition of "mild, moderate and severe" makes it more serviceable and reproducible.

Weakness Distribution

The distribution of weakness is of paramount importance.

Lower Motor Neuron Distribution

Proximal weakness in the limb girdles is usually suggestive of a myopathic process and is often accompanied by weakness of neck flexion or neck extension.

Distal weakness in the small muscles of the hands and feet may suggest a more peripheral neuropathic process.

In between proximal is the weakness corresponding to specific *nerves or nerve roots* (Table 2.1).

A *plexopathy* is suggested if the weakness does not fit the distribution of a single nerve root or single nerve. For example, in high pelvic plexopathy there will be weakness of any two of the iliopsoas, quadriceps, and adductor magnus. If all three are involved, radiculopathy is diagnosed; if only one of the three is weak, this suggests a lesion of the nerve supplying that muscle.

Weakness induced by repetitive exercise suggests end-plate disease—myasthenia.

Upper Motor Neuron Distribution

The pattern of UMN distribution weakness is fairly specific. In the upper limbs, when some movement is retained, rather than in cases with complete paralysis, the weakness will preferentially involve the extensor muscles. Thus there is more weakness in the finger abductors, finger and wrist extensors, elbow extensors, and shoulder abductors than in the corresponding flexors.

In the lower limb the pattern of UMN weakness involves hip flexion, foot and toe dorsiflexion, knee flexion, and thigh abduction.

TABLE 2.1 PERIPHERAL NERVE, ROOT DYSFUNCTION

MOVEMENT	MUSCLE	ROOT	NERVE
Shoulder external rotation	Infraspinatus	C4	Suprascapular
Shoulder abduction	First 10 degrees: supraspinatus Rest of movement: deltoid	C4/5	Suprascapular Axillary
Elbow flexion	Biceps and brachialis	C5	Musculocutaneous
Elbow extension	Triceps	C6/7	Radial
Wrist extension (radial side)	Extensor carpi radialis	C6	Radial
Finger extension	Extensor digitorum	C7	Radial (posterior interosseous)
Finger flexion	Flexor digitorum longus	C8	Median (lateral half) Ulnar (medial half)
Hip flexion	Iliopsoas	L2/3	Nerves to (unnamed)
Hip adduction	Adductors	L2/3	Obturator
Knee extension	Quadriceps	L3/4	Femoral
Ankle extension	Tibialis anterior	L4/5	Deep peroneal (branch of sciatic)
Toe extension	Extensor digitorum brevis (mainly)	L5	Deep peroneal
Toe flexion	Flexor digiti brevis	S1	Tibial (branch of sciatic)
Ankle flexion	Gastrocnemius Soleus	S1	Tibial
Knee flexion	Hamstrings	L5	Sciatic
Thigh abduction	Gluteus medius and minimus	L5	Superior gluteal
Thigh extension	Gluteus maximus	L5	Superior gluteal
Foot pronation	Peroneus	L5	Superficial peroneal
Anal contraction	Sphincter	S2, 3, 4	Pudendal

This table has been designed to help with peripheral localization at the bedside. It details the main testable movements, their agonists, their nerve supply, and segmental innervation. Because there is often segmental overlap, the root levels may not be strictly anatomically correct, but for practical purposes this table serves as a good roadmap for peripheral localization and will almost always suffice for clinical diagnosis.

At times, UMN weakness is more proximal than distal, suggesting a high convexity or watershed lesion of the brain in which the representation of proximal movements in both the upper and lower limbs is in apposition.

Cortical lesions can produce very focal distal weakness and mimic a peripheral nerve lesion.

■ REFLEXES

Tendon Reflexes

Tendon reflexes are elicited by tapping the relaxed tendon close to the joint with the reflex hammer so that its muscle moves.

Generalized areflexia as a physical sign should be taken in context. Some patients have never had elicitable reflexes, which is a normal variant, but depressed to absent tendon reflexes are part of peripheral neuropathy or myopathy. At times, in the presence of severe neuropathy, an inadvertent tap on the muscle away from the tendon itself will result in muscle contraction. This is not a reflex but simply a local myotactic response.

Isolated loss of a single reflex suggests either a lesion of the nerve supplying the effector muscle or a segmental root abnormality. See Table 1.1 for segmental levels.

In UMN dysfunction the reflexes will be increased.

The UMN syndrome consists of hypertonia, weakness in UMN distribution, and hyperreflexia.

Plantar Reflexes

The sole is scraped with a relatively sharp object on its lateral aspect. It is not necessary to continue the stimulus over the ball of the foot. Big toe extension and fanning of the other toes is indicative of a *pyramidal tract* lesion. The extensor plantar response is usually associated with contraction of tensor fascia lata on the lateral aspect of the thigh; sometimes this associated reaction helps to confirm the diagnosis when the plantar response itself is thought to be equivocal.

UMN syndrome is not synonymous with a pyramidal tract syndrome—an isolated lesion of the latter causes weakness, hypotonia, and an extensor plantar response. Hyperreflexia and hypertonia are pathophysiologically related to dysfunction and disinhibition of extrapyramidal descending motor tracts.

■ "GIVE-WAY" WEAKNESS

In "give-way" weakness the patient contracts the muscle being tested only momentarily and then allows the muscle to relax. Give-way can be part of a pain syndrome when the movement itself elicits pain, but in the absence of pain it suggests a psychogenic disturbance.

KEY POINTS

1. Evaluation of weakness is a skill that comes only with practice.
2. The interpretation of the significance of the weakness requires an intimate knowledge of motor anatomy, absent which, attempts at localization will fail.
3. Coexisting signs such as the state of the tendon reflexes or sensory signs help in the diagnosis.

CHAPTER 3

Sensory Examination

Michael Ronthal

■ INTRODUCTION

The symptoms of sensory dysfunction vary according to the sensory pathway involved. A good approach is to separate out the main functional pathways. In the peripheral nerve, large fiber (mainly proprioceptive) versus small fiber (mainly nociceptive) function can be distinguished. Centrally, in the spinal cord the functional division is posterior column system versus the ascending spinothalamic tract. Above the level of the thalamus the distinction is not clearly demarcated, but the posterior part of the insular cortex plays a large role in nociceptive sensation.

Broadly speaking, the subjective sensory complaint points to the pathway, but not always to the site of pathology.

Dysfunction in the proprioceptive pathways leads to the subjective complaint of deep aching, gnawing pain; tight, squeezing garter sensations in the limbs; or nondescript, sometimes bizarre paresthesias. For example, patients may report that their fingers feel swollen or ballooned.

The subjective sensation of nociceptive dysfunction is primarily superficial pain that may be sharp and localized, spontaneous, or reactive, or it may present as feelings of heat or coldness. Itching is a form of nociceptive pain.

■ EXAMINATION

Nociceptive Pathway

A new pin is required for the examination of each patient. A proprietary Neurotip serves us well. This is a small plastic rod with a metal point at one end and a blunt plastic tip at the other, but a new safety pin and sharp broken orangewood stick work as well. The pin should be just sharp enough to elicit the sensation of mild pain but not sharp enough to pierce skin.

The patient must be educated to report subjective sensation. Simply pricking with a pin and asking "do you feel this?" is inadequate because a touch sensation will yield a "yes" response, when in fact pinprick sensation is deficient. Test a normal area first to establish the parameters.

In the face, the three divisions of the trigeminal nerve territory are tested—forehead, check, and chin (Fig. 3.1).

For the body, testing starts at the back of the head (C2). Work downward over the angle of the jaw (C3), shoulder (C4), and lateral upper limb (C5 and 6), and then ascend up the medial side of the upper limb to the axilla (T3). Over the anterior chest wall the approximate level of the nipple line demarcates cervical territory (C4) from thoracic territory (T4). Proceed caudally down the trunk, passing over the lower costal margin (T8) and umbilical level (T10) to the groin (T12/L1). Sensation should also be tested posteriorly and paraspinally (Fig. 3.2).

In the lower limb, testing starts in the upper medial thigh, downward over the medial leg, then the lateral leg, the dorsal aspect of the foot, and the lateral foot and then up the posterior midline of the lower limb to the buttock and perianal region. Loss of pinprick sensation over

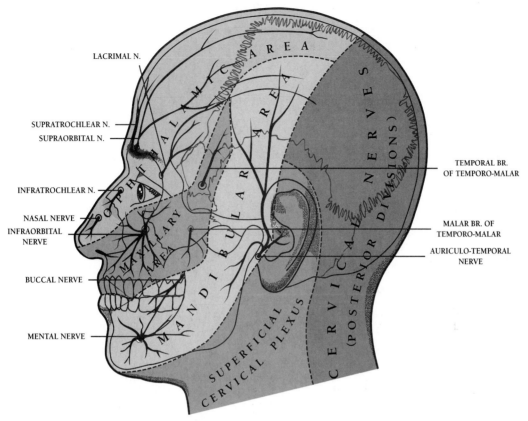

■ FIGURE 3.1 Sensory innervation of the head.

the lateral thigh is never dermatomal because of crowding of dermatomes and almost always is part of a lateral cutaneous femoral nerve syndrome (meralgia).

Having mapped the sensory loss, the likely site of pathology is related to the distribution of anesthesia. The examiner must distinguish nerve lesion, root lesion, tract lesion, or multiples thereof. This requires a detailed understanding of anatomical landmarks (Figs. 3.3–3.5).

Light Touch

A wisp of cotton makes the best sensory tool for light touch. The patient is trained to understand what is being tested. The same anatomical routing is followed as detailed in the discussion of testing of the nociceptive pathway.

Proprioceptive Pathway

Proprioception is tested first at the distal joints. The digit is held by the examiner who grasps it from side to side. The patient, with eyes open, is instructed to report movement as "up" or "down." The patient then closes the eyes. Initial excursions are wide, but for subtle testing only slight movements of the joint are applied by the examiner. In patients with severe proprioceptive loss, more proximal joints can be tested.

Proprioceptive sensation in the skin can be tested by rubbing on an area from distal to proximal or vice versa. The patient, with eyes closed, reports on the direction of movement.

(*Text continues on page 26.*)

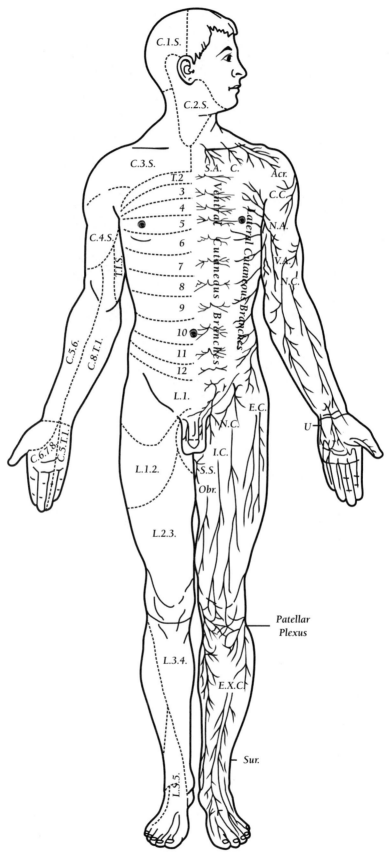

■ **FIGURE 3.2** Dermatomes (*left*) and peripheral (*right*) nerves.

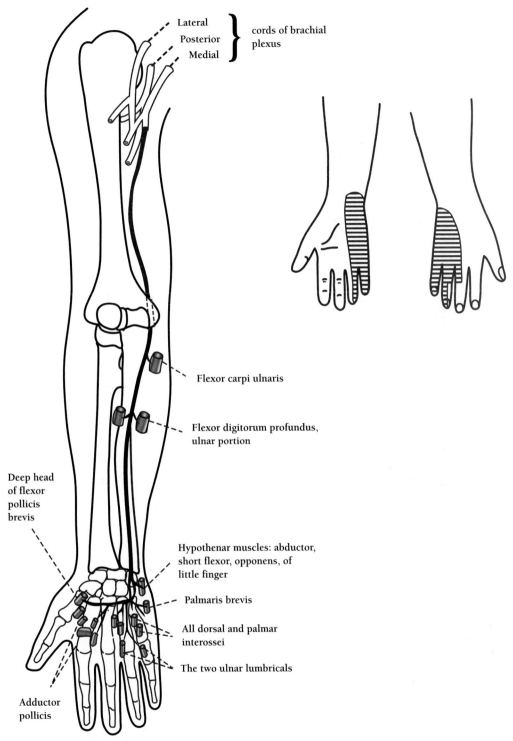

Lateral
Posterior
Medial
} cords of brachial plexus

Flexor carpi ulnaris

Flexor digitorum profundus, ulnar portion

Deep head of flexor pollicis brevis

Hypothenar muscles: abductor, short flexor, opponens, of little finger

Palmaris brevis

All dorsal and palmar interossei

The two ulnar lumbricals

Adductor pollicis

■ **FIGURE 3.3** Ulnar nerve.

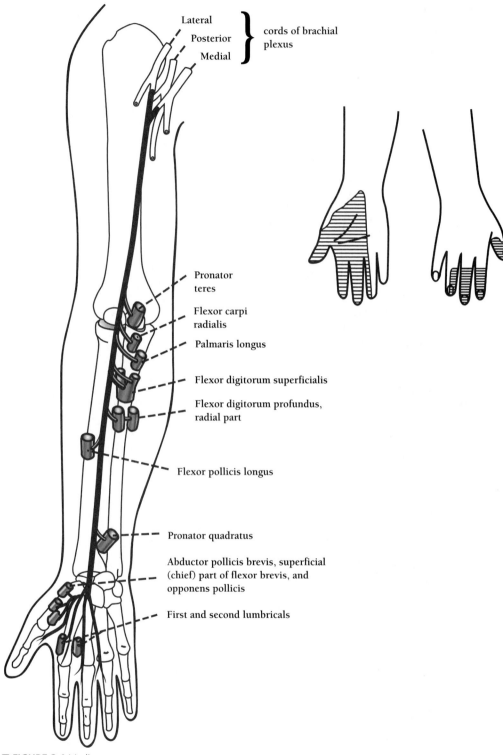

■ **FIGURE 3.4** Median nerve.

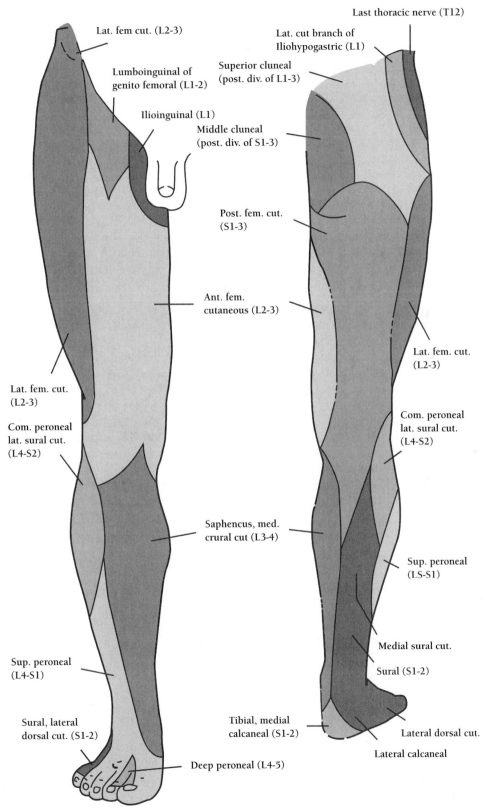

FIGURE 3.5 Cutaneous nerves of the lower limbs.

Vibration Sense

The tuning fork is struck and applied to a bony prominence such as the medial malleolus. The patient reports on perception of vibration. Normally the sensation decays over a short time, and the examiner can compare his or her own perception of vibration in the hand holding the fork with what the patient reports. If vibration fades more rapidly or is absent, as reported by the patient, it is defective.

Localization

Localization depends on the distribution of deficit. It may be in glove or stocking distribution, suggesting a diffuse peripheral neuropathy, or be more discrete, suggesting a single nerve or root dysfunction. A level on the trunk extending caudally to the legs supports the suggestion of a myelopathy. Loss in sacral dermatomes suggests cauda equina localization, whereas saddle sparing suggests central myelopathy. The level of pathology in myelopathic sensory syndromes can be ascertained only by the finding of radiculopathic sensory loss—findings at a simple single level may not help with localization because it could be tract related.

Cortical Sensory Loss

Given normal primary sensation, that is, pinprick, light touch, and proprioception, a defect in recognizing a sensory stimulus is likely to be cortically based. Recognition is "gnosis," and failure of recognition is called agnosia.

Astereognosis is the inability to recognize objects placed in the hand with eyes shut. A coin, key, pencil, paper clip, or comb can be used as the sensory stimulus. Place the object in the patient's hand and ask the patient to identify the object with eyes closed.

More subtle tests of gnosis would be to ask the patient to tell the difference between, say, wool and satin; have the patient compare weights of objects; scratch numbers in the patient's palm and ask the patient to identify them; and touch various areas of the patient's skin with a finger and ask the patient to place his or her (good) forefinger on the exact place stimulated (loss of this function is called autotopagnosia).

Proprioception can also be deficient secondary to a cortical lesion.

KEY POINTS

1. The modalities that can be easily tested are pain (pinprick and temperature), light touch, vibration sense, and position sense.
2. The examination is difficult because the findings are more subjective than objective.
3. The patient needs to be coached to understand exactly what sensation the examiner is testing.
4. Interpretation of the findings requires an excellent knowledge of anatomy.

CHAPTER 4

Gait Disorders

Michael Ronthal

■ INTRODUCTION

Walking is easy—we do it all the time in an unconscious sort of way. Yet, if the gait mechanism breaks down, the consequences may be disastrous.

Of people over the age of 60, 15% have some degree of gait difficulty. Approximately 25% of people over the age of 80 use a mechanical aid for walking. Along with a gait disorder goes the risk for a fall. According to the National Safety Council, the leading cause of death in patients 65 and older is a fall. Accidents are the fifth leading cause of death in people in this age-group; of these, falls account for two thirds of accidental deaths.

Walking is hard-wired in the nervous system. Animals can walk immediately after birth. Humans walk during the first year of life as part of normal development. Newborn infants will produce automatic stepping and placing movements if the sole of the foot is stimulated. Even anencephalic infants will demonstrate automatic walking. Experimentally, decapitated animals can be made to walk on a treadmill. All of this is evidence for the presence of a central spinal pattern generator for walking operating in the absence of higher centers. This central pattern generator can produce a basic locomotor rhythm, but higher centers are required to activate and regulate the rhythm of walking.

There are scattered centers in the brainstem that are activated during walking; by definition, if a region contains neurons that when activated chemically or electrically cause locomotion, that area is called a brainstem locomotor region. These locomotor areas are in turn connected with the cerebellum, basal ganglia, and frontal regions of the brain. The basal ganglia play a role in exploratory behavior and the lateral hypothalamic region in appetitive walking. The medial hypothalamus and central gray matter are recruited in defensive behavior. Such goals are interactive with the motor cortex, and frontal cortical function ranges from a subtle control modification of gait to complete control of locomotor activity. Proprioceptive feedback from the limbs to gait centers regulates their responses.

It is therefore evident that the gait mechanism is complex and scattered over multiple regions of the brain and malfunction at any particular level will result in its own relatively specific gait disorder.

■ CLINICAL EVALUATION OF GAIT DISORDERS IN THE ELDERLY

The complaint "I can't walk" requires meticulous physical examination to pinpoint the functional deficit with a view to further investigation to elucidate the pathology. The history is very rarely sufficient to make the diagnosis, which comes from the clinical examination.

■ GAIT DISORDERS

The causes of gait disorders can be divided into those caused by neurological deficits and those secondary to nonneurological problems.

In the latter category, one should consider a defect of vision, pain, and arthritis, as well as medical problems such as cardiorespiratory failure, angina, postural hypotension, and side effects of drugs. A discussion of these is beyond the scope of this chapter.

Neurological Causes of Gait Disorders

Weakness

The diagnosis of weakness has been discussed in Chapter 2.

Lower Motor Neuron Weakness: In distal lower motor neuron weakness the most prominent sign is foot drop. Because the more proximal muscles, the hip flexors, are intact, the gait is high-stepping, often with an audible slap as of the foot hits the ground.

With predominantly proximal weakness, because the gluteus medius is involved, the gait becomes waddling, with an abnormal pelvic tilt with each step.

Upper Motor Neuron Weakness: Weakness secondary to central disease results in a circumduction gait. Hip flexion is weak, so the often spastic foot drop cannot be compensated for by raising the leg higher. The quadriceps, on the other hand, is relatively spared, which facilitates knee locking, and the patient can bear weight. Often, in association with the circumduction gait there is flexion of the upper limb across the chest.

Deafferentation

Proprioception is tested as described in Chapter 3. Lack of proprioceptive feedback may have a profound effect on gait and when severe can render the patient completely unable to walk. In patients with milder deficits, with each step there is a normal heel strike and then a more pronounced or forcible slap of the sole to the ground. Textbooks often refer to a so-called stamping gait, an attempt to increase sensory feedback, but classic stamping is seldom present.

The Romberg sign is positive. To test for this, the patient is asked to stand with the feet together and the eyes closed. Marked body sway indicates a positive Romberg sign.

Cerebellar Ataxia

Cerebellar signs on examination are described in Chapter 13. Common adjectives used to describe a cerebellar gait include "staggering, reeling, or drunken." Characteristically, there is a wide-based stance with wide-spread legs, and the patient may stagger from side-to-side. Stride length is slightly shortened. Staggering may be brought out by sudden turning. Cerebellar hemisphere dysfunction produces appendicular clumsiness and ataxia. Vermis dysfunction causes trunk ataxia, and patients with superior vermis lesions, as in alcoholic degeneration, present particularly with gait ataxia.

Vestibular Dysfunction

A mismatch in afferent visual, proprioceptive, and vestibular information leads to the complaint of dizziness or loss of balance. A subjective sensation of rotation or spinning is characteristic of vestibular dysfunction, whereas nonvestibular dizziness may be described as light-headedness, floating, or loss of balance.

The gait of vestibular dysfunction progresses from an occasional stumble, to veering, to frank ataxia. With unilateral vestibular dysfunction the patient veers toward the pathological side.

Extrapyramidal Disorders

Extrapyramidal disorders may present with hypokinetic or hyperkinetic movement disorders (see Chapter 13).

Parkinson's Disease: In Parkinson's disease there is paucity of movement, and gait abnormalities are the presenting complaint in approximately 15% of these patients. The gait is narrow-based, and stride length is reduced, leading to a shuffle (*marche a petit pas*). Speed may be increased, leading to the descriptive term "festinating" or hurrying. There is reduced arm swing and a tendency to thoracic kyphosis. The patient is easily displaced backward and may spontaneously take backward steps or even fall (retropulsion). When asked to turn on a dime or about-face, the patient takes many small steps to complete the maneuver. As the disease progresses there is difficulty initiating gait, and the patient may take many small steps on the spot before forward movement ensues (start hesitation). A similar phenomenon may occur when stepping through the portal of a door or attempting to make a sudden turn, when frequent small steps in place without propulsion are seen. When asked to rise from a soft chair, the patient may fall back two or three times before attaining the erect posture.

Varying degrees of Parkinsonian gait are seen in patients with multiple system atrophy in which parkinsonism plays a varying role. In progressive supranuclear palsy, Parkinsonian features and disturbances of ocular motility are seen. Early falling with failure of down gaze is a clue to the diagnosis.

Lower Half Parkinsonism: In lower half parkinsonism, leg movements when walking look to be severely Parkinsonian, but the upper limbs are furiously in movement as if coaxing the patient to walk. This gait is usually caused by subcortical arteriosclerotic dementia (Binswanger's disease).

Hyperkinetic Movement Disorders: In hyperkinetic disorders the extra movements may interfere with gait, leading to scattered and various intrusions that cause the patient to stagger.

Frontal Gait Disorders

The highest centers for the control of gait are in the frontal lobes, and dysfunction there leads to difficulty with initiation and occasional freezing, with or without multiple steps in place. The patient walks on a narrow base with a markedly shortened stride length. There is hesitation on turning. There is disequilibrium and impaired ongoing locomotion.

At times the prime deficit is one of initiation (ignition failure), when the patient hesitates and may take three or four steps on the spot, with the feet barely clearing the floor. Once underway, however, the stride lengthens and foot clearance is normal.

Rarely, profound breakdown in the control of gait results in an ataxic-like gait. The feet may cross or move in a direction inappropriate to the center of gravity, resulting in a bizarre, uncoordinated gait.

When the cause of frontal gait dysfunction is apparent on investigation, for example, hydrocephalus, the dysfunction is regarded as symptomatic, but in approximately 8% to 10% of patients no obvious cause is found and the label "degenerative" or "idiopathic" is appropriate.

Psychogenic Gait Disorder

The Cautious Gait: Murray et al (1969) described the cautious gait as follows: "The walking performance of older men gave the impression of a guarded or restrained type of walking in an attempt to obtain maximum stability and security. The walking of older men resembled that of someone walking on a slippery surface. This is regarded as a compensatory adaptation with an appropriate response to real or perceived disequilibrium."

Fear of Falling: Fear of falling may be exaggerated, but it usually has a rational basis because of prior experience such as a previous fall. The anxiety may be so severe that it could be called a phobia. Such patients, in open spaces, may resort to crawling on hands and knees, and this may culminate in a wheelchair existence. Fear of falling is associated with increased mortality and may be more frequent in women.

Depression: Extreme psychomotor retardation leads to a hypokinetic gait. Depressed patients have reduced stride length and a somewhat lifting motion of the legs.

Psychogenic (Hysterical) Gait Disorder: Astasia-abasia is defined as the inability to stand or walk in the absence of other neurological abnormalities (Jaccoud et al, 1888). Camptocormia is an exaggerated trunk flexion of functional etiology.

Lempert et al (1991) described the following six characteristic features occurring alone or in combination in 97% of their patients with psychogenic gait disorder:

1. Momentary fluctuations of stance and gait, often in response to suggestion.
2. Excessive slowness or hesitation of locomotion incompatible with neurological disease.
3. A "psychogenic" Romberg with a buildup of swaying amplitude after a silent latency, or with improvement by distraction.
4. Uneconomic postures with wastage of muscular energy.
5. "Walking on ice"—characterized by slow, cautious steps with fixed ankle joints.
6. Sudden buckling of the knees usually without falls.

Maintenance of postural control on a narrow base with flailing arms and excessive trunk sway without falling, sometimes called tightrope walking, or excessive slowness and stiffness, are common features.

Confusional State: Asterixis or polymyoclonia, which often accompanies toxic delirium, may cause falls because of sudden loss of tone in the legs or simply an unsteady, swaying gait. Even without the movement disorder, confused patients often have a wandering/broad-based gait probably on the basis of a lack of attention.

Because the physiological control of normal walking is complex and operates at multiple levels of the nervous system, it is rare for the patient's history to pinpoint the cause. The examiner should have in mind a differential diagnosis of the possible causes of gait disorder and then by careful physical examination drill down to an anatomical or pathophysiological explanation for the deficit. This anatomical diagnosis in turn dictates further investigation.

KEY POINTS

1. The history, however meticulous, almost never gives the diagnosis.
2. Nonneurological causes should be excluded.
3. The diagnosis comes only by virtue of a meticulous clinical examination.
4. The examination pinpoints which domains are at fault—weakness, proprioception, cerebellar coordination, vestibular, extrapyramidal, or frontal.
5. If no cause is apparent, consider a psychogenic diagnosis.

■ **SUGGESTED READINGS**

General Reference

Ronthal M. *Gait Disorders*. Boston: Butterworth-Heinemann, 2002.

Falls in the Elderly

Cummings RG, Miller PJ, Kelsey JL, et al. Medications and multiple falls in elderly people: the St. Louis OASIS study. *Age Ageing* 1991;20:455–461.
Kapoor WN. Syncope in older persons. *J Am Geriatr Soc* 1994;42:426–436.

Lipsitz LA, Nyquist RP, Wei JY. Postprandial reduction in blood pressure in the elderly. *N Eng J Med* 1983;309:81–83.

Lipsitz LA, Jonsson PV, Kelley MM, et al. Causes and correlates of recurrent falls in the ambulatory frail elderly. *J Gerontol Med Sci* 1991;46:M114–M122.

Nevitt MC, Cummings SR, Kidd S, et al. Risk factors for recurrent nonsyncopal falls. *JAMA* 1989;261:2663–2668.

Rubenstein LR, Robbins AS, Schulman BL, et al. Falls and instability in the elderly. *J Am Geriatr Soc* 1988;36: 266–278.

Sattin RW, Lambert Huber DA, DeVito CA, et al. The incidence of fall injury events among the elderly in a defined population. *Am J Epidemiol* 1990;131:1028–1037.

Tideiksaar R. Falls in the elderly. *Bull NY Acad Med* 1988;64:145–163.

Tinetti ME, Speechley M, Ginter SF. Risk factors for falls among elderly persons living in the community. *N Eng J Med* 1988;19:1701–1707.

Walker JE, Howland J. Falls and fear of falling among elderly persons living in the community: occupational therapy interventions. *Am J Occup Ther* 1991;45:119–122.

Physiology of Gait

Dickinson MH, Farley CT, Full RJ, et al. How animals move: an integrative view. *Science* 2000;288:100–106.

Dietz V. Neurophysiology of gait disorders: present and future applications. *Electroencephalogr Clin Neurophysiol* 1997;103:333–355.

Drew T, Jiang W, Kably B, et al. Role of the motor cortex in the control of visually triggered gait modifications. *Can J Physiol Pharmacol* 1996;74:426–442.

Graham-Brown T. The fundamental activity of the nervous centers. *J Physiol* 1914;48:18–46.

Grillner S, Parker D, El Manira A. Vertebrate locomotion: a Lamprey perspective. *Ann NY Acad Sci* 1998;860:1–18.

Jordan LM. Initiation of locomotion in mammals. *Ann NY Acad Sci* 1998;860:83–93.

Kiehn O, Kjaerulff O. Distribution of central pattern generators for rhythmic motor outputs in the spinal cord of limbed vertebrates [review]. *Ann NY Acad Sci* 1998;860:110–129.

McCrea DA. Neuronal basis of afferent-evoked enhancement of locomotor activity. *Ann NY Acad Sci* 1998;860: 216–225.

Mori S, Matsui T, Kuze B, et al. Cerebellar-induced locomotion: reticulospinal control of spinal rhythm generating mechanism in cats. *Ann NY Acad Sci* 1998;860:94–105.

Mori S, Matsuyama K, Kohyama J, et al. The constituents of postural and locomotor control systems and their interaction in cats. *Brain Dev* 1992;14S:S109–S120.

Sherrington CS. *The Integrative Action of the Nervous System.* New Haven, CT: Yale University Press, 1906.

Shik ML, Orlovsky GN. Neurophysiology of locomotor automatism. *Physiol Rev* 1976;56:465.

Whelan PJ. Control of locomotion in the decerebrate cat. *Prog Neurobiol* 1996;49:481–515.

Weakness

Messina C. Pathophysiology of muscle tone. *Funct Neurol* 1990;5:217–223.

Ronthal M. Weakness. In: Samuels M, ed. *Office Practice of Neurology.* New York: Churchill Livingstone, 1996.

Younger DS. Differential diagnosis of progressive flaccid weakness. *Semin Neurol* 1993;13:241–246.

Walshe FMR. The Babinski plantar response, its form and its physiological and pathological significance. *Brain* 1956; 79:529–556.

Deafferentation

Collins WF, Nulsen FE, Randt CT. Relationship of peripheral nerve fiber size and sensation in man. *Arch Neurol* 1960;3:381–385.

Cook AW, Browder EJ. Function of posterior columns in man. *Arch Neurol* 1965;12:72–79.

McCloskey DI. Kinesthetic sensibility. *Physiol Rev* 1978;58:763–820.

Cerebellar Ataxia

Bird TD. Hereditary ataxia overview. Available at http://www.ncbi.nlm.nih.gov/bookshelf/br.fcgi?book=gene&partid= 1138#ataxias. Accessed May 30, 2008.

Brennan RW, Bergland RM. Acute cerebellar hemorrhage: analysis and clinical findings and outcome in 12 cases. *Neurology* 1977;27:527–532.

Bronstein AM, Hood JD, Gresty MA, et al. Visual control of balance in cerebellar and Parkinsonian syndromes. *Brain* 1990;113:767–779.

Gilman S, Bloedel JR, Lechtenberg R. *Disorders of the Cerebellum.* Philadelphia: FA Davis, 1981.

Hallett M, Stanhope SJ, Thomas SL, et al. Pathophysiology of posture and gait in cerebellar ataxia. In: Shimamura M, Grillner S, Edgerton VR, eds. *Neurobiological Basis of Human Locomotion.* Tokyo: Japan Scientific Societies Press, 1991.

Vestibular Dysfunction

Baloh RW, Honrubia V, Jacobson K. Benign positional vertigo: clinical and oculographic features in 240 cases. *Neurology* 1987;37:371–378.

Bender MB. Oscillopscia. *Arch Neurol* 1965;13:204–213.

Buttner-Ennever JA. Vestibular oculomotor organization. In: Fuchs AF, Becker W, eds. *The Neural Control of Eye Movements*. Amsterdam: Elsevier, 1981.

Dix M, Hallpike C. The pathology, symptomatology, and diagnosis of certain common disorders of the vestibular systems. *Ann Otol Rhinol Laryngol* 1952;61:987–1016.

Drachman DA, Hart CW. An approach to the dizzy patient. *Neurology* 1972;22:323–334.

Fregley AR. Vestibular ataxia and its measurement in man. In: Kornhuber HH, ed. *Handbook of Sensory Physiology VI*, Part 2. New York: Springer Veralag, 1974.

Fukuda T. The stepping test: two phases of the labyrinthine reflex. *Acta Otolaryngol* 1959;50:95–108.

Leigh RJ, Zee DS. *The Neurology of Eye Movements*. New York: Oxford University Press, 1999.

Magarian GJ. Hyperventilation syndromes: infrequently recognized common expressions of anxiety and stress. *Medicine* 1982;61:219–236.

Extrapyramidal Disorders

Calne DB, Chu N-S, Huan CC, et al. Manganism and idiopathic parkinsonism: similarities and differences. *Neurology* 1994;44:1583–1586.

Cummings JL. Depression and Parkinson's disease: a review. *Am J Psychiatry* 1992;149:443–454.

Feany MB, Dickson DW. Neurodegenerative disorders with extensive tau pathology: a comparative study and review. *Ann Neurol* 1996;40:139–148.

Fitzgerald PM, Jankovic J. Lower body parkinsonism: evidence for a vascular etiology. *Mov Disord* 1989;4:249–260.

Graybiel AM, Aosaki T, Flaherty AW, et al. The basal ganglia and adaptive motor control. *Science* 1994;265:1826–1831.

Jankovic J. Parkinsonian syndromes. In: Kurlan R, ed. *Treatment of Movement Disorders*. Philadelphia: Lippincott Williams & Wilkins, 1995.

Krusz JC, Koller WC, Ziegler DK. Historical review: abnormal movements associated with epidemic encephalitis lethargica. *Mov Disord* 1987;2:137–141.

Langston JW, Ballard PA, Tetrud JW, et al. Chronic parkinsonism in humans due to a product of meperidine analogue synthesis. *Science* 1983;219:979–980.

Levy R, Hazrati LN, Herrero MT, et al. Reevaluation of the functional anatomy of the basal ganglia in normal and parkinsonian states. *Neuroscience* 1997;76:335–343.

Litvan I, Agid Y, Goetz C, et al. Accuracy of the clinical diagnosis of corticobasal degeneration: a clinicopathological study. *Neurology* 1997;48:119–125.

Litvan I, Campbell G, Mangone CA, et al. Which clinical features differentiate progressive supranuclear palsy (Steele-Richardson-Olszewski syndrome) from related disorders? A clinicopathological study. *Brain* 1997;120:65–74.

Obeso JA, Rodriguez MC, DeLong MR. Basal ganglia pathophysiology: a critical review. *Adv Neurol* 1997;4:3–18.

Rebeiz JJ, Kolodny EH, Richardson EP. Corticodentatonigral degeneration with neuronal achromasia. *Arch Neurol* 1968;18:20–26.

Steele JC, Richardson JC, Olszewski J. Progressive supranuclear palsy: a heterogenous degeneration involving the brainstem, basal ganglia and cerebellum with vertical gaze and pseudobulbar palsy, nuchal dystonia and dementia. *Arch Neurol* 1964;10:333–359.

Frontal Gait Disorders

Adams RD, Fisher CM, Hakim MD, et al. Symptomatic occult hydrocephalus with "normal" cerebrospinal fluid pressure. *N Engl J Med* 1965;273:117–126.

Black PM. Idiopathic normal-pressure hydrocephalus: results of shunting in 62 patients. *J Neurosurg* 1980;52:371–377.

Borgesen SE, Gjerris F, Sorensen SC. Intracranial pressure and conductance to outflow of cerebrospinal fluid in normal-pressure hydrocephalus. *J Neurosurg* 1979;50:489–493.

Katzman R, Hussey F. A simple constant infusion manometric test for measurement of CSF absorption. *Neurology* 1970;20:534–544.

Nitz WR, Bradley Jr, WG, Watanabe AS, et al. Flow dynamics of cerebrospinal fluid: assessment with phase-contrast velocity MR imaging performed with retrospective cardiac gating. *Radiology* 1992;183:395–405.

Nutt JG, Marsden CD, Thompson MD. Human walking and higher-level gait disorders, particularly in the elderly. *Neurology* 1993;43:268–279.

Stolze H, Kuhtz-Buschbeck JP, Drucke H, et al. Comparative analysis of the gait disorder of normal pressure hydrocephalus and Parkinson's disease. *J Neurol Neurosurg Psychiatry* 2001;70:289–297.

Walker JE, Howland J. Falls and fear of falling among elderly persons living in the community: occupational therapy interventions. *Am J Occup Ther* 1991;45:119–122.

Wikkelso C, Andersson H, Blomstrand C, et al. The clinical effects of lumbar puncture in normal pressure hydrocephalus. *J Neurol Neurosurg Psychiatry* 1982;45:64–69.

Psychogenic Gait Disorder

Arfken CL, Lach HW, Birge SJ, et al. The prevalence and correlates of fear of falling in elderly persons living in the community. *Am J Public Health* 1994;84:565–570.

Bhala RP, O'Donnell J, Thoppil E. Phobic fear of falling and its clinical management. *Phys Ther* 1982;62:187–190.

Elble RJ, Hughes L, Higgins C. The syndrome of senile gait. *J Neurol* 1992;239:71–75.

Jette A, Assmann S, Peterson EW. Fear of falling and activity restriction: a survey of activities and fear of falling in the elderly (SAFE). *J Gerontol B Psychol Sci Soc Sci* 1998;53:P43–P50.

Keane JR. Hysterical gait disorders: 60 cases. *Neurology* 1989;39:586–589.

Lempert T, Brandt T, Dieterich M, et al. How to identify psychogenic disorders of stance and gait: a video study in 37 patients. *J Neurol* 1991;238:140–146.

Marks I, Bebbington P. Space phobia: syndrome or agoraphobic variant? *Med J* 1976;2:345–347.

Murray MP, Kory RC, Clarkson BH. Walking patterns in healthy old men. *J Gerontol* 1969;24:169–178.

Sloman L, Berridge M, Homatidis S, et al. Gait patterns of depressed patients and normal subjects. *Am J Psychiatry* 1982;139:94–97.

Stickler GB, Cheung-Patton A. Astasia abasia: a conversion reaction: prognosis. *Clin Pediatr (Phila)* 1989;28:12–16.

CHAPTER 5

The Neurogenic Bladder

Michael Ronthal

■ INTRODUCTION

The first order of business in diagnosing bladder symptoms is to make the distinction between urological and neurological pathophysiology. Local pathology such as outlet obstruction or stress incontinence must be excluded before the neurological dysfunction is defined. At times the symptoms can be the same or similar; urgency and frequency could be due to cystitis rather than central nervous system (CNS) dysfunction, and retention could be due to bladder outlet obstruction or, say, cauda dysfunction. The urine must be examined in conjunction with the physical examination.

This chapter will deal, for the most part, with the neurogenic bladder and will begin with the "ground rules" for diagnosis, followed by a review of the physiology and pathophysiology of micturition.

■ HISTORY

Enquiry should be made as to bladder sensation, frequency of micturition, nocturia, hesitancy, intermittency, pain, and dysuria as part of the general medical and neurological history. Overt blood in the urine clearly implies a urological problem. A review of the patient's medication is mandatory. The presence of a gait disorder of any magnitude is strongly suggestive of a neurogenic basis for the symptoms.

Normal bladder sensation progresses in a continuum of gradually increasing intensity and unpleasantness from the first sensation of bladder filling, through the first desire to void, to a strong desire to void.

Urinary incontinence is defined by the International Continence Society as an involuntary loss of urine that is objectively shown and a social hygiene problem. Incontinence is present in 20% of women over the age of 40.

Urgency, which is an abnormal symptom, is either present or absent without a graduated increase in symptomatology and is defined as "the complaint of a sudden compelling desire to pass urine which is difficult to defer." If there is involuntary loss of urine in the setting of urgency, urgency incontinence is suggested and implies detrusor hyperactivity. Loss of urine when coughing or straining suggests nonneurologic stress incontinence.

Micturition in a healthy adult with a bladder capacity of about 500 mL is likely to be approximately once every 3 to 4 hours; the physiological rate of bladder filling is about 2 mL per minute. Many normal individuals will have at most one episode of nocturia, and most usually have none.

Hesitancy and intermittency usually imply outlet obstruction, but hesitancy can be the symptom of detrusor/sphincter dyssynergy—the fundus of the bladder contracts on a closed sphincter.

Micturition should be painless, perhaps even slightly pleasant!

Any medication with anticholinergic effects can cause outlet symptoms, particularly in men. These include the tricyclic antidepressants and many of the neuroleptic agents, muscle relaxants, and sympathomimetics.

■ EXAMINATION

Because bladder symptoms can be part of pathology at multiple sites in the nervous system, a detailed neurological examination must be performed. The mental status screen helps to diagnose frontal lobe disorders; parkinsonism is manifest by slowness; posterior fossa pathology by ataxia and cranial nerve signs; myelopathy by spastic, weak legs or loss of position sense; and cauda equina pathology by loss of ankle reflexes, saddle sensory loss, and poor sphincter tone. Finally, the bladder may be involved in autonomic neuropathy and postural hypotension, or lack of sweating may be the clues.

■ DIAGNOSIS

The physiology of bladder function is complex and diagnosis can be difficult at the bedside, but some general principles are helpful. In general, central pathology can be likened to the upper motor neuron syndrome with spasticity—translated to the bladder this means a low-capacity, high-pressure system manifested by urgency, frequency, and urgency incontinence. This has been called detrusor overactivity or overactive bladder syndrome (International Continence Society). The syndrome could be idiopathic, but only by exclusion.

Lack of bladder sensation leads to a large, flabby bladder, with overflow incontinence sometimes labeled a "tabetic bladder." The cause may be autonomic neuropathy, dorsal root ganglionopathy, or myelopathy. Acute cauda equina syndromes such as those caused by herpes simplex or massive disc herniation cause retention with or without sensory loss.

Acute spinal cord injury causes retention until an "automatic bladder" establishes itself by activation of suppressed or dormant C-fiber reflexes.

If bladder dysfunction occurs in the setting of spinal cord or cauda syndromes, whatever the pathology, a sense of urgency is injected into the management, which becomes an emergency. Many of the long-term complications of paraplegia are urological, and if treated early, might be avoided.

■ INVESTIGATION

If a clearly defined site of pathology is suggested after the initial clinical examination, imaging studies should be performed and the cerebrospinal fluid should be examined if the imaging is negative.

If the site of pathology or the symptoms are unclear, further urodynamic studies will help to define the problem; however, urodynamics give information only as to bladder function and not etiology. The urodynamic evaluation may guide further neurological workup.

■ BLADDER PHYSIOLOGY

The functions of the bladder are only two—storage and emptying. The system is in storage mode for more than 99% of the time. As in all neurological functions there are both central and peripheral components that work synergistically to support normal bladder dynamics (Fig. 5.1).

Central Control

Suprapontine Centers

The highest center for motor control is cortex, more specifically the frontal cortex. In humans, positron emission tomography shows activation of the right dorsolateral prefrontal cortex during micturition. The right anterior cingulate shows decreased blood flow when the subject is not able to micturate despite a full bladder.

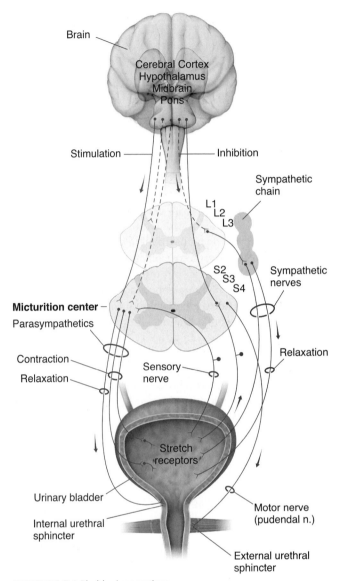

■ **FIGURE 5.1** Bladder innervation.

The physiological purpose of normal bladder sensation is to provide information to the brain about bladder filling so that the voiding reflex can be kept under voluntary control. One should be able to decide when and where to void. Bladder sensation as investigated by activation magnetic resonance imaging shows activity in the insula bilaterally for normal bladder filling sensations, shifting anteriorly as the sensation becomes stronger and more unpleasant. Activity is also seen in the basal ganglia, periaqueductal gray (PAG), and anterior cingulate.

Pontine Centers

The pontine micturition center consists of two groups of cells. The medial, or M-region, in the medial part of the dorsolateral pons, projects to the intermediolateral cell column and the parasympathetic preganglionic bladder motor neurons, which innervate the detrusor. The M-region is sometimes called Barrington's nucleus.

Neurons in the lateral part of the dorsolateral pons, the L-region, project to Onuf's nucleus in the sacral cord. Onuf's nucleus is the motor nucleus containing the anterior horn cells innervating the sphincters.

The M-region is likely the site of activation of micturition, and the L-region is important for continence. Onuf's nucleus is inhibited during micturition so that the bladder contracts on an open sphincter.

A brainstem mechanism by which the bladder is switched from one mode of activity to another is the likely source of control of micturition. The PAG receives sensory input from the lumbosacral spinal cord and projects to the pontine micturition center, and PAG neurons activate the premotor interneurons in the M-region, initiating micturition.

The striatum and thalamus interact with the pontine micturition center and PAG, respectively, but the exact physiology has not yet been worked out.

Peripheral Mechanisms

The striated external urethral sphincter is part of the pelvic floor and innervated by the pudendal nerve. Motor neurons to the urethral sphincter are located in the ventrolateral part of Onuf's nucleus in the ventral horn at S1–S2.

The smooth muscle detrusor is innervated by postganglionic parasympathetic fibers that originate in the sacral intermediolateral cell group in the spinal cord at S2–S4, and their axons reach the bladder via the pelvic nerve.

Receptors in the bladder wall send afferent signals in the pelvic and hypogastric nerves, which respond during slow filling or during the micturition contraction. These receptors are described as in series tension receptors. Apart from the classic parasympathetic activity discussed previously, sensory discharge in bladder afferents coincide with rhythmic contractions in the bladder autonomous activity. Autonomous activity involves local propagating waves of contraction and stretch intrinsic to the bladder wall. The significance of this system is not yet elucidated, but it holds out the hope of generating new drugs that may control sensations of urgency, leaving micturition itself unaffected.

The clinical significance of motor sympathetic bladder innervation of the bladder neck region is unknown, but its activity prevents retrograde ejaculation. Alpha-adrenergic blockers are helpful in outlet obstruction.

■ URODYNAMICS

Cystometry

Cystometry is the recording of pressure/volume relationships in the bladder. The detrusor pressure is derived by subtracting the intra-abdominal pressure measured by a rectal line from the intravesical pressure measured by a urethral catheter.

The bladder is filled via a double-lumen catheter by an infusion pump at approximately 2 to 10 mL per minute. The patient reports the sensation of a normal desire to void (300 mL), a strong desire, and finally a sense of urgency. Pressures can be measured during filling and voiding. The normal male voids at pressures of 40 to 60 cm H_2O. A pressure/volume graph can be constructed.

Solid-state transducers have led to the introduction of ambulatory urodynamics, with patients able to continue their normal daily routine and keep a voiding diary.

Uroflometry

The patient voids into a receptacle with a rotating disc at its base. This generates a uroflow curve, which is a graphic representation of the rate at which urine is voided.

A discontinuous or fractionated curve is seen in detrusor/sphincter dyssynergia.

Residual Volume

The residual volume after micturition can be measured by catheter or an ultrasound scan. Up to 100 mL of residual volume is acceptable in spinal cord disease.

Electromyography

Sphincter electromyography (EMG), recording from the striated muscle of urethral sphincter or anal sphincter, yields information about detrusor/sphincter synergy. Denervation activity may be seen in cauda equina lesions. In patients with multiple system atrophy (MSA) there is degeneration of Onuf's nucleus and the test can help with diagnosis because there is no denervation in simple Parkinson's disease. Young women with urinary retention, often in the setting of polycystic ovaries, show complex repetitive discharges and decelerating bursts thought to be due to ephaptic transmission (Fowler's syndrome). Before this finding, these patients were thought to have psychiatric bladder dysfunction.

■ DISEASE ENTITIES CAUSING NEUROGENIC BLADDER DYSFUNCTION

Because the control of bladder function has input from so many levels of the nervous system, a neurogenic bladder can be part of pathology at multiple sites. Only a few entities will be discussed.

In frontal lobe disorders, whatever the pathology, the usual finding is of detrusor overactivity. Occasionally, retention is seen. The syndrome of normal-pressure hydrocephalus has incontinence as part of a triad of dementia, gait disorder, and bladder dysfunction. Detrusor overactivity is usually the bladder dysfunction.

Three months after hemispheric strokes in one series, 53% of patients had significant urinary complaints—nocturnal frequency in 36%, urge incontinence in 29%, and difficulty voiding in 25%. Urinary incontinence within 7 days of stroke onset is a prognosticator of poor outcome. Bladder symptoms can occur in as many as 50% of patients with brainstem strokes, more likely with hemorrhage.

In Parkinson's disease, urinary symptoms occur late in the illness. Early symptoms suggest the alternative diagnosis of MSA.

In spinal cord disease, urgency and urgency incontinence, often with a large residual resulting from an element of dyssynergia, is common, whatever the cause. Severe dyssynergia suggests a thoracic spinal cord lesion. Approximately 75% of patients with multiple sclerosis have spinal cord involvement; therefore demyelination should be considered in the differential diagnosis of myelopathy with bladder dysfunction. In acute spinal cord lesions there is retention, but after weeks to months an automatic bladder can be established by activation of new C fiber activity; hyperactivity of this reflex bladder can be a problem.

In cauda equina syndromes there is saddle sensory loss caused by damage to S2–S4 roots, with loss of voluntary control of anal and urethral sphincters. The detrusor is decentralized, and sympathetic innervation may be preserved.

In diabetes with neuropathy there is impaired detrusor contractility, reduction of urinary flow rate, and increased postmicturition volume with reduced bladder sensation.

■ TREATMENT

Even though the cause of the neurogenic bladder dysfunction has been elucidated and treated, many patients will continue to have symptoms.

Anticholinergics are used for detrusor hyperactivity but can cause dry mouth and constipation. Oxybutynin was the standby drug, but tolterodine has fewer side effects. Use of 1-deamino-8-D-arginine vasopressin (DDAVP) at night may reduce urinary production and allow for a better sleep pattern.

Intravesical capsaicin has been used for intractable detrusor hyperreflexia because it is toxic to C fibers.

Some men prefer an external latex condom sheath to medication, which is acceptable provided there is no significant residual.

Botulinus toxin injected into the detrusor muscle is symptomatic for detrusor hyperactivity, and the injections can last as long as 9 months.

Clean intermittent catheterization at least twice a day for incomplete emptying with a large residual volume or inability to void is preferable to an indwelling catheter, which is more likely to become infected. Bacteriuria is present in 50% of patients performing clean intermittent catheterization, but symptomatic infection is less likely. Some patients may be physically unable to comply and will require help.

A sacral extradural nerve stimulator is sometimes suggested. It lessens detrusor instability, probably by stimulating pelvic afferents.

In patients with complete spinal cord transection a nerve root stimulator may improve urinary continence, and posterior rhizotomy is often combined with the stimulator to increase bladder capacity.

■ PSYCHOGENIC URINARY DYSFUNCTION

Psychogenic bladder dysfunction was a fairly popular diagnosis in the past. The aphorism was that retention without obvious cause was likely to be psychogenic, whereas incontinence was likely to be organic. More sophisticated investigations have whittled down the number of patients thought to have nonorganic bladder dysfunction, and many young women with retention are now diagnosed with Fowler's syndrome after sphincter EMG.

Disturbances of bladder function have been related to anxiety, depression, phobias, dementia, and schizophrenia.

Psychogenic urinary dysfunction (PUD) is a diagnosis of exclusion and is usually accompanied by obvious psychological/psychiatric features. It is classified as psychosomatic dysfunction. The workup must be extensive and negative and should include urodynamics and imaging. In one series of 2300 patients investigated in a urodynamic laboratory, only 0.7% of patients with bladder symptoms were thought to have psychogenic symptoms.

PUD has been labeled variously as mental disorder caused by toileting or as a urinary dysfunction caused by a mental disorder. A more colorful label "bashful bladder syndrome" refers to the inability to void in public restrooms (paruresis). This is classified as a social phobia in the *Diagnostic and Statistical Manual of Mental Disorders,* fourth edition.

KEY POINTS

1. Urological bladder dysfunction must be differentiated from neurological bladder dysfunction.
2. Acute or subacute bladder symptoms of neurological origin should be treated as an emergency.
3. The history and physical examination can be amplified by urodynamic testing. In general, CNS dysfunction affecting bladder function causes urgency and urgency incontinence.
4. Treatment is primarily that of the prime neurological pathology aided by symptomatic bladder treatment.

■ **SUGGESTED READINGS**

Abrams P. Describing bladder storage function: overactive bladder syndrome and detrusor overactivity. *Urology* 2003;62(5 suppl 2):28–37.

Chaib TC, Steers WD. Neurophysiology of micturition and continence. *Urol Clin North Am* 1996;23:221–236.

DasGupta R, Fowler CJ. What neurologists need to understand outside their own speciality. *Pract Neurol* 2008;9:98–105.

Fowler CJ. Neurological disorders of micturition and their treatment. *Brain* 1999;122:1213–1231.

Gillespie JI. The autonomous bladder: a view of the origin of bladder overactivity and sensory urge. *BJU Int* 2004;93:478–483.

Griffiths D. Imaging bladder sensations. *Neurourol Urodyn* 2007;26:899–903.

Hammelstein P, Soifer S. Is "shy bladder syndrome" (paruresis) correctly classified as a social phobia? *J Anxiety Disord* 2006;20:296–311.

Macaulay AJ, Stern RS, Holmes DM, et al. Micturition and the mind: psychological factors in the etiology and treatment of urinary symptoms in women. *Br Med J (Clin Res Ed)* 1987;294:540–543.

Sakakibara R, Uchiyama T, Awa Y, et al. Psychogenic urinary dysfunction: a uro-neurological assessment. *Neurourol Urodyn* 2007;26:518–524.

Scientific Committee of the First International Consultation on Incontinence. Assessment and treatment of urinary incontinence. *Lancet* 2000;355:2153–2158.

Selius BA, Subedi R. Urinary retention in adults: diagnosis and initial management. *Am Fam Physician* 2008;77:643–650.

Thakar R, Stanton S. Management of urinary incontinence in women. *BMJ* 2000;321:1326.

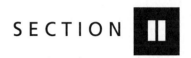

Behavioral Neurology

CHAPTER 6

The Neurological Mental Status Examination

David B. Robinson • Daniel Z. Press

■ INTRODUCTION

Behavioral neurology is an essential complement to the psychiatric approach for evaluating cognition and behavior. Both disciplines seek to more fully understand the most complex of human behaviors, thoughts, and abilities and to apply that knowledge helping those impaired by diseases affecting those functions.

Neuropathology has always been fundamental to the neurologist's understanding of the link from structure to function. The psychiatric approach uses a mental status examination describing insight, judgement, and the like; the behavioral neurology approach parallels the general neurological strategy by determining the location of dysfunction, based on the pattern of cognitive deficits. Localization then assists with narrowing the differential diagnosis.

Focal pathologic conditions such as strokes, tumors, or traumatic brain injury have given way to the *lesion method* for correlating structure to function. Focal cognitive signs and symptoms can be just as useful and precise for localization as weakness or visual loss. Multifocal or degenerative illnesses can also cause a combination of behavioral, cognitive, and other neurological manifestations that, while less attributable to a single anatomical correlate, can aid in diagnosis and treatment.

This section on behavioral neurology is organized around the general functional geography of the four lobes, with an emphasis on disease processes manifesting in dysfunction in one or more of these regions. Topics covered will be weighted according to their relative exposure potential in a clinical setting.

■ CORTICAL ORGANIZATION

Some principles can help in forming a construct for brain-behavior relationships. Cognitive functions are subserved by networks of brain regions, so although these rules oversimplify the complexity of cognitive function, they have clinical utility (Figs. 6.1 and 6.2).

- Motor systems are mostly **anterior to the central sulcus**.
- Sensory systems are mostly **posterior**.
- Each has a primary cortex, as well as nearby association cortices.
- Semantic knowledge is usually inferior—from occipital to temporal lobe (the "what" pathway) and visuospatial and orienting are in the occipital to parietal lobes (the "where" pathway) (Figs. 6.2 and 6.3).
- **Cerebral dominance** (lateralization of function)—many functions are asymmetrically represented by hemisphere.
  - **Left hemisphere**—language, praxis, calculation.
  - **Right hemisphere**: face recognition, prosody, visuospacial function.
  - Non–right-handed individuals sometimes do not conform to lateralization rules.

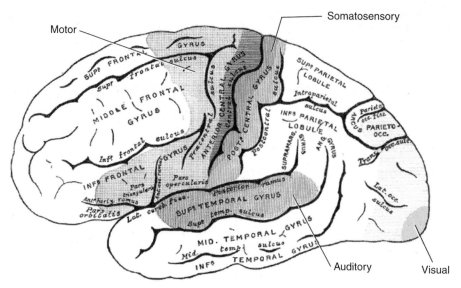

FIGURE 6.1 Primary sensory and motor regions, secondary association regions in lighter shading. (From Gray H. *Anatomy of the Human Body*. Philadelphia: Lea and Febiger;1918.)

■ ELEMENTS OF THE HISTORY AND PHYSICAL EXAMINATION

Cognition and behavior are the most plastic of brain functions. Because of this, complaints and examination findings must be considered in the setting of developmental, educational, and social history, as well as any previous evidence of cortical damage or dysfunction. Critical areas to explore include learning disabilities, special educational interventions, work history, medication usage, history of head trauma, and family history of cognitive disorders. When patients' cognitive

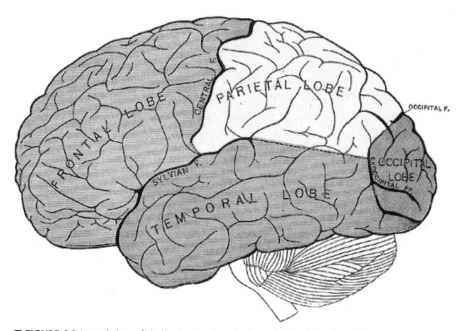

FIGURE 6.2 Lateral view of the brain showing the boundaries of the four lobes.

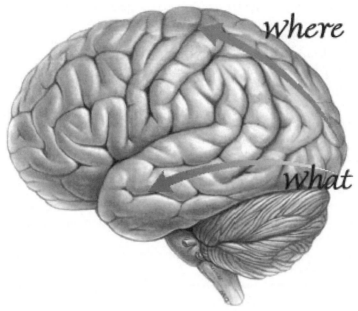

■ FIGURE 6.3 General organization of visual processing commonly referred to as the "what" and "where" pathways: what is it? Where and how is it moving?

deficits limit their ability to convey historical information, additional information from family and caregivers is critical.

Safety screening is another important element of the history, and information about driving and cooking concerns (burning food, small car dents) can help prevent future disaster.

Screening tools, such as the Folstein Mini-Mental Status Exam, can be useful in staging patients with dementia, but more sensitive and detailed testing is required to determine the type of process causing a cognitive impairment. This cognitive testing is often done in the office, but detailed neuropsychological testing, which often takes 3 to 4 hours to conduct by a trained neuropsychologist, is sometimes required where deficits are subtle and careful quantification is necessary.

■ OVERVIEW OF THE NEUROLOGICAL MENTAL STATUS EXAMINATION

The goal of the mental status examination is to determine the specific nature of any deficits in cognitive function, to determine the regional basis for the deficits, and to use this localization to aid in diagnosis and treatment. No detailed testing of higher cortical functions can be performed if there is significant impairment in alertness or attention. Alertness refers to the level of consciousness, ranging from comatose (unresponsive to even noxious stimuli), to stuporous/obtunded (responds only briefly to noxious stimuli), to drowsy, and finally to alert. A functional description, such as "the patient arouses only briefly to noxious stimulation, then drowses off after seconds," is preferable to a jargon term, such as "obtunded," where the definition may not be uniformly applied. Attention refers to the ability to maintain a coherent stream of thought or action. Simple attention can be tested by having the person perform a digit span task. Complex attention refers to a higher level of manipulation of information, such as reporting the months of the year backward or digit span backward. Other components of attention, such as inhibition, can be tested with motor "go–no go" tasks.

Once alertness and attention have been assessed, a detailed testing of language, visuospatial function, memory, and executive function can be performed. Language testing involves determining language production, comprehension, and repetition. Visuospatial function involves determining ability to copy a complex figure, perceive space completely via line bisection, and describe a detailed scene. Executive function refers to the ability to monitor and switch between tasks fluidly. Although difficult to completely assess at the bedside, tasks such as verbal fluency and planning a clock tap into executive function. Other functions, such as praxis, or the ability to perform a learned motor task, are tested only under specific circumstances and described in detail under the corresponding neuroanatomical region.

KEY POINTS

1. The anatomy relevant to this section has a general organization which aids in the conceptualization of how disease states produce predictable patterns of behavioral or cognitive deficits.
2. The patterns include primary input and output regions with nearby association areas, functions which are typically lateralized and other functions which have localization value.
3. The neurologists' mental status test can help rule out neurological causes of diseases presenting with psychiatric features.

CHAPTER 7

Frontal and Parietal Lobe Syndromes

David B. Robinson • Daniel Z. Press

As the most voluminous portion of the brain's four lobes, the frontal lobes continue to myelinate throughout the second decade. The disproportionate size of the adult human frontal lobe compared with that of other mammals or even children reinforces the idea that the frontal lobes facilitate living in a socially demanding environment. Impairment of functions such as planning, complex decision making, and inhibiting inappropriate impulses are the functions most relevant to this review.

A useful approach differentiates the function of three main anatomical regions of the cortex using an anterior view of the brain. In practice, many patients may have symptoms referable to more than one of these three regions or may display only one of the symptoms, suggestive of a single region (Table 7.1).

Diseases affecting the white matter of the frontal lobes may also demonstrate combinations of the clinical characteristics listed previously. In addition to frontotemporal dementia, a degenerative disorder directly impairing frontal gray matter, the differential of such illnesses is broad and includes (but is not limited to) multiple sclerosis, chronic hydrocephalus, and vascular disease. Degenerative diseases affecting the frontal lobes are discussed further in Chapter 9, The Dementias.

Supportive signs and symptoms suggesting frontal lobes dysfunction should be sought and documented whether present or absent. These include Broca's aphasia on the left and occasionally aprosodia on the right, frontal eye field involvement (hemineglect, gaze deviation/preference away from lesion), and, in larger lesions, hemiparesis.

Pathological reflexes seen in frontal lesions (frontal release signs) are easily elicited with practice. These include the grasp (a tendency to squeeze anything placed in the palm), palmomental (scratching the palm from wrist toward thumb causes a contraction of the mentalis on the same side), snout (tapping the lips leads to a pursing of the mouth), and glabellar reflexes (an inability to suppress closing the eyes when forehead is tapped).

■ PARIETAL LOBE FUNCTION

Parietal lobe damage can produce an interesting array of clinical deficits and, because several parietal functions are highly lateralized, they are exceptionally helpful for localization. In this section we'll discuss focal syndromes, though it should be noted that more diffuse processes (e.g., Alzheimer's disease) can preferentially affect the parietal lobes.

   Aphasia is an acquired disorder of language and is often highly localizable (Fig. 7.1). Language impairments should affect *all* output modalities (writing as well as speech, for example). In the general population about 95% to 99% of right-handers and 70% of left-handers have left cerebral dominance of language, placing language function in the left hemisphere in about 95% of people (depending on which study you reference).

TABLE 7.1

REGION (FUNCTION)	DISEASES	COG TEST	CLINICAL OBSERVATIONS
DLPFC (working memory, attention)	Depression Sleep disorders Encephalopathy Schizophrenia Tumors Strokes	Go–no go Trails B Verbal fluency Serial 7's, MOYR	**Major features:** Poor response inhibition (perseveration) Environmentally bound behaviors **Impairments in:** Working memory and executive function Sustained attention Set shifting Judgment
OFC (emotional modulation)	Trauma (associated anosmia) Tumors FTD	Observation Rating scales Cognitive testing often normal	**Major features:** "Pseudopsychopath" Syndrome of acquired sociopathy: tactless, inappropriate, impulsive Easily distracted, lability of emotional regulation **Impairments in:** Knowing social boundaries Controlling high-risk behavior
mPFC (initiation and monitoring)	NPH ACA strokes Hydrocephalus Tumors Acute-unilateral Chronic-bilateral	Stroop observation	**Major features:** Bradyphrenia Abulia: apathy and impaired initiation *Decreased* motor, cognitive, and emotional activity *Akinetic mutism (coma vigil):* most severe form of abulia *Complete absence* of initiation—patients appear awake and alert but have a paucity of movement and essentially no verbal output

ACA, anterior cerebral artery; DLPFC, dorsolateral prefrontal cortex; mPFC, medial prefrontal cortex (includes anterior cingulate and supplementary motor area); OFC, orbital frontal cortex.

Evaluation of aphasia should include comprehension, naming, repetition, reading and writing, as well noting spontaneous speech. If indicated, hearing aids and glasses should be worn during evaluation (Table 7.2).

Neglect is another clinical deficit caused by parietal lesions. It is a disorder of attention, and affects perceptual hemispace, including external as well as personal space. Right parietal lesions are most often the cause, in another example of lateralization. The oversimplified underpinning of this is that the right hemisphere attends to all of space, while the left only monitors the right. When more subtle, neglect in various sensory modalities may only be elicited through *extinction* by *double simultaneous stimulation*.

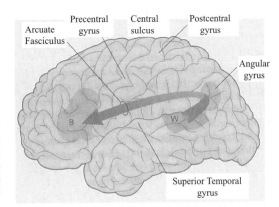

■ FIGURE 7.1 Anatomy helps with an understanding of the classification of aphasias. Consider the following task: repeating a spoken phrase verbally. The input travels posteriorly from auditory cortex to Wernicke's area, through the arcuate fasciculus, to Broca's area anteriorly for language output, and finally to the articulatory speech production centers.

TABLE 7.2 APHASIA TYPES

APHASIA TYPE (LOCALIZATION)	FLUENCY	NAMING	AUDITORY COMPREHENSION	REPETITION	PRESENTATION
Broca's (Broca's area, frontal operculum)	** poor	*poor	fair	* poor	Telegraphic speech non-fluent, effortful, slow Short phrase length Often aware of deficit and frustrated. Often with hemiparesis
Wernicke's (Wernicke's area, near primary auditory Cortex)	good	*poor	**poor	*poor	Normal rhythm and phrase length, with Paraphasic errors. Neologisms Poor self monitoring *jargon aphasia*
Conduction (Interruption of the arcuate fasciculus)	good	poor	fair	**poor	Auditory comprehension is near normal, and oral expression is fluent with occasional paraphasic errors. Repetition ability is poor.
Global	poor	poor	poor	poor	Most severe- no language function
Transcortical sensory	good	mod –severe	**poor	good	Like Wernicke's aphasia, but repetition ability remains intact.
Transcortical motor	poor	**mild –severe	mild	good	Like Broca's aphasia, but repetition ability remains intact.
Transcortical mixed	poor	**poor	**poor	fair	Similar deficits as in global aphasia, but repetition ability remains intact.
Anomic	good	**mod –severe	mild	mild	Difficulty with naming. Present in all aphasia to some degree. grammatic, yet empty, speech.

CHAPTER 8

Temporal and Occipital Lobe Syndromes

David B. Robinson • Daniel Z. Press

■ TEMPORAL LOBE

Dysfunction of the temporal lobes accounts for several types of amnesia, aphasia, and the agnosias. The anatomy is a bit more complex conceptually than that of the other lobes because the cortex extends into the inferior surface and medial regions of the brain, and because limbic structures are so closely structurally related.

Amnesia

Amnesia, in the most general sense, is memory dysfunction. Memory can be divided along different characteristics. Memory for information within conscious awareness is termed *explicit* while information outside of awareness is termed *implicit*. In general, explicit information is termed declarative and it can be further subdivided into episodic memory, recall of specific events, and semantic memory, recall of facts, or knowledge. In contrast to declarative memory, procedural memory refers to changes in the ability to perform tasks as a result of experience. If declarative memory answers "what" queries, procedural memory deals with "how" to do tasks. Table 8.1 presents a clinically and conceptually useful classification system.

Diseases affecting these systems invariably involve the related anatomy and are listed in the following section by type of memory impaired (Table 8.2).

Tumors, strokes, hemorrhages, and other focal disease can affect all memory types as well, depending on the location of the dysfunction.

Two frequently encountered syndromes involving memory are **transient global amnesia** and **Korsakov syndrome**.

Clinically, **transient global amnesia** presents with patient disorientation and repetitive questioning on the patient's part to solve that disorientation. It usually lasts hours, and patients should not have any recollection of that time later. Although vascular and epileptic theories both exist for the etiology, sequelae are typically minimal and recurrence is uncommon. A thorough workup is nevertheless indicated, although if negative, treatment is not indicated.

Patients with **Korsakov syndrome** seem conversationally normal but are unable to retain new information. They tend to guess and confabulate responses rather than deny their knowledge. Thiamine deficiency often presents acutely with Wernicke encephalopathy, with Korsakov syndrome occurring later. The nutritional imbalance is often due to the patient's preference for the calories contained in ethanol to the exclusion of anything else. Pathologically, microhemorrhages occur in mammillary bodies and the medial dorsal nucleus of the thalamus, both parts of the Papez circuit (Fig. 8.1). While treatment of thiamine deficiency does not often reverse acute Wernicke encephalopathy, for Korsakov syndrome it will not reverse the damage.

TABLE 8.1 AMNESIA CLASSIFICATION

MEMORY TYPE (DEFINITION) AND DURATION	ANATOMY	EXAMPLES	AWARENESS
Episodic (events and experiences); minutes to years	Medial temporal lobes, anterior thalamic nucleus, mammillary bodies, fornix	The food eaten for dinner Current events Recounting the plot of a movie	Explicit Declarative
Semantic (encyclopedic, general knowledge); minutes to years	Inferolateral temporal lobes	Naming the longest river in the United States Identifying relative size—an elephant or a mouse? Identifying color— such as color of flamingoes	Explicit Declarative
Working (actively rehearsed or manipulated); seconds to minutes	Phonological: PFC, Broca and Wernicke Spatial: PFC, visual association areas	Phonological: Keeping a phone number in head while dialing Visuospatial: Mentally following a route Mental rotation	Explicit Declarative
Procedural (automated improvement); minutes to years	Basal ganglia, cerebellum, supplementary motor area	Riding a bike Driving a car with a standard transmission Playing an instrument	Implicit Nondeclarative

Modified from Budson AE, Price BH. Memory dysfunction. *N Engl J Med* 2005;352:692–699.

Agnosia

Agnosia is an impairment in recognition, and visual agnosia is the most common type. Visual **agnosias** are typically classified into apperceptive and associative types. In the **apperceptive** type, patients can demonstrate full function of all elementary aspects of visual perception— shapes, colors, angles, and depth, yet they remain unable to recognize, match, or point to named objects. It is most often encountered clinically as a recovery phase of cortical blindness.

TABLE 8.2 MEMORY TYPE IMPAIRED

MEMORY TYPE	DISEASE STATES
Episodic	**Alzheimer disease**, mild cognitive impairment (amnestic type), Lewy body dementia, encephalitis, frontotemporal dementia, transient global amnesia, Korsakoff syndrome, concussion, traumatic brain injury, seizures, hypoxic ischemic event, medication side effects, temporal lobe surgery, multiple sclerosis, vascular dementia
Semantic	**Semantic dementia**, Alzheimer disease, herpes encephalitis, traumatic brain injury
Procedural	**Parkinson disease, Huntington disease, progressive supranuclear palsy**
Working	Normal aging, vascular dementia, Parkinson disease, frontal variant of frontotemporal dementia, Alzheimer disease, dementia with Lewy bodies, multiple sclerosis, traumatic brain injury, medication effects, attention deficit disorder, schizophrenia

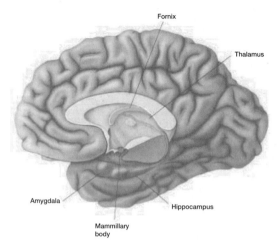

■ FIGURE 8.1 The Papez circuit underlies memory formation. The hippocampus (*Alzheimer's, Herpes encephalitis*) receives sensory information from primary cortices and projects to the mammillary bodies of the hypothalamus (*Korsakov's*) via the fornix. From there, it connects to the anterior thalamic nucleus, cingulate cortex (*ACA strokes*), enterrhorhinal cortex, then back to the hippocampus. The amygdala contributes emotional valence. Damage to any portion can cause amnesia. (*Italics indicate associated pathologies*).

Patients with **associative** agnosia have an impairment of recognition for visually presented stimuli. They can physically describe, copy, and even pick an item from a group. They still cannot describe the function of the item or name it unless given a nonvisual cue to bypass the visual recognition pathways, such as hearing a bell for a phone or touching a key. Of note, this is not aphasia; another sensory input would not be helpful if it were. This type has been aptly described as a normal perception stripped of its meaning.

Associative agnosia may display uneven loss for some categories more than others and result in a **category specific agnosia**. Anatomically, the regions affected represent the "what" pathway or the inferolateral temporal lobe. They correlate from anterior to posterior with information about people, then animals, and tools. These regions are affected in herpes simplex and limbic encephalitis, in semantic dementia, and after traumatic brain injury.

Finger agnosia and **prosopagnosia** are two other types of agnosia. The first is an element of **Gerstmann syndrome** and localizes to the left angular gyrus. Patients cannot name or identify fingers by name. **Prosopagnosia** is face blindness and involves lesions to the fusiform face area, typically on the right, although it often requires bilateral lesions to be clinically significant. In its most severe form, patients cannot recognize faces, familiar or not. If asked to describe the gender of a face, they may use cues such as a beard for hints but otherwise could not perform the task. They often rely on other cues, such as voices. More frequently, recognition is only somewhat impaired and becomes evident when a face is seen only briefly or belongs to someone who is not well known to the patient.

Temporal Lobe Epilepsy

Temporal lobe epilepsy resulting from mesial temporal sclerosis is a common cause of seizures, typically the complex partial type. Seizures should be considered in anyone who describes olfactory hallucinations (typically unpleasant); feelings of intense emotion such as fear, terror, or, rarely, pleasure; a rising feeling in the gut; feeling "unable to describe it"; and having lost time. Less commonly, affected people describe déjà vu, Jamais vu, depersonalization, or intense religious experiences (ecstatic seizures).

An interesting observation regarding a personality type rarely exhibited by individuals with temporal lobe epilepsy, called Geschwind syndrome (or interictal personality syndrome), has led to speculation of historical figures such as Vincent Van Gogh being such afflicted. The syndrome includes hyperreligiosity, altered sexuality (often hyposexuality, but sometimes hypersexuality), hypergraphia (either written or painting productivity), irritability, and bradyphrenia.

Damage to bilateral temporal poles can give rise to **Kluver Bucy syndrome**, a clinical mix of hyperorality, agnosia, hyperexploration of the environment, inappropriate sexual behavior, and (from involvement of the amygdala) heightened docility or placidity and loss of fear.

■ OCCIPITAL LOBES

Hallucinations, visual distortions, and illusions are encountered quite frequently clinically and often have a neurological basis. Not surprisingly, the occipital lobe is usually involved in visual phenomena.

Visual hallucinations can be seen in delirium and withdrawal from medications or alcohol, but can also be seen in **Lewy body dementia** and **Charles Bonnet syndrome**. In the former, the hallucinations are part of a clinical picture that helps suggest the typical manifestations of the disease. The hallucinations are often well formed—frequently people or animals—and often have no emotional element; they are sometimes even welcomed or enjoyed. The hallucinations are often triggered by either anticholinergic or dopaminergic medications, such as dopamine agonists.

Charles Bonnet syndrome can be thought of as phantom sight (similar to phantom limb pain) and occurs in people whose vision is becoming or has become impaired. Typically, they experience fully formed hallucinations, especially later in the day when the amount of light decreases. This is considered a benign condition and often responds to better lighting situations (patients can even carry a flashlight at night to make images vanish).

Migraines with visual auras can produce simple visual hallucinations involving shapes, lines, and flashes of light. Seizures originating from the occipital cortex are similarly poorly formed and more elemental in appearance. Occasionally, seizures can produce an effect known as **pallinopsia**. People report continuation of a previously viewed object superimposed in a new visual location, like a visual echo.

Cortical blindness from bilateral occipital lesions (from anoxia, carbon monoxide poisoning, or bilateral PCA infarcts) often presents with other intact elements of the visual system. The light reflex is normal, and patients will sometimes be able to react to approaching objects. Amazingly, patients often acutely deny the disability, a type of agnosognosia called **Anton's syndrome**, and will sometimes confabulate with direct questioning about visual stimuli ("what color is my hair," "am I wearing glasses").

Alexia without agraphia occurs when the right occipital lobe is damaged, and, in addition, the posterior portion of the corpus callosum. This produces the odd combination of the ability to write, but an inability to read. This includes reading what the person has written just minutes before.

KEY POINTS

1. An understanding of general memory definitions and classification can help with localization and improved differential building.
2. The temporal lobes house much of the memory circuit as well as extensive connections to visual pathways for knowledge, and thus local disease can cause agnosias and amnesias.

■ **SUGGESTED READINGS**

Budson AE, Price BH. Memory dysfunction. *N Engl J Med* 2005;352:692–699.

Cummings JL, Trimble MR. *Concise Guide to Neuropsychiatry and Behavioral Neurology (Concise Guides)*, 2nd ed. Arlington, VA: American Psychiatric Publishing; 2002.

Feinberg TE, Farah MJ. *Behavioral Neurology and Neuropsychology*, 2nd ed. New York: McGraw-Hill Professional; 2003.

CHAPTER 9

The Dementias

Daniel Z. Press • David B. Robinson

■ INTRODUCTION

Dementia is the broad term for a set of brain disorders characterized by a loss of cognitive function sufficient to interfere with the tasks of daily life. There are several different causes of dementia, with Alzheimer's disease being the most frequent. The specific cognitive realms that are impaired in dementia vary from patient to patient and depend in part on the specific cause of dementia. They generally include memory and often include impaired language (with naming problems or aphasia), visuospatial function, judgment, executive function, and difficulty with motor skills (apraxia). The rate of dementia increases with age, but it differs from normal aging in that at least half of all centenarians (those living to 100) do not have dementia. Further, rare genetic forms of dementia can occur as early as the 30s.

■ EPIDEMIOLOGY

The main risk factor for dementia is age. The prevalence of dementia doubles for every 5 years after the age of 60. Approximately 2% of those 65 to 70 years of age will have dementia, but this increases to approximately 14% of those age 80 to 85 years. The estimated prevalence varies depending on the definition and ascertainment mechanism, but between 2 million and 5 million people in the United States likely are currently affected. The prevalence does not markedly differ between genders. Other risk factors depend on the type of dementia. For instance, in Alzheimer's disease, risk factors include a family history (particularly of first-degree relatives who developed the disorder before the age of 70), vascular risk factors (e.g., diabetes and untreated hypertension), limited education, and a history of significant head trauma.

■ TYPES OF DEMENTIA

There is no clear consensus on the prevalence of the various forms of dementia. In general, AD underlies between 60% and 70% of dementia. The next most frequent causes include dementia with Lewy bodies (or Parkinson's-related dementia), vascular-related cognitive impairment, and frontotemporal dementia, with each accounting for approximately 5% to 15%. Less frequent causes of dementia include alcohol-related dementias, normal pressure hydrocephalus, acquired immunodeficiency syndrome (AIDS)-dementia complex, Huntington's disease, and Creutzfeldt-Jakob disease (Table 9.1).

■ ALZHEIMER'S DISEASE

Symptoms, Signs, and Imaging

Alzheimer's disease (AD) is the most common form of dementia in the elderly; its prevalence increases dramatically with age, doubling for every 5 years after the age of 60. Clinically, it presents with insidious onset and gradual progression of short-term memory loss. In general, social graces are preserved. In addition to memory, patients have problems with visuospatial function

TABLE 9.1 CLINICAL, PATHOLOGICAL, AND IMAGING FINDINGS IN THE MOST COMMON FORMS OF DEMENTIA

	AD	DLB	FTD	VCI
Cognitive Features	Early impairment of declarative memory	Early impairment in attention and visual-spatial skills	Behavioral changes and executive function deficits	Executive function deficits, depression
Fluctuations	+	+++	−	+
Neuropsychiatric Features				
Visual hallucinations	+	+++; persistent, and early in disease course	−	
Delusions	++	+++	++	
Depression	++	+++		++
Apathy	++	++	+++ (late)	++
Disinhibition	+	+	+++ (early)	+
Extrapyramidal Motor Symptoms	Mild and only late in disease, paratonia (gegenhalten) and axial symptoms. Absence of rest tremor	Pronounced rigidity and bradykinesia; may be similar severity to PD, rest tremor in roughly 50%	Rare but can occur in FTDP	Impaired gait, axial signs, and upper motor neuron signs
Neuropathology	Dense, neuritic plaques, neurofibrillary tangles, sparing of primary sensory-motor cortex	Cortical and subcortical lewy bodies, frequent comorbid AD changes with plaques>tangles	Lobar degeneration, sometimes with Tau+ inclusions, often lacking distinctive histology	White matter changes, cortical strokes, ±AD changes
Neuroimaging	Neocortical atrophy sparing primary sensory-motor cortices, hippocampal atrophy	Similar to AD, though sometimes with sparing of medial temporal lobes. Impaired DA activity on f-Dopa PET	Focal atrophy of frontal or temporal lobes	White matter changes, cortical infarcts

AD, Alzheimer's disease; DLB, dementia with Lewy bodies; FTD, frontotemporal dementia; FTDP, frontotemporal dementia with Parkinsonism; PD, Parkinson's disease; PET, positron emission tomography; VCI, vascular cognitive impairment.

(such as learning their way around in new environments), word finding (with anomia for low-frequency words), and complex motor functions (apraxia). Several mental status batteries have been developed to help in the diagnosis, with the Mini-Mental Status Examination being the most widely used. Unfortunately, it has relatively poor sensitivity, with particular difficulty in diagnosing highly educated patients and those early in the course of the disease. It is also not specific for AD versus other conditions. Other batteries with higher sensitivity and specificity include the Blessed Dementia Rating Scale and Addenbrooke's Cognitive Examination Battery. Diagnosis relies on clinical examination, although brain imaging should be performed both to rule out other conditions and to determine the pattern of atrophy. In AD, imaging generally reveals atrophy in the medial temporal lobes and in temporal-parietal cortex. Advanced imaging techniques, such as positron emission tomography (PET), are rarely indicated clinically but can be useful, particularly in patients with early-onset disease or in whom the clinical presentation is atypical.

Pathophysiology

The pathological hallmarks of AD are neuritic plaques and neurofibrillary tangles. The plaques, found primarily in neocortical regions, are extracellular deposits containing a form of amyloid that is 40 to 42 amino acids in length. Tangles are intracellular neuronal inclusions containing hyperphosphorylated tau protein that initially appear in the entorhinal cortex and the hippocampus. The amyloid hypothesis is the dominant theory for the pathophysiology of AD. This hypothesis states that the deposition of amyloid is the primary inciting event and that molecules of amyloid form dimers and oligomers, finally leading to amyloid plaques. Amyloid is cleaved from an amyloid precursor protein by the successive actions of two enzymes—beta secretase and gamma secretase. The deposition of amyloid triggers a cascade of events, including excitotoxicity and inflammation. This causes downstream changes in tau, leading to its hyperphosphorylation and deposition in tangles.

The primary evidence for the amyloid hypothesis arises from genetic studies. A very small percentage of patients with AD have autosomal dominant mutations in genes, including the amyloid precursor protein and gamma secretase, which lead to excessive deposition of amyloid, causing AD.

Treatment

Treatment aims at improving behavioral and cognitive symptoms. As of yet, no treatments have proved to be disease modifying. Medications that can improve cognitive symptoms include the cholinesterase-inhibitors donepezil, rivastigmine, and galantamine and the glutamate antagonist memantine. The cholinesterase inhibitors have significant cholinergic side effects, such as nausea, vomiting, and diarrhea. Although their benefit is modest, they are effective from early in the disease through the advanced stages. Memantine is primarily recommended in moderate to advanced stages.

Certain behavioral symptoms can respond to medication. Symptoms of depression respond to serotonin reuptake inhibitors. Delusions and hallucinations can respond to atypical neuroleptics. Agitation, which occurs in approximately 50% of patients, can represent several different processes from a superimposed delirium resulting from infection to disorientation, depression, frightening delusions, or sleep disturbance. Medications such as donepezil or atypical neuroleptics are effective for only a subset of patients with agitation. It is critical to determine the cause by determining preceding events, recent changes in environment, alterations in sleep, presence of fever, or other signs of a superimposed illness. Other symptoms, such as hoarding, social withdrawal, and disorientation respond much better to behavioral strategies.

■ LEWY BODY DEMENTIAS

Symptoms and Signs

The LBDs lie at the interface between PD and AD. The core features are cognitive decline, Parkinsonism (rigidity, bradykinesia, and/or tremor), visual hallucinations, and fluctuations in attention. A controversial and somewhat arbitrary distinction can be made between PD dementia, in which motor symptoms precede cognitive impairment by at least 1 year, and DLB, in which dementia occurs within 1 year of motor symptoms. Both conditions have nearly identical clinical symptoms, pathology, and response to medication.

Core Features

Cognitive Profile: The cognitive profile of DLB has similarities to that of AD. Both diseases impair memory, naming, visuospatial function, and executive/frontal lobe function. Patients with DLB often have more severe deficits in attention, verbal fluency, visuospatial ability, and frontal-subcortical performance, with disproportionate cognitive slowing on timed tasks.

Parkinsonism: The majority of patients with DLB have the motor symptoms of Parkinsonism, which closely mirror those of idiopathic PD. Rigidity and bradykinesia are present in approximately 90% of both PD and DLB. Resting tremor is somewhat less common in DLB, present in 55% compared to 85% of patients with PD. The Parkinsonian symptoms of DLB are usually mild. These symptoms are levodopa-responsive but generally do not require treatment, and patients are at high risk for developing visual hallucinations when treated.

Fluctuations in Attention: Patients with DLB frequently show marked variations in cognitive performance and level of alertness that can be discerned by caregivers. Fluctuation occurs early in the course of the disease and is often a prominent symptom, affecting 80% to 90% of patients at some point. The depth of the fluctuations can range from episodes of simple daytime sleepiness or mild impairments in concentration to episodes of wakeful unresponsiveness, or "going blank."

Visual Hallucinations: Approximately 80% of patients with DLB have visual hallucinations, and typically these occur early in the disease course. Visual hallucinations are very rare in AD, and their presence is highly suggestive of DLB. The hallucinations are often vivid, colorful, three-dimensional images of mute people or animals and resemble those seen as a side effect of excessive dopaminergic stimulation in patients with idiopathic PD. Some degree of insight into the nature of the hallucinations is generally present, but this recedes over the course of the disease. The hallucinations are not typically threatening and may upset the caregiver more than the patient. Apathy, anxiety, and depression also occur frequently in DLB.

Pathophysiology

The underlying pathology of LBD is identical to that of PD, with both cortical and subcortical Lewy bodies, neuronal inclusions containing alpha-synuclein, and ubiquitin. In LBD, the distribution of Lewy bodies is greater in the cerebral cortex, but they can also be found in the substantia nigra, similar to PD.

Patients with LBD have a marked cholinergic deficit in addition to a dopamine deficiency. Clinically, dopamine-blocking agents, such as haloperidol, can cause a life-threatening condition akin to neuroleptic malignant syndrome. Anticholinergic medications can also worsen cognition. Conversely, treatment with cholinesterase inhibitors can markedly improve cognition and resolve visual hallucinations.

Treatment

Both cognitive and behavioral symptoms often respond to cholinesterase inhibitors, with rivastigmine having proven efficacy in PD dementia. Cholinesterase inhibitors can also lessen hallucinations. When neuroleptics are required to manage hallucinations, only low doses of highly atypical agents such as quetiapine and clozapine should be used. Numerous deaths have been reported after use of typical neuroleptics, such as haloperidol. In managing the motor symptoms of Parkinsonism, low doses of levodopa are preferable to dopamine agonists. Anticholinergics should be strongly avoided because they will worsen both cognition and hallucinations.

■ VASCULAR COGNITIVE IMPAIRMENT

The relationship between vascular disease and cognition is complex, and the term "vascular cognitive impairment" (VCI) captures this better than the older term, "vascular dementia." There are at least three prominent ways that vascular disease can impair cognition. First, a cortical stroke can cause a focal cortical syndrome such as aphasia or neglect, which, depending on the definition used, may meet the definition of dementia (e.g., with language difficulty and memory problems for words that interfere with day-to-day function). Second, vascular disease often causes subcortical white matter changes that lead to impaired executive function, depression, and difficulty with complex tasks, although rarely leading to a severe dementia. Third, vascular disease interacts synergistically with AD, such that a small amount of vascular disease and a relatively mild plaque and tangle burden causes much more cognitive impairment.

The management of VCI involves aggressively treating vascular risk factors to prevent progression. Both cholinesterase inhibitors and memantine show some efficacy in treating VCI. The comorbid depression, however, tends to be resistant to medication.

■ FRONTOTEMPORAL DEMENTIAS

The frontotemporal dementias (FTDs) are a series of dementias marked by focal atrophy in specific lobes of the brain, while sparing other lobes, particularly early in the disease process. Typically, the age of onset is much younger than in AD, with a peak in the 50- to 60-year age-group. For patients developing dementia before the age of 60, FTD and AD are of roughly equal prevalence, whereas in those older than 80, AD is far more prevalent than FTD. Approximately 15% of the time, FTD is familial, with autosomal dominant transmission; the remaining cases are sporadic. Pathologically, some patients will have tau-positive intraneuronal inclusions. Recently, mutations in the gene coding for the protein progranulin have been found in many pedigrees of FTD. The three most common forms of FTD are a behavioral variant, a variant termed primary progressive aphasia, in which a progressive language production impairment develops, and a variant called semantic dementia, in which the meanings of words (semantics) are lost. Selective serotonin reuptake inhibitors (SSRIs) can help with some of the behavioral symptoms, although there is no effective disease-modifying therapy for FTD (Fig. 9.1).

■ HUNTINGTON'S DISEASE

Huntington's disease (HD) is an autosomal dominant condition causing choreiform movements (jerky, irregular, and rapid involuntary movements of the face or extremities), altered behavior, and dementia. Behavioral symptoms include personality changes, depression, and psychosis. Peak age of onset is between 35 and 50 years. It is caused by an expansion of the trinucleotide sequence CAG on chromosome 4 (4p.16.3), which codes for the protein huntingtin. In most, the CAG sequence repeats fewer than 20 times. In patients, the repeats vary in size from 36 to 121, with higher repeat numbers correlating with earlier onset and more rapid progression. HD can show genetic "anticipation," with an increase in repeat size when inherited paternally, leading to an earlier age of onset. Genetic diagnosis by measuring repeat size is available both for diagnosis in patients and for prediction in asymptomatic carriers. Extensive genetic counseling is required in assisting potential carriers in deciding whether to be tested. Both the movement disorder and the behavioral symptoms can respond to dopamine-blocking agents, such as haloperidol. Dopamine blockers can lead to tardive dyskinesia, so treatment is generally used only when the chorea or behavioral symptoms are disabling.

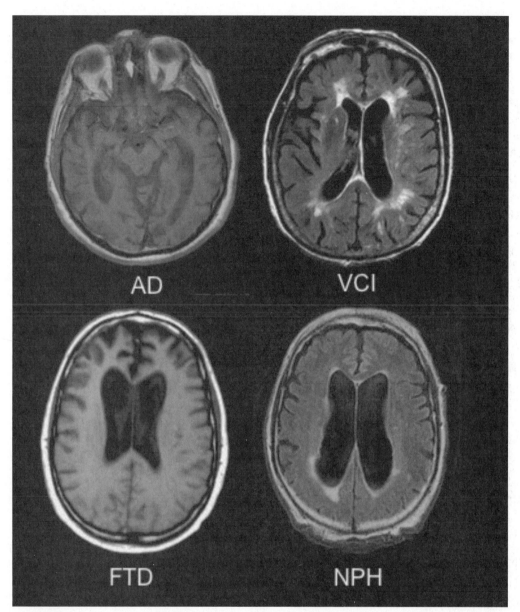

■ **FIGURE 9.1** Representative MR images demonstrating the characteristics of different dementias. In Alzheimer's disease (AD), there is particular atrophy of the medial temporal lobes in addition to lateral temporal-parietal cortex, with sparing of occipital cortex and primary sensory-motor cortex. In frontotemporal dementia (FTD) there is focal atrophy of either the frontal lobes (in this example) or the temporal lobes. In vascular cognitive impairment (VCI) there are often a combination of medial temporal lobe atrophy and significant white matter changes. In normal pressure hydrocephalus (NPH) there is marked dilatation of the ventricles without significant cortical atrophy.

■ NORMAL PRESSURE HYDROCEPHALUS

Normal pressure hydrocephalus (NPH) is a clinical triad of gait disorder, urinary incontinence, and cognitive decline related to hydrocephalus but in the absence of markedly elevated intracranial pressure. Approximately 50% of patients with clinically diagnosed NPH will improve after shunt surgery. The gait disorder varies and can include a wide base, often with short steps and shuffling. Gait initiation can also be impaired, termed "magnetic gait." Urinary urgency and incontinence are due to loss of central inhibition centers. With progression of the disease, a lack of concern for incontinence develops. The cognitive deficits generally occur after the gait dysfunction and are characterized by a "subcortical" pattern, with slowed responses but the absence of significant aphasia, apraxia, or visuospatial impairment. Imaging shows moderate to severe ventriculomegaly in the absence of cerebral atrophy. Both frontal and temporal horns are expanded, without atrophy of the hippocampus.

The primary challenge in NPH is in accurately diagnosing it and determining who will benefit from shunting. A spinal tap with removal of 40 to 50 mL of cerebrospinal fluid (CSF) is the most useful test, with a clear improvement in gait strongly predicting a positive response to shunting. Unfortunately, the absence of a response to a spinal tap does not rule out NPH. Clinical factors favoring a good response to shunting include presentation with gait disturbance before cognitive impairment, a mild and brief history of cognitive impairment, a known cause of NPH (previous subarachnoid hemorrhage or meningitis), and a positive response to a spinal tap. Factors favoring a poor response include predominance of dementia, MRI showing marked cerebral atrophy, and widespread white matter changes on MRI. Additional tests include monitoring intracranial pressure to look for occurrence of oscillations in pressure (B-waves), lumbar CSF infusion tests to measure compliance of the ventricular system, and placement of a lumbar drain to lower CSF pressure for 2 to 3 days. Unfortunately, the tests have variable predictive value and the more informative tests, such as pressure monitoring and placing a lumbar drain, have considerable morbidity.

■ CREUTZFELDT-JAKOB DISEASE

Creutzfeldt-Jakob disease (CJD) is an extremely rare disorder, with an incidence of approximately 1 in 1 million. It generally presents with a rapidly progressive dementia over weeks to months. In addition to focal cognitive impairment, patients frequently develop myoclonus, particularly when startled. The pathological entity that causes CJD has not been proven, but the consensus is that the misfolding of a prion protein is the causative agent. The disease is most often sporadic, but rare autosomal dominant genetic forms can occur. Variant CJD can arise from the consumption of beef contaminated by bovine spongiform encephalopathy, a related prion disease. The diagnosis is supported by specific electroencephalographic findings of sustained biphasic or triphasic periodic sharp wave complexes, MRI abnormalities of high T1 signal in the basal ganglia and high signal in the cortical gyri on diffusion weighted imaging, and CSF changes with elevated 14-3-3 protein. There is no proven therapy for CJD, though clinical trials are under way.

KEY POINTS

1. The dementias are a diverse group of neurodegenerative disorders leading to impairments in cognitive function and behavior.
2. Our understanding of their various pathophysiologies is increasing rapidly.
3. Misfolding and aggregation of proteins into inclusions underlie the most common forms of dementia.
4. Treatment currently is aimed primarily at symptomatic reduction, but future advances should yield disease-modifying therapies.

■ SUGGESTED READINGS

Brown P. Transmissible spongiform encephalopathy in the 21st century: neuroscience for the clinical neurologist. *Neurology* 2008;70:713–722.

Collins SJ, Sanchez-Juan P, Masters CL, et al. Determinants of diagnostic investigation sensitivities across the clinical spectrum of sporadic Creutzfeldt-Jakob disease. *Brain* 2006;129(Pt):2278–2287.

Cummings JL. Alzheimer's disease. *N Engl J Med* 2004;351:56–67.

Galpern WR, Lang AE. Interface between tauopathies and synucleinopathies: a tale of two proteins. *Ann Neurol* 2006;59:449–458.

Hachinski V. The 2005 Thomas Willis Lecture: stroke and vascular cognitive impairment: a transdisciplinary, translational and transactional approach. *Stroke* 2007;38:1396.

McKeith IG, Dickson DW, Lowe J, et al. Diagnosis and management of dementia with Lewy bodies: third report of the DLB Consortium. *Neurology* 2005;65:1863–1872.

Pasquier F, Fukui T, Sarazin M, et al. Laboratory investigations and treatment in frontotemporal dementia. *Ann Neurol* 2003;54(suppl 5):S32–S35.

Reisberg B, Doody R, Stèoffler A, et al. Memantine in moderate-to-severe Alzheimer's disease. *N Engl J Med* 2003;348:1333–1341.

Rogers SL, Farlow MR, Doody RS, et al. A 24-week, double-blind, placebo-controlled trial of donepezil in patients with Alzheimer's disease. Donepezil Study Group. *Neurology* 1998;50:136–145.

Sink KM, Holden KF, Yaffe K. Pharmacological treatment of neuropsychiatric symptoms of dementia: a review of the evidence. *JAMA* 2005;293:596–608.

Vanneste JA. Diagnosis and management of normal-pressure hydrocephalus. *J Neurol* 2000;247:5–14.

CHAPTER 10

Confusion

Sean I. Savitz

■ INTRODUCTION

Confusion is defined as the inability to maintain a coherent stream of thought or action. The level of consciousness is reduced in confusional states, and this can be the predecessor of stupor or coma if the underlying cause is not found and reversed. Confusion presents a unique challenge in acquiring the history. In patients who are confused, the organ system that is required to report on symptoms (the central nervous system [CNS]) is itself impaired. For that reason, clinicians must obtain most of the historical information from caregivers and family members. Although this poses an extra level of challenge in acquiring accurate historical information, the history is important to determine the correct diagnosis. Often an acute confusional state is superimposed on a dementia, and demented patients are particularly vulnerable to become confused, given an appropriate precipitant. This syndrome has been called "beclouded dementia." The diagnosis of delirium is missed in up to 40% to 60% of those affected, and its presence indicates a worse prognosis with higher hospital readmission rates and 30-day mortality, especially if untreated.

■ PSYCHOLOGY OF ATTENTIONAL SYSTEMS

Attentional mechanisms function at a subconscious level to allow for normal cognitive and motor function.

Selectivity: To permit effective learning, humans must pay attention to selective stimuli and ignore other surrounding stimuli. In evolutionary terms, the predator must follow the trail of its prey while disregarding other distracting stimuli in its environment.
Coherence: This implies the ability to maintain selective attention over time.
Distractibility: The degree to which the focus of attention is disrupted and shifted to other coincident and simultaneous stimuli.
Universality: The monitoring system must register as many environmental stimuli as possible.

■ PATHOPHYSIOLOGY AND ANATOMY OF CONFUSION

The attentional matrix is regulated at the cortical level by a distributed network of neurons in the parietal and frontal lobes. Diffuse thalamocortical connections regulated by the reticular formation project to and activate the cortex. The right hemisphere is dominant for the overall attentional matrix, and structural causes of confusion are mainly right-sided. Confusion results from disruption in the attentional matrix at the cortical or subcortical level.

■ ETIOLOGY

Causes of confusion can be subdivided into three large categories:

1. Primary insults to the CNS (e.g., seizures, ischemic stroke, intracranial hemorrhage, or meningitis)

TABLE 10.1 RISK FACTORS FOR CONFUSION IN HOSPITALIZED PATIENTS

RISK FACTOR	RELATIVE RISK (RANGE)
Use of physical restraints	4.4 (2.5–7.9)
Malnutrition	4.0 (2.2–7.4)
>3 Medications added	2.9 (1.6–5.4)
Use of bladder catheter	2.4 (1.2–4.7)
Any iatrogenic event	1.9 (1.1–3.2)

2. Systemic toxic-metabolic conditions impairing global CNS function (systemic infections, hypoxia, hypotension, renal failure, or hepatic failure)
3. The effect of medications or other intoxicants

When confusion develops in hospitalized patients, it generally occurs in those with predisposing risk factors (Inouye, 1996). A severe insult can cause confusion even in patients at low vulnerability, but a relatively mild insult can trigger it in those with multiple risk factors (Table 10.1).

■ CLINICAL FEATURES

Confused patients are inattentive and distractible. Patients cannot interact with the examiner in an orderly, goal-directed, and coherent fashion. On the motor side, there is often a history of difficulties with sequential goal-directed movements.

The cognitive signs may include some or all of the following: agitation, playful behavior or unconscious humor, use of occupational jargon, and paramnesia. There may also be hallucinations, ideas of reference, and disorientation. Patients are usually amnestic for the event on recovery.

The presence of asterixis and or polymyoclonia strongly supports the notion of an intoxication.

KEY FEATURES
1. Acute onset and fluctuating course
2. Inattention
3. Distractibility
4. Disorganized thinking

Differentiating Confusion from Dementia

A history of preexisting cognitive deficits points to an underlying dementia, but this may be impossible to determine at the time of confusion. Poor attention, especially with fluctuations, suggests a confusional state (Table 10.2).

Workup

Obtaining the History

Because of the confusional state, the patient cannot give a good consecutive history. It is important to ask focused questions, such as whether the patient has a headache, has recently used drugs, or has had fevers, but all history should be confirmed with a caregiver.

Every effort should be made to contact a caregiver if none is present with the patient. The task may require some detective work, but it is crucial.

TABLE 10.2 CAUSES OF CONFUSION

Primary CNS causes
Meningitis/encephalitis
Stroke (primarily right MCA or occipital)
Seizures (postictal state or partial seizures)
Head trauma
Secondary CNS causes
Infections, especially UTI, pneumonia or septicemia
Hypoxia or acidosis
Hypoperfusion (CHF, shock, etc.)
Hypoglycemia
Renal failure
Hepatic failure
Toxins (carbon monoxide, heavy metals)
Medications
Alcohol
Narcotic analgesics
Opiates
Amphetamines
Anticholinergic drugs (especially diphenhydramine)
Drug withdrawal syndromes

CHF, congestive heart failure; CNS, central nervous system; MCA, major coronary artery; UTI, urinary tract infection.

It is critical to determine the medications that the patient is taking and whether any have changed recently. An accurate determination often requires calls to the patient's pharmacy or requests to have the family bring in all the medication bottles.

Inquire about the timing of the episode, previous episodes, and the suddenness of onset. Also determine whether there has been baseline confusion previously; associated symptoms, such as fever, shortness of breath, headache, abnormal motor activity; or use of drugs of abuse or pain medications or recent drug withdrawal.

Physical Examination

The goal is to determine whether there are signs pointing toward a primary CNS disorder versus a systemic, metabolic, or drug disorder. Focal signs on examination (e.g., hemiparesis, field cut, Babinski sign) suggest a structural brain lesion; meningeal signs are worrisome for meningitis or subarachnoid hemorrhage. Asterixis (flapping of the outstretched hand) and scattered myoclonic jerks suggest a toxic-metabolic disorder.

■ IDENTIFYING ALARMING CLINICAL FEATURES

Confusion is a sign of major CNS dysfunction and signifies a serious pathology, either within or outside of the brain, especially if the onset has been acute. Several investigations are required to determine the cause, and certain symptoms will suggest which tests should be performed first. In the end, a wide array of investigations may be necessary (Table 10.3).

TABLE 10.3 INVESTIGATING ALARMING FEATURES

ALARMING CLINICAL FEATURES	IF PRESENT, CONSIDER . . .	TESTS
Fever or hypothermia	Meningitis, sepsis	Spinal tap
Abnormal motor activity or history of epilepsy	Seizures, either status epilepticus or postictal state	EEG
Stiff neck or other meningeal signs	Meningitis or subarachnoid hemorrhage	Neuroimaging/spinal tap
Headache	ICH, meningitis, mass lesion	Neuroimaging/spinal tap
Shortness of breath	Hypoxia (CHF, pneumonia, PE)	Radiograph, sputum analysis, CT angiography
Diaphoresis, tremors	Hypoglycemia	Glucose
Neglect or visual field loss, or hemiparesis	Ischemic stroke	Neuroimaging
Ataxia, nystagmus	Wernicke's encephalopathy	Neuroimaging
History of seizures	Nonconvulsive status or postictal state	EEG
Pain on urination or re-catheterization	UTI or urosepsis	Urine and blood cultures
History of insulin requirement	Hypoglycemia or hyperglycemia	Glucose
Recent use of sleep medication	Anticholinergic or sedative	Serum and urine toxicology
Recent falls	Trauma, ICH (in particular SDH)	Neuroimaging
History of memory problems	Underlying dementia	

CHF, congestive heart failure; CT, computed tomography; EEG, electroencephalography; ICH, intracranial hemorrhage; PE, pulmonary embolism; SDH, subdural hematoma; UTI, urinary tract infection.

■ DIAGNOSTIC APPROACH

The diagnostic approach to confusion varies depending on the temporal course (Fig. 10.1). An onset over hours to days suggests delirium, whereas a gradual onset over months suggests dementia. Further, when delirium develops in a previously well elderly patient, there is an increased likelihood of an underlying dementia predisposing to confusion. When onset is recent, a search for the underlying reversible, possibly life-threatening cause is urgent. It is helpful to divide the causes of confusion into primary CNS events, secondary CNS events in which the CNS dysfunction is due to a systemic problem, and drug effects. Confusion is a reason to admit the patient to the hospital for a complete workup.

The risk factors can be divided into those that can be modified (maximizing environmental cues, minimizing medication changes, limiting sleep disturbances, minimizing visual and auditory impairments) and those that are not easily modified (underlying dementia or other neurodegenerative disease).

■ MANAGEMENT

The primary goal of management is to determine the cause of the confusional state and treat appropriately. Symptomatic treatment often requires a sitter who will prevent wandering. A quiet, nonstimulating environment can have a calming effect. Ambient noise, bright lights, and other distracting stimuli should be toned down. Agitation requires drug therapy. Atypical antipsychotics are preferable, including low doses of quetiapine (Seroquel). Trazodone (Desyrel) has become favored for its sleep-promoting effects with minimal sequelae.

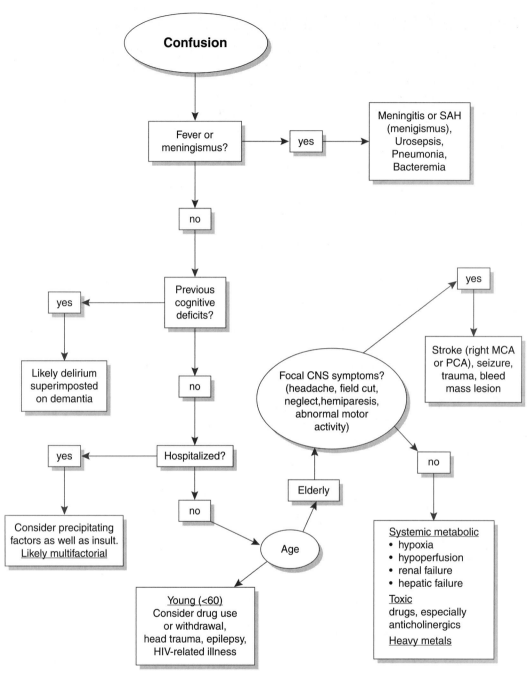

■ **FIGURE 10.1** Diagnostic algorithm for confusion.

■ PROGNOSIS

At least some of the symptoms of delirium can persist for 6 months or longer in up to 80% of patients. Those who develop delirium during a hospital stay are much more likely to require long-term institutional care, with 43% residing in an institution at 6 months. The 1-month mortality for those with delirium as an inpatient is approximately 14%, significantly higher than controls even when accounting for comorbid conditions. Although delirium is frequently completely reversible, it is often the harbinger of more serious and chronic cognitive deficits.

KEY POINTS

1. The confused patients' ability to communicate and provide useful history can fluctuate markedly. Be sure to get ancillary information from other caregivers and, when in doubt, test at different times.
2. Do not assume that confusion has been long-standing in a patient who appears "demented." It is better to err on the side of assuming there is a treatable delirium present, even on patients with chronic cognitive deficits.
3. Delirium and dementia often coexist. Determining whether an underlying dementia is present is nearly impossible in the setting of a delirium. Appropriate testing and interventions should be planned after the causes of the confusion have been treated.

■ SUGGESTED READINGS

American Psychiatric Association (1998). Delirium: Practice Treatment Guideline. Available at: http://www.psychiatry-online.com/pracGuide/pracGuideTopic_2.aspx. Accessed July 10, 2008.

Brown TM, Boyle MF. Delirium. *BMJ* 2002;325:644–647.

Cole MG, Primeau FJ. Prognosis of delirium in elderly hospital patients. *CMAJ* 1993;149:41–46.

Francis J. Recognition and evaluation of delirium. In: Rose BD, ed. *UpToDate*. Wellesley, MA: UpToDate, 2003.

Francis J, Kapoor WN. Delirium in hospitalized elderly. *J Gen Intern Med* 1990;5:65–79.

Francis J, Kapoor WN. Prognosis after hospital discharge of older medical patients with delirium. *J Am Geriatr Soc* 1992;40:601–606.

Francis J, Martin D, Kapoor WN. A prospective study of delirium in hospitalized elderly. *JAMA* 1990;263:1097–1101.

Inouye SK. Delirium in hospitalized older patients: recognition and risk factors. *J Geriatr Psychiatry Neurol* 1998;11:118–125, discussion 157–158.

Inouye SK, Charpentier PA. Precipitating factors for delirium in hospitalized elderly persons: predictive model and interrelationship with baseline vulnerability. *JAMA* 1996;275: 852–857.

Lewis LM, Miller DK, Morley JE, et al. Unrecognized delirium in ED geriatric patients. *Am J Emerg Med* 1995;13:142–145.

Rahkonen T, Luukkainen-Markkula R, Paanila S, et al. Delirium episode as a sign of undetected dementia among community dwelling elderly subjects: a 2 year follow up study. *J Neurol Neurosurg Psychiatry* 2000;69:519–521.

CHAPTER 11

Pathological Laughter and Crying

Josef Parvizi

■ INTRODUCTION

Most psychiatrists are familiar with disorders of emotional *experience* such as the prototypical mood disorders, including major depressive or bipolar disorders. Psychiatrists are also aware of disorders in which patients suffer from labile emotions that fluctuate rapidly from one extreme to another, such as in borderline personality disorder. However, many are unfamiliar with the problem of inappropriate emotional *expression*, a condition in which the patient has uncontrollable bouts of laughter or crying or both without an underlying mood or personality disorder. An affected individual exhibits episodes of laughter and/or crying without an apparent motivating stimulus or in response to stimuli that would not have elicited such an emotional response before the onset of their underlying neurological disorder.

■ ETIOLOGY

The problem in this condition is not an excessive emotional response resulting from labile feelings or a pervasive problem of mood. The problem is a pathologically lowered threshold for the expression of laughter or crying or both. The threshold is so low that the response can be pathologically exaggerated or inappropriate for the context in which it occurs. Patients with this problem have proper knowledge about the cognitive and social norms of the moment, and they are aware that their emotional response is out of proportion to their feeling. The problem is that they appear unable to adjust the type and extent of the emotional display to the contextual information due to lesions along the network connecting cortical and subcortical structures (Fig 11.1).

■ HISTORICAL CONTEXT

Historically, this condition was referred to as *pseudobulbar affect*. In the 1880s, Hermann Oppenheim (the father of German neurology) and Ernst Siemerling described exaggerated laughing and crying in patients with pseudobulbar palsy, a disease in which lesions along the pathways to the brainstem (i.e., the *bulb*), rather than in the brainstem nuclei themselves (hence *pseudobulbar*), cause an upper motor neuron pattern of weakness in the cranial nerve muscles. Patients with pseudobulbar palsy are usually unable to close their eyes, elevate the corners of their mouth, swallow, chew, or move their tongue when they are asked to do so. Oppenheim observed that these patients exhibited involuntary spells of uncontrollable laughter and crying, which in physical character involved symmetrical movements of the face and lips with normal lacrimation and vocalization. In other words, they were unable to move their facial muscles to command but they could move the same muscles involuntarily. This exaggerated emotional response in patients with pseudobulbar palsy was termed *pseudobulbar affect*.

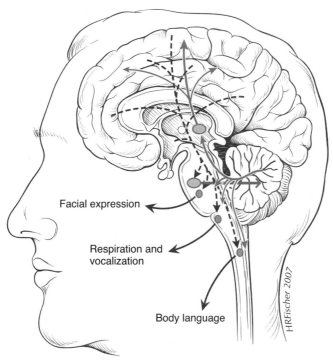

Facial expression

Respiration and
vocalization

Body language

H.R.Fischer 2007

■ **FIGURE 11.1** Corticobulbar tracts and emotional expression. Pathological emotional expression is caused by lesions along the corticobulbar tract, which encompasses projections from the motor cortices and limbic structures to the brainstem nuclei involved in emotional expression. Higher order association areas of the cerebral cortex also send projections along the corticobulbar tract to the nuclei of the basis pontis, from which they are relayed to the cerebellum. In return, the cerebellum has the anatomical means to project onto the same brainstem and cortical structures.

■ CLINICAL FINDINGS

Subsequent clinical observations have shown pseudobulbar affect in various neurological disorders. Among them are traumatic brain injury (5% to 11%), multiple sclerosis (10%), amyotrophic lateral sclerosis (30% to 40%), Parkinson disease (3% to 5%), the noncerebellar type of multiple system atrophy (MSA, ~3%), and the cerebellar type of MSA (~37%). Patients with stroke in the descending white matter (especially in the basis pontis or internal capsules) do also suffer from the condition (11% to 34%). Besides neurological causes of pathological laughter and crying (PLC), toxins and chemicals such as alcohol or nitrous oxide (i.e., laughing gas) can cause a reversible and short-lasting version of pseudobulbar affect.

It is important to note that pseudobulbar affect does not need to be accompanied by the classic features of pseudobulbar palsy. In fact, most of the time, clinicians will not find typical features of pseudobulbar palsy in patients suffering from pseudobulbar affect. Therefore, authors have used terms other than pseudobulbar affect to describe this clinical condition. Terms such as "emotional incontinence," "pathological laughter and crying," "emotional lability," or "emotionalism" have been used to describe the condition of inappropriate laughing or crying response in these patients. In essence, all of these terms refer to variations of the same problem. Because the condition is pathological and involves laughing and crying (and not all the other emotions), the term pathological laughter and crying is the closest descriptor of the phenotype of this condition.

What kind of laughing or crying is pathological? There are individual differences in expressing emotions, and each person has an idiosyncratic *affective style*. Not everything triggers the same emotional response in every person. Some people laugh aloud and others rarely go beyond a quiet smile in a given situation. Each person's affective style depends on factors such as cultural background, personality trait, and education in a broad sense. What we call a pathologically exaggerated emotional display in one culture may not qualify as pathological in another culture. Regardless of these variables, PLC is a problem because it is abnormal from the patient's own point of view. This abnormal condition becomes pathological when the frequency or the severity of the problem is so abnormal that it causes social handicap and psychological suffering.

■ DISTINGUISHING PATHOLOGICAL LAUGHTER AND CRYING FROM MOOD DISORDERS

Mood-Incongruent Pathological Laughter and Crying

How can PLC be distinguished from mood disorders? It is important to ask the patient about the issue of mood congruency. On one side of the spectrum, that is, mood-incongruent PLC, the emotional display of laughter or crying is totally incongruent with the patient's underlying mood or feeling. The act of laughing and crying in these patients will resemble automatisms in epilepsy or tics in Tourette's disorder. In this form of the condition, the patient is aware of the inappropriateness of the emotional display and is often embarrassed by it, but reports that the intense affective response occurs involuntarily—out of control and out of "will." The patient may even report that the affective display is contradictory to the emotional valence of the stimulus and to the context in which it occurs. For instance, a patient may start laughing aloud each time after hearing sad news. The emotional response in these patients can also switch in form from pathological laughing to pathological crying or vice versa. The incongruence between emotional expression and emotional experience in these cases makes it easy for a clinician to distinguish this form of PLC from prototypical mood disorders.

Mood-Congruent Pathological Laughter and Crying

At the other end of the spectrum, that is, mood-congruent PLC, the condition becomes more difficult to discern from a mood disorder. In this variant, the emotional display is congruent with the mood of the patient, *but* the emotional expression is pathologically exaggerated in intensity, frequency, or duration compared to what the patient feels. For example, unlike a patient with depression, a patient with pathological crying does not complain of sadness, but comes with a complaint of now crying to stimuli that would never elicit such response before. For instance, a patient reported that he had begun crying out of his control every time he relayed slightly sad telephone messages to his wife. Unlike patients with mood disorders, these patients are often surprised by how easily they go into tears or laughter without feeling sad enough to cry or happy enough to laugh. Patients' caregivers often allude to their impression that the patient's emotional display does not seem to be "coming from the heart."

■ DIAGNOSIS

One might think that a clinician will not have a problem making a correct diagnosis, even at the mood-congruent end of the spectrum. Studies suggest that this is unfortunately not the case. Clinicians often misdiagnose cases of PLC as depression or bipolar disease. It is important to note that the problem of PLC in both mood-congruent and mood-incongruent forms of the condition is a paroxysmal (i.e., moment-to-moment) problem, unlike mood disorders that are characterized by pervasive and sustained changes in emotional experience. Even in the mood-congruent form of PLC, the pathological emotional display is short-lasting and its course does not parallel changes of the baseline mood. It has been estimated that about 50% to 70% of patients with PLC also suffer from depression. Even if a patient suffers from both PLC and a mood disorder, the clinician will be able to dissect these two problems from each other. For instance, in one of our series of patients with PLC, paroxysmal spells of inappropriate laughing occurred in patients who had a sustained and pervasive sadness and other vegetative signs of depression.

There are several diagnostic scales to rate the severity of mood disorders. There are at least two scales that have been used to rate the severity of PLC (Table 11.1). However, the diagnosis of PLC is clearly a bedside one and a single screening question is sufficient to lead the physician

TABLE 11.1 RATING SCALES FOR THE SEVERITY OF PATHOLOGICAL LAUGHTER AND CRYING

PLACS: Pathological Laughter and Crying Scale (Robinson et al, 1993)*	**Scale** Rarely = 0 Occasionally = 1 Quite often = 2 Frequently = 3	1. Have you recently experienced sudden episodes of laughter in the past 2 weeks? 2. Have you recently experienced sudden episodes of crying in the past 2 weeks? *If the patient has experienced pathological laughter, the next 8 questions are pursued. Otherwise the patient is instructed to skip to question 11.* 3. Have the episodes of laughter occurred without any cause in your surroundings? 4. Have the episodes of laughter lasted for a long period of time? 5. Have the episodes of laughter been uncontrollable by you? 6. Have the episodes of laughter occurred as a result of feeling of happiness? 7. Have the episodes of laughter occurred in excess of feeling of happiness? (rate the ones disproportionate to mood) 8. Have the episodes of laughter occurred as a result of feeling of sadness? 9. Have the episodes of laughter occurred with any emotions other than happiness or sadness (nervousness, anger)? 10. Have the episodes of laughter caused you any distress or social embarrassment? *If the patient has experienced pathological crying, the next 8 questions are answered.* 11–18: Repeat questions 3–10 for episodes of crying.
NS-LS: Center for Neurological Studies Lability Scale†	**Scale** Never = 1 Rarely = 2 Occasionally = 3 Frequently = 4 Most of the time = 5	1. There are times when I feel fine one minute, and then I'll become tearful the next over something small or for no reason at all. 2. Others have told me that I seem to become amused very easily or that I seem to become amused about things that really aren't funny. 3. I find myself crying very easily. 4. I find that even when I try to control my laughter I am often unable to do so. 5. There are times when I won't be thinking of anything happy or funny at all, but then I'll suddenly be overcome by funny or happy thoughts. 6. I find that even when I try to control my crying I am often unable to do so. 7. I find that I am easily overcome by laughter.

*In the study of patients with ischemic brain injury, the PLACS score ranged from 11 to 15 in patients with PLC, whereas in patients with traumatic brain injury with PLC, the PLACS score ranged from 9 to 22 (mean 13.6, SD 4.6).

†In a study of 46 patients with amyotropic lateral sclerosis with pseudobulbar affect a cutoff score of 13 provided a sensitivity of 0.84 and a specificity of 0.81. In a subsequent study of 90 patients with multiple sclerosis (50 with PBA), a cutoff of 17 provided a combination of both high sensitivity (0.94) and high specificity (0.83).

toward correct diagnosis. The clinician must ask the patient or the caretaker about the presence of frequent laughing or crying or both. Once the answer is confirmatory, other routine questions are warranted to discern whether the patient's uncontrollable episodes of laughing or crying are a paroxysmal problem or a pervasive and sustained problem. A mood disorder and PLC can occur simultaneously in the same patient.

■ THERAPEUTIC OPTIONS

Once the diagnosis is made, one can choose from several therapeutic options, even though none of the medications are approved by the Food and Drug Administration for this condition. Of interest, most of the therapeutic options for PLC are the ones that are used for mood disorders. Tricyclic antidepressants (TCA), such as amitriptyline 60 mg daily and nortriptyline 100 mg daily, and selective serotonin reuptake inhibitors (SSRIs), such as sertraline 50 mg daily, fluoxetine 20 mg daily, citalopram 10 to 20 mg daily, and paroxetine 10 to 40 mg daily, have been reported in the literature to be effective in treatment of PLC. Although the same medication works for both mood disorders and PLC, it is remarkable that the beneficial effect of these medications on PLC is very rapid (i.e., within days of treatment initiation) and occurs in response to doses less than those usually needed for the treatment of mood disorders.

The fact that there are treatment options should not necessarily make the clinician immediately prescribe one for every patient with PLC. PLC does not need to be treated in all patients. For example, one patient with pathological laughing caused by multiple system atrophy thought that her frequent laughing, even though inappropriate in a social context, was an excellent way for her to cope with her fatal and devastating neurological disorder. One should be cautious and prescribe treatment only if the patient's problem is so severe that it causes additional social handicap or psychological suffering.

KEY POINTS

1. PLC is known by many different names.
2. PLC is a problem of generating an inappropriate emotional expression in the absence of a commensurate feeling.
3. PLC can be treated with the same medications that are used for the treatment of mood disorder.
4. PLC is more common than you might think.

■ SUGGESTED READINGS

Parvizi J, Anderson SW, Martin C, et al. Pathological laughter and crying: a link to the cerebellum. *Brain* 2001;114: 1708–1719.

Parvizi J, Arciniegas DB, Bernardini GL, et al. Diagnosis and management of pathological laughter and crying. *Mayo Clin Proc* 2006;81:1482–1486.

Poeck K. Pathological laughter and crying. In: Frederiks JAM, ed. *Clinical Neuropsychology.* New York: Elsevier, 1985:219–225.

Robinson RG, Parikh RM, Lipsey JR, et al. Pathological laughing and crying following stroke: validation of a measurement scale and a double-blind treatment study. *Am J Psychiatry* 1993;150:286–293.

Smith RA, Berg JE, Pope LE, et al. Validation of the CNS emotional lability scale for pseudobulbar affect (pathological laughing and crying) in multiple sclerosis patients. *Mult Scler* 2004;10:679–685.

Wild B, Rodden FA, Grodd W, et al. Neural correlates of laughter and humour. *Brain* 2003;116:2111–2138.

Wilson SAK. Some problems in neurology. II: Pathological laughing and crying. *J Neurol Psychopathol* 1924; IV:299–333.

CHAPTER 12

Brief Overview of Neuropsychological Assessment

Nancy K. Madigan • Sara J. Hoffschmidt

■ INTRODUCTION

The field of clinical neuropsychology is a specialization within clinical psychology that emphasizes study of the brain/behavior relationships and assessment of cognitive functioning. By providing objective, quantifiable data regarding a patient's deficits, evaluation results are often a critical component of diagnosis and treatment planning. Patients appropriate for neuropsychological evaluation vary greatly in functional level and present with a wide variety of medical, neurological, and psychiatric problems. At the core of the neuropsychological evaluation are empirically developed assessment tools that have been standardized on neurologically intact individuals. The patient's performance on tests is compared to age- and education-matched norms to obtain a profile of his or her intellectual, cognitive, and affective/personality functioning. In addition to clinical interview and formal testing, key components of neuropsychological assessment include diagnostic formulation and communicating recommendations to both the patient and referring clinician.

■ INDICATIONS FOR TESTING

There are several reasons why a neuropsychological assessment may be of use to the clinician, including assistance with differential diagnosis, treatment planning, and documentation of cognitive deficits to aid in eligibility for services. In addition, characterization of the client's cognitive strengths and weaknesses can be reassuring and therapeutic for the patient, especially for the "worried well" or those who may have an undiagnosed learning disorder. The referring clinician should understand the kinds of questions that may be realistically addressed by neuropsychological testing. Table 12.1 provides a summary of indications for testing and several examples of referral questions.

Although neuropsychological evaluation may be useful in addressing such referral questions, one often-cited limitation relates to ecological validity, or the degree to which test performance predicts real-life behavior and functioning. For example, a patient's adaptive or compensatory behavior in daily living may exceed what might be expected on the basis of the patient's test deficits. Further, neuropsychological assessment can provide an accurate picture of current functioning, but it may not be as useful for problems in which ongoing assessment is needed for the most accurate diagnosis (e.g., complex, emerging psychiatric disorders). Finally, sociocultural factors can affect or limit the validity of testing, including English as a second language, limited educational opportunity (which often correlates with neuropsychological performance), lack of normative data for a particular ethnic population, and cultural differences in symptom presentation.

TABLE 12.1 INDICATIONS FOR TESTING AND EXAMPLE REFERRAL QUESTIONS

INDICATIONS FOR TESTING	EXAMPLES
• Differential diagnosis	• Progressive dementia versus depression in the elderly • Dementia subtype (e.g., frontal temporal, vascular, Lewy body disease, Alzheimer's) • Mild cognitive impairment versus normal aging • Objective assessment of attention deficit hyperactivity disorder and learning disorders • Evidence of cognitive impairment secondary to medical illness (e.g., seizures, brain injury, demyelinating illnesses, stroke)
• Treatment considerations	• Aid in determining appropriate medications, as well as medication efficacy and toxicity • Appropriateness for cognitive remediation • Use and application of relevant compensatory strategies • Formal academic or workplace accommodations
• Baseline testing and prognosis	• Improvement in acute conditions (e.g., head injury, stroke) • Decline in deteriorating conditions (e.g., dementia)
• Issues of capacity	• Objective evidence of cognitive dysfunction to aid in determining competency • Eligibility for services (e.g., documentation of mental retardation, disability evaluations, educational accommodations) • Safety considerations in those with dementia
• Forensic evaluation	• Objective assessment of suboptimal performance (e.g., malingering, possible embellishment of cognitive deficits) via symptom validity measures • Evidence of cognitive dysfunction in traumatic brain injury

■ FUNDAMENTALS OF THE NEUROPSYCHOLOGICAL EVALUATION

Assessment Process

Diagnostic Interview

This important component of the evaluation involves obtaining pertinent medical, educational, social, and psychiatric history. Essential to the diagnostic formulation is historical information, which provides the context for examining the patient's test performance. In addition to interviewing the patient, the neuropsychologist makes efforts to obtain collateral information from a family member, as well as pertinent patient records (e.g., medical evaluations, school reports, and work assessments).

Behavioral Observations

Notes regarding patient behavior are made and incorporated into the final evaluation report. In addition to general physical appearance, aspects of speech, movement/activity, mood, interpersonal comportment, judgment, and insight are described. Behavioral observations also include an assessment of the validity of test results based on the patient's level of effort, motivation, and cooperation.

Formal Testing

Outpatient evaluations typically are a minimum of 3 to 4 hours in duration, although briefer assessments are common for bedside evaluations. In addition to tests directly administered by the examiner to the patient, the evaluation also may include paper-and-pencil and computer-based measures.

Cognitive Abilities and Domains Assessed

Once the referral question and the goals of the evaluation are identified, the battery of measures to be administered is determined. Neuropsychological tests must meet criteria for adequate psychometric (e.g., reliability, validity, sensitivity) and normative properties. Historically, there have been two primary approaches to neuropsychological testing. In the "fixed battery" approach, a standard set of tests is administered to all patients. The chief advantages of the fixed battery method include a rigorous, quantitative foundation and increased reliability; critiques of this approach focus on its lengthiness and its potential for limiting more individualized, in-depth assessment of specific areas of concern. Contrasting with the fixed battery approach is the "Boston process" approach, in which a qualitative, hypothesis-driven emphasis allows the clinician to select different measures over the course of the evaluation. This method may provide greater understanding of the individual's specific complaints, with a focus on application of results to life circumstances. In practice, most contemporary neuropsychologists elect to use a "flexible battery" approach, in which core measures are administered and additional tests are added based on clinical observation and the patient's initial performance.

The selected battery of tests may be administered by the neuropsychologist or by a well-trained testing technician, although test interpretation is always completed by a neuropsychologist. Test measures assess intellect, attention, executive functions, memory, language, visual-spatial skills, motor functions, academic skills, effort and motivation, and mood and personality. Within each cognitive domain, specific abilities are assessed. For instance, components of attention include sustained attention/vigilance, divided attention, and processing speed. The executive functioning domain encompasses mental flexibility, impulse control, planning, organization, problem solving, and abstraction. Within memory testing, encoding, retrieval, and retention of newly learned visual and verbal material is evaluated. Language assessment concentrates on comprehension and expression (e.g., naming and word retrieval) abilities. Visual perception and visual spatial functions are examined via complex visual discrimination tasks and visual construction measures. Many test measures are multifactorial, requiring multiple cognitive abilities for successful performance; in this way, such measures may more closely approximate real-life situations. A general summary of the neuropsychological domains assessed, their presumed neuroanatomical correlates (when appropriate), and commonly used tests are provided in Table 12.2.

Diagnostic Formulation and Differential Diagnosis

After completion of test administration, measures are scored and the individual's performance is compared to the appropriate normative sample. The patient's cognitive strengths and deficits are examined. Given the pattern of performance seen, dysfunction in underlying brain substrates can then be inferred to aid in treatment planning and to clarify the patient's diagnosis.

Neuropsychologists are often asked to use their knowledge of the distinguishing characteristics and cognitive profiles associated with subtypes of dementia to assist with differential diagnosis. Although the *Diagnostic and Statistical Manual of Mental Disorders,* fourth edition, stipulates that memory impairment is the essential feature in the diagnosis of dementia, there are cognitive findings specific to various diagnostic groups. For example, a common referral question is to determine the extent of which an individual's memory complaints are secondary to depression versus dementia. Depression can result in cognitive impairment and can also co-occur with dementia; thus, serial assessment is often necessary to follow the course of an illness and clarify the diagnosis. In addition to documentation regarding the severity of cognitive deficits present, evaluation of the individual's functional impairment in daily life can aid in the differentiation of cognitive difficulties seen in normal aging versus those indicative of mild cognitive impairment (MCI) or dementia. For MCI, determining whether the impairment is primarily amnestic (deficits in new learning and memory) versus nonamnestic (deficits in

TABLE 12.2 SUMMARY OF COGNITIVE FUNCTIONS AND DOMAINS ASSESSED, THEIR PRESUMED NEUROANATOMICAL CORRELATES, AND EXAMPLE TEST MEASUREMENTS

FUNCTIONS AND DOMAINS ASSESSED AND NEUROANATOMICAL CORRELATES	EXAMPLE TEST MEASUREMENTS
Estimated premorbid intellectual functioning	Wechsler Test of Adult Reading; National Adult Reading Test
Current intellectual functioning	Wechsler Adult Intelligence Scale III (WAIS-III), Wechsler Intelligence Scale for Children–IV (WISC-IV), Stanford-Binet Intelligence Scales-V (SB5)
Attention and concentration Prefrontal cortex and cortical/subcortical projections to frontal regions	Conners' Continuous Performance Test–2, Symbol Digit Modalities Test, Cancellation Test, Trail Making A, WAIS-III Digit Span, WMS-III Spatial Span, Paced Auditory Serial Addition Test
Executive functioning Prefrontal cortex	Wisconsin Card Sort Test, Tower of London Test, Ruff Figural Fluency Test, Stroop Test, Trail Making B, WAIS-III Similarities, Delis-Kaplan Executive Function System (D-KEFS)
Learning and memory *Encoding and retrieval:* Prefrontal cortex and projections to frontal regions *Consolidation:* hippocampus	Wechsler Memory Scale III (WMS-III), California Verbal Learning Test II, Rey-Osterrieth Complex Figure Test, Brief Visuospatial Memory Test–Revised, Rey Auditory Verbal Learning Test, Recognition Memory Test, Buschke Selective Reminding Test
Language Frontal-temporal, parietal-temporal	Boston Naming Test, Controlled Oral Word Association Test, Token Test, Boston Diagnostic Aphasia Examination, Peabody Picture Vocabulary Test–Third Edition
Visual spatial functions Parietal, parietal-occipital	Rey-Osterrieth Figure Copy, WAIS-III Block Design, Hooper Visual Organization Test, Benton Judgment of Line Orientation
Fine motor Premotor, primary motor	Grooved Pegboard Test, Finger Tapping Test
Academic skills	Woodcock Johnson Tests of Achievement–III, Wide Range Achievement Test 4, Nelson Denny Reading Test, Wechsler Individual Achievement Test–II (WIAT-II)
Effort and motivation	Green Word Memory Test (WMT), Test of Memory Malingering (TOMM), Rey Fifteen-Item Test
Mood and personality	Beck Depression Inventory–2, Beck Anxiety Inventory, Geriatric Depression Scale, Minnesota Multiphasic Personality Inventory–2 (MMPI-2)

attention, visual spatial functions, or language) can be useful in predicting the possible course of the illness and its outcome (i.e., progression to a particular dementia subtype). Typical neuropsychological test profiles and distinguishing characteristics in the more common dementia subtypes are described in Table 12.3.

Recommendations and Feedback

Once the nature and extent of deficits are determined and a conditional diagnosis is made, a comprehensive report is prepared. In addition to the patient history and test findings, the report includes recommendations and suggestions for treatment. For example, evaluation results may direct choice of medication, type of therapeutic intervention, work and learning accommodations, lifestyle changes, and compensatory cognitive strategies. The evaluating

TABLE 12.3 DISTINGUISHING CHARACTERISTICS AND COGNITIVE DYSFUNCTION IN COMMON DEMENTIA SUBTYPES

DEMENTIA TYPE	COMMON COGNITIVE FINDINGS	CLINICAL AND BEHAVIORAL FINDINGS
Alzheimer's disease	• Deficits in memory consolidation/storage, with evidence of rapid forgetting (poor recognition) • Deficits in language (naming)	• Intact social comportment • Frequent repetition of questions or stories
Lewy body dementia	• Deficits in attention and executive functioning • Deficits in visuospatial ability • Preserved language (naming) • Preserved memory early in the course of the illness	• Fluctuations in attention/alertness • Recurrent visual hallucinations • Parkinsonism
Frontal-temporal dementia	• Deficits in attention and executive functioning • Preserved memory early in the course of the illness	• Personality changes typically occur early in the course of the illness • Disinhibited, impulsive behavior • Age of onset typically in fifties and sixties
Vascular dementia	• Deficits in attention, processing speed, and executive functioning • Deficits in memory encoding and retrieval with intact storage (recognition)	• Personality changes typically occur later in the course of the illness • History of cardiovascular risk factors

neuropsychologist may also recommend additional medical workup and re-evaluation for monitoring of cognitive status. After providing a written report, implications of the results and recommendations are reviewed with the patient, family members, or referring clinician.

KEY POINTS

1. Indications for neuropsychological testing include differential diagnosis, treatment recommendations, establishing cognitive baseline, issues of capacity, and forensic evaluation.
2. The key components of the neuropsychological evaluation include a diagnostic clinical interview, behavioral observation, and cognitive assessment using standardized test measures.
3. Cognitive domains assessed include estimated intellect, attention and concentration, executive functioning, learning and memory, language, visuospatial functions, psychomotor skills, academic skills, and mood and personality.
4. Once testing is completed, diagnostic formulation and treatment recommendations are generated.

■ **SUGGESTED READINGS**

Feinberg TE, Farah MJ, eds. *Behavioral Neurology and Neuropsychology*, 2nd ed. New York: McGraw-Hill, 2003.

Heilman KM, Valenstein E, eds. *Clinical Neuropsychology*, 4th ed. New York: Oxford University Press, 2003.

Kaplan E. A process approach to neuropsychological assessment. In: Boll T, Bryan BK, eds. *Clinical Neuropsychology and Brain Function: Research, Development, and Practice*. Washington, DC: American Psychological Association, 1992.

Kolb B, Whishaw IQ. *Fundamentals of Human Neuropsychology*, 5th ed. London: Worth Publishers, 2003.

Lezak MD. *Neuropsychological Assessment*, 4th ed. New York: Oxford University Press, 1995.

Mesulam MM. *Principles of Behavioral and Cognitive Neurology*, 2nd ed. New York: Oxford University Press, 2000.

Nelson AP, O'Connor M. Adult neuropsychological assessment. In: Koocher GP, Norcross JC, Kocher GP, Norcross JC, Hill III SS, eds. *Psychologists' Desk Reference,* 2nd ed. New York: Oxford University Press, 2005.

Snyder PJ, Nussbaum PD, eds. *Clinical Neuropsychology: A Pocket Handbook for Assessment.* Washington, DC: American Psychological Association, 1992.

Strauss E, Sherman EMS, Spreen O. *A Compendium of Neuropsychological Tests: Administration, Norms and Commentary*, 3rd ed. New York: Oxford University Press, 2006.

Walsh K. *Neuropsychology: A Clinical Approach*, 3rd ed. New York: Churchill Livingstone, 1994.

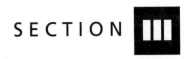

Specific Disease Entities by Neurological Category

CHAPTER 13

Movement Disorders

Ludy C. Shih • Daniel Tarsy

■ INTRODUCTION

Movement disorders comprise a group of conditions characterized by abnormal movements and postures. These disorders are commonly conceptualized in the context of causing either excessive movements (hyperkinetic disorders) or a paucity of movement (hypokinetic disorders) (Table 13.1). Elements of the history and examination that are helpful in the evaluation of a movement disorder often include observations of the distribution of body parts involved, symmetry, velocity, rhythm, and whether the movement changes with respect to specific tasks, posture, or aggravating or ameliorating factors. It is important to recognize that an abnormal movement or posture may be described as an isolated symptom or as part of a larger syndrome in which other abnormal movements or neurological signs may be present. This chapter will focus on enabling recognition of specific movement disorder phenomenology, as well as key diagnostic and therapeutic considerations.

■ HYPOKINETIC DISORDERS

Hypokinetic disorders, which are also known as akinetic-rigid syndromes, cause considerable disability because of decreased or slowed spontaneous movement, also known as hypokinesia or bradykinesia, rigidity, and postural instability. Tremor is commonly associated with akinesia and rigidity and is discussed separately later. The most common cause of these signs is idiopathic Parkinson's disease, but they also occur in other forms of parkinsonism, including drug-induced parkinsonism, vascular parkinsonism, and a group of neurodegenerative disorders collectively referred to as atypical parkinsonism when they are commonly accompanied by other neurological signs.

Idiopathic Parkinson's Disease

Idiopathic Parkinson's disease (PD) is the most common of the akinetic-rigid syndromes, presents in middle to late life, and affects approximately 0.3% of the entire population of industrialized countries and 1% of all persons over the age of 60 years. The diagnosis of clinically probable PD requires the presence of at least two of the cardinal features of the disease—resting or postural tremor, rigidity, and bradykinesia. Patients often initially present with complaints of tremor, usually accompanied by unilateral or asymmetrical clumsiness and slowness of one hand and sometimes the leg on the same side, best demonstrated during finger- or foot-tapping maneuvers. Other features typically seen in parkinsonism include reduced voice volume or facial expression that are frequently mistaken for depression, a stare with reduced eye-blink frequency, slowing in routine activities of daily living, hesitation arising from deep chairs, flexed posture, and shuffling gait (Fig. 13.1A). As the disease progresses, signs of akinesia and postural disturbance predominate. Progressive mutism, dysphagia, severe gait disturbance, freezing, and falls resulting from loss of postural reflexes may eventually produce severe disability. A particularly severe form of

TABLE 13.1 HYPOKINETIC AND HYPERKINETIC DISORDERS

Hypokinetic disorders
  Idiopathic Parkinson's disease
  Diffuse Lewy body disease
  Atypical parkinsonism
    Progressive supranuclear palsy
    Multiple system atrophy
    Corticobasal degeneration
  Secondary parkinsonism
    Wilson's disease
    Cerebrovascular disease with multiple small infarcts
    Anoxic encephalopathy
    Normal pressure hydrocephalus
    Drug-induced parkinsonism
    Head trauma
    Brain tumor
    Arteriovenous malformation
    Postencephalitic parkinsonism
    Acquired hepatocerebral degeneration

Hyperkinetic disorders
  Tremor
  Chorea
  Dystonia
  Dyskinesia
  Athetosis
  Ballism
  Myoclonus
  Tics
  Stereotypy
  Akathisia
  Hemifacial spasm
  Stiff person syndrome

flexed posture of the trunk and upper limbs often associated with more advanced PD is shown in Figure 13.1B.

In addition to the prominent motor disability in PD, there are significant nonmotor manifestations as well, including a high rate of psychiatric comorbidity, such as depression, anxiety, and cognitive dysfunction ranging from mild impairment to dementia. Depression is the most common neuropsychological condition affecting patients with PD and may in fact precede motor symptoms of PD by several years. Although only approximately 5% of patients with PD meet criteria for moderate to severe depression, 45% to 50% of patients with PD meet criteria for mild depression. Anxiety disorders are considerably less common but also can be an important comorbidity, especially in patients who experience significant motor fluctuations. Obsessions and compulsions are a potentially devastating complication of antiparkinson medication, specifically dopamine agonists such as pramipexole and ropinirole. Reports of dopamine agonist–induced pathological gambling, hypersexuality, eating and shopping compulsions, and punding (a stereotyped behavior characterized by repetitive handling of mechanical objects), have all led to greater scrutiny and surveillance while caring for patients with PD on these drugs. Psychosis in the form of visual hallucinations is also commonly triggered by antiparkinson medication but when present spontaneously may signal the presence of dementia with Lewy bodies (DLB), with its distinctive visuospatial impairments and burden of microscopic PD pathology in the visual cortex. The distinction from PD-related dementia (PDD) is controversial; however, typically its diagnosis is made when time of onset of cognitive symptoms occurs within a year of developing motor symptoms of PD.

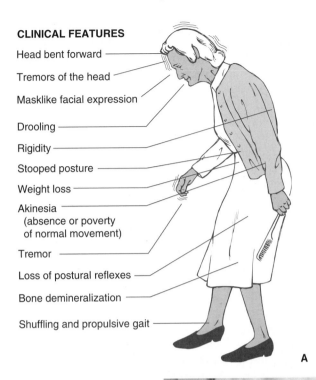

CLINICAL FEATURES

Head bent forward

Tremors of the head

Masklike facial expression

Drooling

Rigidity

Stooped posture

Weight loss

Akinesia
(absence or poverty
of normal movement)

Tremor

Loss of postural reflexes

Bone demineralization

Shuffling and propulsive gait

A

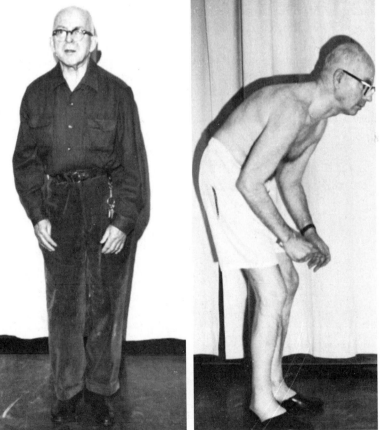

B

■ **FIGURE 13.1 A.** Several motor and nonmotor features of parkinsonism result in a typical appearance in moderate to advanced cases of Parkinson's disease (PD). **B.** A particularly severe form of flexed posture of the trunk and upper limbs often associated with more advanced PD.

The motor symptoms and signs of PD arise from dysfunction in the basal ganglia, which include the substantia nigra pars compacta and pars reticulata, subthalamic nucleus, thalamus, caudate nucleus, putamen, and globus pallidus. Collectively, this group of structures is thought to be responsible for the automatic execution of learned motor plans. The hallmark pathological finding in the brains of patients with PD is degeneration of dopaminergic neurons projecting from the substantia nigra to the striatum, consisting of the caudate and putamen. Lewy bodies, which are eosinophilic intracytoplasmic neuronal inclusions containing insoluble proteins, are found in areas of neuronal degeneration, particularly in the substantia nigra. Protein aggregation in the form of alpha-synuclein is thought to be possibly neurotoxic and to play a presently unclear role in neurodegeneration. Dopamine is released from the axon terminals of substantia nigra pars compacta neurons in the striatum on two populations of striatal neurons, which initiate neurotransmission through a direct and an indirect pathway through the globus pallidus, both of which facilitate striatum-pallidal-thalamocortical interactions in the control of movement. As a result of degeneration of nigral dopaminergic neurons, projections from the substantia nigra to the striatum are reduced in PD. As a result, the indirect pathway is disinhibited and the direct pathway is inhibited, both leading to enhanced pallidal-thalamic inhibition followed by reduced thalamocortical facilitation. The net functional effect of this cascade is inhibition of motor function. Pathological changes are also found in other areas of the brain, including the brainstem, cortex, and autonomic ganglia. These changes result in noradrenergic, serotonergic, and cholinergic depletion with corresponding symptoms, including autonomic dysfunction, depression, and dementia. The early appearance and predominance of the latter in some cases results in the related disorder DLB.

Dopaminergic therapy has been the mainstay of medical treatment of PD. Treatment options consist of dopamine replacement with levodopa, dopamine agonists, and inhibition of dopamine metabolism (Table 13.2). However, nonmotor aspects of PD, including depression, anxiety, sleep disorders, urinary incontinence, constipation, orthostatic hypotension, psychosis, and visual hallucinations are managed with medications that are used for these conditions in other disorders. One important exception lies in the use of neuroleptics for psychosis, because patients with PD who are given D2-receptor blockers are exquisitely sensitive to these medications and experience a profound worsening of motor function. Acceptable alternatives include quetiapine

TABLE 13.2 PHARMACOLOGICAL TREATMENT FOR PARKINSON'S DISEASE

Anticholinergic drugs
  Trihexiphenidyl
  Benztropine

Dopamine agonists
  Pramipexole
  Ropinirole
  Rotigotine
  Cabergoline

Dopamine replacement
  Carbidopa/levodopa

Monoamine oxidase inhibitors
  Selegiline
  Rasagiline

Catechol *O*-methyltransferase inhibitors
  Tolcapone
  Entacapone

Glutamate antagonists
  Amantadine

and clozapine, which are relatively weak dopamine-receptor blockers. In patients with advanced PD, motor fluctuations to levodopa treatment and levodopa-induced dyskinesias may become prominently disabling, even with best medical therapy. Deep brain stimulation (DBS) of the subthalamic nucleus is often beneficial in relieving cardinal motor symptoms, reducing motor fluctuations, and reducing dyskinesias by reducing the need for levodopa.

The prognosis of PD is quite variable because of variable rates of progression in individual patients. Generally speaking, patients with PD are able to enjoy symptomatic motor benefit from oral medications for many years and later from DBS surgery. Mortality in PD depends on degree of motor dysfunction, as well as other comorbidities, but patients generally continue to have a favorable response to medical or surgical therapy 10 to 20 years after symptom onset. Efforts are currently underway to identify agents capable of slowing down or halting the neurodegenerative process.

Atypical Parkinsonism

In addition to the presence of akinesia, rigidity, and postural disturbance, there are a number of clinical features that, when present, may signify atypical parkinsonism (Table 13.3). This is particularly true if symmetrical and midline motor manifestations appear early in the clinical course. Useful clues that may suggest other forms of parkinsonism are the presence of pyramidal tract signs, cerebellar ataxia, nystagmus, oculomotor abnormalities, early and severe dementia, frontal release signs, sensory findings, or prominent autonomic disturbances early in the illness.

Multiple System Atrophy

Parkinsonian syndromes resulting from multiple system atrophy (MSA) are typically the most difficult to distinguish on clinical grounds from idiopathic Parkinson's disease. MSA is a group of disorders that share similar underlying neuropathology but exhibit a spectrum of variable and evolving neurological findings that differ depending on when the patient is seen in the course of the disease. For example, MSA-P may resemble idiopathic PD but is typically more rapidly progressive and only transiently or poorly responsive to levodopa. MSA-C features cerebellar ataxia early in the course, followed by varying degrees of parkinsonism. MSA-A features prominent orthostatic hypotension and bladder dysfunction. Although MSA also produces multiple sites of nervous system involvement, dementia is notably absent. Pyramidal tract findings, including hyperreflexia and the Babinski sign, may be present in any of the subtypes.

TABLE 13.3 FEATURES SUGGESTIVE OF ATYPICAL PARKINSONISM

Rapid disease progression
Early postural instability and falls
Poor or transient response to levodopa
Pyramidal signs
Cerebellar signs
Orthostatic hypotension
Bladder incontinence and impotence
Early dysarthria or dysphagia
Slowing or paralysis of saccadic eye movements
Supranuclear gaze palsy
Early or severe dementia
Visual hallucinations not related to medication
Apraxia

The pathophysiology of MSA is similar to that of PD in that alpha-synuclein is found in regions of neuronal loss and gliosis, earning its classification as a synucleinopathy. However, in contrast to PD, alpha-synuclein–containing Lewy bodies are not present and neurodegeneration involves loss of striatal neurons rather than nigral neurons. Glial cytoplasmic inclusions are found in dying neurons. Other areas involved may include the pontine and olivary nuclei in the cerebellar-predominant form of MSA, autonomic ganglia, and intermediolateral cell column of the spinal cord in patients with MSA with severe autonomic dysfunction.

Management with antiparkinson medications is often tried, with temporary and limited success. Approximately 30% of patients with MSA may be levodopa-responsive for several years before demonstrating the more typical lack of levodopa-responsiveness that characterizes most forms of atypical parkinsonism. Progressive autonomic dysfunction, motor disability, and predisposition to aspiration pneumonia are main causes of death. The average time from diagnosis to death is 9 to 10 years.

Progressive Supranuclear Palsy

Progressive supranuclear palsy (PSP) is best known for paralysis of voluntary vertical and horizontal gaze, although the ocular findings do not necessarily appear early in the course of the illness. The oculomotor nuclei are preserved, and this gaze impairment can be overcome by oculocephalic head maneuvers that produce normal reflex eye movements. Initial eye findings may be subtle and limited to impaired saccadic movements. Supranuclear gaze palsy predominantly impairs downward more than upward gaze, but also affects horizontal gaze. Other eye findings may include blepharospasm, impaired voluntary eyelid opening, and square-wave jerks. Unlike in PD, postural instability and falls are the most common initial symptoms in PSP. Other early symptoms include generalized slowing, visual complaints, sleep disturbance, and personality change. Besides postural instability, other features that may distinguish PSP from PD include prominent axial rigidity and pseudobulbar palsy with spastic dysarthria, dysphagia, and emotional release. Cognitive decline is typically frontal in type, and it has been proposed that a frontal assessment battery test may distinguish PSP from other forms of parkinsonism. There is often a characteristic, astonished-appearing facial expression produced by the prominent stare, upper eyelid retraction, frontalis creases, and impaired voluntary gaze that is considerably different from the facial masking of PD.

PSP is characterized histologically by the presence of neurofibrillary tangles, consisting of aggregated tau microtubule–associated proteins, which are similar to those found in Alzheimer's disease, corticobasal ganglionic degeneration, and Down's syndrome. Neuronal death and gliosis are found prominently in substantia nigra, subthalamic nuclei, and brainstem nuclei, along with cortical atrophy. Management is largely supportive, because lack of levodopa-responsiveness is usually the rule, particularly with respect to early falls. Amantadine, which has dopaminergic and antiglutamatergic properties, has been shown in small, uncontrolled clinical trials to confer some benefit. Although cholinergic deficits are quite prominent in PSP, treatment with cholinesterase inhibitors has not offered any benefit in the cognitive domain. Nonpharmacological treatment largely consists of supportive care for swallowing dysfunction and lack of mobility. Death occurs at an average of 5 to 10 years from diagnosis.

Other Forms of Parkinsonism

Other causes of secondary parkinsonism include exposure to dopamine-depleters, dopamine-receptor blockers such as neuroleptics or metoclopramide, cerebrovascular disease with multiple small deep infarcts, anoxic encephalopathy, normal pressure hydrocephalus, head trauma, brain tumor, arteriovenous malformation, postencephalitic parkinsonism, and acquired hepatocerebral degeneration. Of these etiologies, of particular importance to the psychiatrist is that of neuroleptic-induced parkinsonism, which may occur with both typical and atypical newer generation antipsychotics. Parkinsonism from these drugs is typically reversible with removal of the offending agent, but may take up to several months to occur.

Depending on the distribution of pathology, acquired brain disorders that cause parkinsonism are usually associated with dementia, corticospinal tract findings, pseudobulbar palsy, or gait ataxia. Dementia early in the clinical course is a useful clue that one is dealing with secondary parkinsonism. Parkinsonism may occur in association with a number of other primary, degenerative neurological disorders, such as familial olivopontocerebellar atrophy, Huntington's disease, pallidal degenerations, corticobasal ganglionic degeneration, Alzheimer's disease, Pick's disease, basal ganglia calcification, Creutzfeldt-Jakob disease, Wilson's disease, and several metabolic and storage diseases of the nervous system. Wilson's disease, which is reviewed later, is an especially important diagnostic consideration because neurological signs are often reversible with proper treatment. Differentiation of these secondary disorders from idiopathic PD is usually assisted by the rest of the neurological history and examination, supplemented in many cases by laboratory and imaging studies.

KEY POINTS

1. There are many causes of hypokinetic-rigid syndromes, which include idiopathic PD, atypical parkinsonism, and drug-induced parkinsonism.
2. The cardinal signs and symptoms of PD include resting or postural tremor, rigidity, and bradykinesia.
3. Other nonmotor manifestations of PD commonly include depression, psychosis, sleep disorders, autonomic dysfunction, and cognitive impairment.
4. The mainstay of treatment for PD includes dopamine agonists, monoamine oxidase inhibitors, levodopa, and DBS in cases in which motor complications arise from dopaminergic medications.
5. Atypical parkinsonism should be suspected when one of the following is present: pyramidal tract signs, cerebellar ataxia, nystagmus, oculomotor abnormalities, early and severe dementia, frontal release signs, sensory findings, or prominent autonomic disturbances.

■ HYPERKINETIC DISORDERS

Tremor

Tremor is defined as an involuntary rhythmic oscillation of a body part produced by alternating contractions of agonist and antagonist muscle groups. Tremor occurs in a variety of conditions, as well as in normal healthy patients. The body parts involved, tremor frequency, and particular postures in which tremor is observed are criteria by which tremor is classified. Tremor may involve the arms, legs, head, jaw, lips, tongue, or voice. Resting tremor occurs when the limbs are completely at rest (which sometimes requires being in a relaxed, supine position) and subsides with any action or maintenance of a fixed posture. Postural tremor is typically elicited with the arms extended horizontally in front of the body. Action tremor, which is also known as kinetic tremor, can be observed during any goal-directed activity, such as writing, drinking, or bringing the limb to a target. Intention tremor is a specific form of action tremor, which worsens as the limb approaches its intended target.

Essential Tremor

Essential tremor is the most common type of tremor. A defining characteristic is that tremor is nearly always the sole clinical manifestation. Tremor is typically postural and kinetic, but in rare cases and when particularly severe, may also occur at rest. The distal upper extremities are the most commonly affected sites, but tremor of the head, voice, trunk, and lower extremities may also be present. In the upper extremities, tremor becomes immediately apparent when the arms are held outstretched and typically increases at the end of goal-directed movements such as drinking from a glass or finger-to-nose testing. Head tremor may be vertical or horizontal and, although usually associated with upper extremity or voice tremor, may be the predominant manifestation of essential tremor in some patients. Although often familial, essential tremor occurs sporadically in 40% of cases. Familial studies to date support the idea that it is transmitted in an autosomal dominant manner with variable onset and penetrance.

Essential tremor is thought to be centrally generated via the thalamus and the inferior olives. This is in part based on observations that thalamotomy successfully alleviates tremor and that thalamic and inferior olivary neuron firing frequency closely parallel that of tremor in the affected body part. Abnormal cerebellar function may also contribute to increased synchrony of thalamic and inferior olivary firing, which in turn may be responsible for increased thalamocortical coupling that results in tremor.

First-line therapeutic agents in essential tremor include propranolol and primidone. Other beta-adrenergic blockers may be used effectively, but the best available evidence exists for propranolol. Dosing starts at 40 mg twice daily and is increased as tolerated to a maximum of 320 mg daily or until treatment benefit is reached. If tremor is not well controlled, the addition of primidone, an anticonvulsant drug that is metabolized to phenobarbital, is started at 25 mg nightly and increased slowly to a maximum of 250 mg daily in two divided doses or given at night. Adverse effects of propranolol include hypotension, bradyarrhythmia, and depression. Primidone frequently causes somnolence, less commonly ataxia, especially in high doses, and nausea and vomiting in occasional patients. A slow dose titration upward is useful to help the patient develop tolerance to the drug. Other drugs used in the treatment of essential tremor include benzodiazepines, such as alprazolam and clonazepam, and other anticonvulsants, such as topiramate and gabapentin. Clozapine has some antitremor activity but is not commonly used for this purpose because of the small risk of agranulocytosis. Head and voice tremor are less responsive to oral medication but may be relieved with botulinum toxin injections. Directed injections of cervical muscles or vocal cords can lead to symptomatic improvement in most patients but requires repeated visits because the duration of effectiveness is usually limited to about 3 months.

Essential tremor is usually slowly progressive and results in significant bilateral postural and action tremor of the upper extremities in many patients. In some patients for whom tremor is disabling and poorly responsive to medications, DBS of the ventralis intermedius nucleus of the thalamus can be dramatically helpful in alleviating tremor.

Parkinsonian Tremor

The most common cause of tremor that occurs at rest is PD. This is most evident when the affected body part is supported and completely at rest and disappears or at least temporarily dampens during voluntary activity. Because of its suppression with activity, it usually produces less functional disability than postural-action or intention tremors. In most cases, rest tremor produces disability by its undesirable cosmetic effect and social embarrassment. Rest tremors characteristically fluctuate in amplitude and may disappear and reappear depending on the degree of relaxation, if the patient feels under public observation, or related to unknown factors. In PD, tremor usually appears first in one upper extremity and later spreads to involve the ipsilateral lower limb, followed in some cases by the contralateral side. Leg or foot tremor is more commonly due to PD than essential tremor. When the tremor is limited to distal muscles of the hand it often produces a characteristic "pill rolling" appearance. Tremor frequency is usually 4 to 6 Hz. When it increases in severity, it may become more continuous, larger in amplitude, and more proximal in distribution, but tremor frequency remains constant. The face, lips, and jaw may be involved, but unlike in essential tremor or cerebellar disease, PD only rarely produces head tremor.

Management of resting tremor usually consists of dopaminergic therapy or anticholinergic drugs. Resting tremor often responds to dopaminergic medications to a lesser degree than other features of parkinsonism. The anticonvulsant zonisamide is sometimes helpful for resting tremor. Prognosis for parkinsonian tremor is variable. In some individuals, resting tremor is present early in the course of the disease but subsides as the disease advances. In others, a tremor-predominant form of PD is present, with otherwise mild bradykinesia, rigidity, or gait disorder. This form of PD usually has a good prognosis for relatively slow progression and little disability.

Wilson's Disease

Wilson's disease is an autosomal recessive disease that leads to hepatic, neurological, and psychiatric dysfunction. Clinical features vary depending on age of onset. In childhood, hepatic dysfunction may be the sole manifestation. In adult-onset cases, neurological symptoms are more common and early signs may include parkinsonism, tremor, dystonia, or chorea. Tremor appears to be the most common movement disorder in these patients and is highly variable in its manifestations. It can be a resting, postural, action, or, commonly, a mixed tremor. Dysarthria, cerebellar dysfunction, dystonia, and gait abnormalities may also be present. Psychiatric manifestations of Wilson's disease are variable and include personality changes such as irritability or impulsiveness, depression, and suicidal ideation. Kayser-Fleischer rings are always evident with slit-lamp examination.

Wilson's disease is caused by a mutation in the *ATP7B* gene, encoding for a copper-transporting adenosine triphosphatase. Copper is typically processed in the liver, where hepatocytes incorporate copper into ceruloplasmin, which can then be excreted via the biliary system for excretion. In Wilson's disease, copper elimination is dysfunctional, leading to copper accumulation in the liver, eyes (resulting in the characteristic Kayser-Fleischer rings), and brain, among other organs. Brain magnetic resonance imaging (MRI) reveals areas of basal ganglia T2 hyperintensities, often surrounded by T2 hypointensity, which is thought to be due to copper deposition. Diagnosis is made by detection of reduced serum ceruloplasmin and elevated 24-hour urinary copper level. In some cases, liver biopsy to demonstrate elevated hepatic copper content is necessary to make the diagnosis.

Management of Wilson's disease focuses on restoring normal levels of systemic copper by reducing dietary copper intake; inhibiting intestinal copper absorption with potassium, zinc, or tetrathiomolybdate; or with copper-chelation therapy, usually with penicillamine. In cases of fulminant hepatic failure, liver transplantation is necessary.

Cerebellar Tremor

Cerebellar tremors may be either postural-action or intention in type and, in severe cases, may spill over to occur at rest. They are relatively low in frequency at 3 to 4 Hz and are associated with ataxia and dysmetria. Titubation of the head and neck may be present and is distinguished from essential head tremor by the presence of other cerebellar findings. Intention tremor is due to disturbances of the cerebellar outflow projection system, which is mediated by the dentate nucleus and superior cerebellar peduncles. This large-amplitude tremor typically increases in severity as the body part moves closer to its target, in contrast to postural-action tremors, which either remain constant throughout the range of motion or increase after terminal fixation. These tremors are large in amplitude because of involvement of proximal muscles and are sometimes difficult to distinguish from severe cerebellar ataxia and dysmetria, which are usually also present. Nonetheless, the frequent association with ataxia, dysmetria, titubation, and other cerebellar signs is common and supports the idea of a cerebellar origin of intention tremor. The most common causes of cerebellar tremor are multiple sclerosis, midbrain trauma, and stroke. Degenerative diseases of the dentate nucleus and cerebellar outflow pathways, severe forms of essential tremor, Wilson's disease, hepatocerebral degeneration, and mercury poisoning may also produce intention tremor. Rubral tremor (or Holmes' tremor) is due to lesions of the dentatothalamic projection system running through and near the red nucleus, which typically produce a combination of rest, postural-action, and intention tremor.

Medical treatment of cerebellar tremor is largely ineffective, although propranolol, clonazepam, carbamazepine, tetrahydrocannabinol, and trihexyphenidyl have been used either alone or in combination with at best only modest benefit. In disabling cases of tremor, DBS of the ventralis intermedius nucleus of the thalamus is undertaken and is helpful in approximately half of cases.

Rubral Tremor

Rubral tremor, also known as Holmes' tremor, refers to tremor that occurs after midbrain injury in the vicinity of the red nucleus as a result of lesions of the superior cerebellar peduncle subserving the rubro-olivo-cerebello-rubral loop and substantia nigra rather than the red nucleus, for which it is named. This is a mixed tremor that is constant, occurs at rest, and commonly increases with goal-directed activity.

Management of rubral tremor is difficult, although some success has been reported with levodopa, clonazepam, anticholinergic drugs, and treatment of the underlying cause. Prognosis depends on the underlying syndrome.

Physiological Tremor

All individuals have a very low-amplitude, high-frequency tremor of about 10 to 12 Hz that is not visible under ordinary circumstances. Physiological tremor results from a combination of mechanisms, including intrinsic motor neuron firing rates, suprasegmental influences on motor unit firing patterns, stretch reflex oscillations, and peripheral beta-adrenergic mechanisms. Enhanced physiological tremor is the most common cause of postural tremor. Many factors increase physiological tremor, most by the common mechanism of increased sympathomimetic activity. Common drugs that increase adrenergic activity include alpha- and beta-adrenergic agonists such as terbutaline, isoproterenol, salmeterol, and epinephrine; amphetamines; tricyclic antidepressants; levodopa; nicotine; and xanthines, such as theophylline and caffeine. Anxiety, excitement, fright, muscle fatigue, hypoglycemia, alcohol and narcotic withdrawal, thyrotoxicosis, fever, and pheochromocytoma also enhance physiological tremor by adrenergic mechanisms. Miscellaneous toxic causes of increased physiological tremor with unknown mechanisms include lithium, corticosteroids, selective serotonin reuptake inhibitors, immunodepressants, sodium valproate, selective serotonin reuptake inhibitors, immunodepressants, amiodarone, mercury, lead, and arsenic. Since enhanced physiological tremor is the most common cause of postural-action tremor, it is apparent that a medical rather than primary neurological cause for postural-action tremor is responsible in most cases.

KEY POINTS

1. Essential tremor is the most common movement disorder. It is characterized by the presence of a postural and action tremor of the hands, head, or voice without other neurological features.
2. First-line therapy of essential tremor includes primidone and propranolol. Other treatment options include benzodiazepine, topiramate, gabapentin, and, in medication-refractory tremor, DBS of the ventralis intermedius nucleus of the thalamus.
3. Parkinsonian tremor is characterized by an asymmetrical, often unilateral, resting tremor of the upper extremity. It can be resistant to dopaminergic medications, and anticholinergics and zonisamide have been helpful in such cases.
4. Tremor is the most common movement disorder associated with Wilson's disease, a treatable copper elimination defect of the liver. Tremor type can be variable in its presentation.
5. Cerebellar tremor is often described as a low-frequency, intention-type tremor that worsens as the limb approaches the target. This type of tremor is difficult to treat either medically or surgically.
6. Enhanced physiological tremor has a multitude of causes, most commonly toxic.

Chorea

The term *chorea* is derived from the Greek word meaning "dance" and is used to refer to an involuntary movement disorder characterized by randomly appearing irregular, purposeless, jerky movements of various portions of the body, extremities, and face. The character, location, and duration of individual movements are unpredictable, although individual patients usually exhibit a certain repertoire of recurrent abnormal movements and postures that become stereotyped and characteristic for them. Later in the course, in some choreiform disorders, unsteady gait, abnormal postures of the arms and hands while walking, and impaired balance may become prominent. Examination may reveal a wide variety of involuntary movements of the face, extremities, and trunk. In mild chorea, involuntary movements may be infrequent, of small amplitude, and relatively isolated, giving an appearance difficult to distinguish from fidgetiness, myoclonus, or tics. Like many hyperkinetic movements, some choreic movements can be partly suppressed or successfully obscured by incorporation into semi-purposeful movements. In more advanced chorea, movements occur nearly continuously and appear to spread fluidly from site to site over the body.

The differential diagnosis of chorea in the adult is broad and includes a large number of hereditary, degenerative, and acquired disorders (Table 13.4).

Huntington's Disease

The most well-known cause of chorea is Huntington's disease, an inherited neurodegenerative condition causing atrophy of caudate and putamen, which is inherited in an autosomal dominant manner. Carriers of an unstable CAG trinucleotide expansion in the huntingtin gene

---

TABLE 13.4 CAUSES OF CHOREA

Drug-induced
  Neuroleptics (tardive dyskinesia)
  Cocaine
  Amphetamines
  Antiparkinson drugs
  Anticonvulsants

Vascular
  Basal ganglia lacunar infarction
  Subthalamic nucleus infarction or hemorrhage

Systemic
  Sydenham's chorea
  Acquired hepatolenticular degeneration associated with chronic liver disease
  Systemic lupus erythematosus
  Phospholipid antibody syndrome
  Hyperthyroidism
  Hypoparathyroidism
  Acute electrolyte imbalance

Hereditary
  Wilson's disease
  Benign familial chorea
  Neuroacanthocytosis
  Metabolic disorders
  Paroxysmal choreoathetosis
  Huntington's disease

Other
  Senile chorea

greater than 36 repeats are highly likely to become symptomatic from the disease. Penetrance is thought to be nearly complete, especially with repeat sizes greater than 40. Sporadic cases occasionally occur but are presumed more to be the result of incomplete information concerning family history rather than new mutations. Age of onset inversely correlates with number of trinucleotide repeats and, in a phenomenon known as anticipation, each successive generation that inherits the disorder usually has a higher number of trinucleotide repeats and an earlier age of onset than the previous generation. Clinical features are notable for reduced facial expression with superimposed involuntary facial movements. Abnormal movements and postures of the trunk may include arching of the back, flexion and extension of the trunk, stretching of the neck, shoulder shrugging, and rocking of the pelvis. Abnormal limb movements can be distributed proximally or distally and may include sudden and sustained twisting or hyperextension postures of an arm or leg. Respiratory dyskinesia may produce irregular breathing, grunting noises, and air gulping. Motor impersistence is particularly common in Huntington's disease and is manifest by inability to maintain a strong grip or keep the tongue protruded for more than several seconds. Disability in Huntington's disease is due not only to the involuntary movements but to other, nonchoreic neurological symptoms, which include dysarthria, gait disturbance, dementia, and psychotic disturbances.

Neuropsychiatric abnormalities are seen in almost all patients with Huntington's disease, and personality changes, including irritability, impulsivity, dementia, and major affective disorder, are common. These result in suicide in a small percentage of cases. Psychosis is a frequent complication and is usually treated with neuroleptics. The dopamine-depleter tetrabenazine, which is commonly used as an antichorea drug, can worsen depression, akathisia, and sedation in these patients.

The pathology of Huntington's disease includes neuronal death and gliosis in the caudate and putamen. Subcortical and cortical atrophy is also present. Intranuclear and intracytoplasmic inclusions are seen in striatal and cortical neurons, which stain for the mutant huntingtin protein as well as ubiquitin and proteosomal elements, which are thought to be necessary for proper protein degradation, which is defective in HD. Based on basal ganglia circuitry models, reduced striatal output leads to excessive inhibition of the subthalamus. As a result, subthalamic excitation of internal globus pallidus is reduced, leading to enhanced thalamocortical motor activity.

Management consists of symptomatic treatment of the choreiform movements, which includes dopamine-receptor blockers, such as neuroleptics or tetrabenazine. Affective symptoms are treated with antidepressants and anxiety states with serotonin reuptake inhibitors or benzodiazepines. Neuroprotective trials are currently under way, but no agents have demonstrated definite clinical efficacy. Most patients survive between 10 and 25 years from onset, with the rate of progression not clearly correlated with CAG repeat length.

Tardive Dyskinesia

Tardive dyskinesia (TD) may be differentiated from other choreiform disorders by the presence of more repetitive, stereotyped movements that predominantly but not exclusively involve muscles of the face, mouth, and tongue. Oral, facial, and lingual dyskinesias are especially conspicuous in elderly patients. These may include protruding and twisting movements of the tongue; pouting, puckering, or smacking movements of the lips; retraction of the corners of the mouth; bulging of the cheeks; chewing movements; and blepharospasm. Dyskinesias of the extremities also occur, such as twisting, spreading, and "piano-playing" finger movements; tapping foot movements; and dystonic extensor postures of the toes. Abnormal movements are often more dystonic than choreic, and the lack of progression, together with absence of other motor abnormalities such as motor impersistence, dysarthria, and gait ataxia, help to distinguish TD from Huntington's disease. TD must be distinguished from stereotyped movements and psychotic mannerisms associated with chronic schizophrenia, as well as spontaneous orofacial dyskinesias, which often occur in elderly individuals. Stereotyped movements in schizophrenia are usually less rhythmic, more stereotyped and complex, and not choreoathetotic or dystonic. Spontaneous oral dyskinesias in the elderly are often associated with edentulism and dementia.

TD may appear as early as 1 to 6 months after dopamine-receptor blocker exposure, such as neuroleptics or certain antiemetic medications, such as prochlorperazine and metoclopramide. TD has been seen with both older and newer generation neuroleptics, with the notable exceptions of quetiapine and clozapine; reports following exclusive exposure to these agents are extremely rare and have usually been reported in patients who were also treated with older generation neuroleptics. Onset is insidious and most commonly occurs while the patient is receiving a dopamine-receptor blocker. However, TD also commonly appears after a reduction in dose, after switching to a less potent neuroleptic, or after discontinuation of a neuroleptic. This "unmasking" effect is due to removal of the hypokinetic effects of neuroleptics, which frequently causes a delay in recognition of TD. Withdrawal dyskinesia usually disappears within several weeks of dopamine blocker discontinuation but should be considered to be a precursor to more persistent forms of TD.

The pathophysiology of TD is unclear, but a generally accepted hypothesis is that chronic dopamine blockage leads to upregulation of dopamine receptors, which are more sensitive to nascent dopamine release.

Management consists of cessation of the offending drug. If movements are not reduced, dopamine-receptor blockers can be used to ameliorate symptoms, preferably with quetiapine or clozapine. However, clozapine carries a 1% risk of agranulocytosis that must be weighed against any possible benefit and is also associated with other adverse effects, such as weight gain, sedation, and drooling. Clonazepam is a useful alternative and may produce mild symptomatic benefit. The dopamine-depleter tetrabenazine may be used but carries a risk of exacerbating preexisting depression. Currently, tetrabenazine is not yet available in the United States.

The estimated risk of developing TD has been reported in several epidemiological studies. Cumulative incidence of TD is estimated to be 5% after 1 year, 27% after 5 years, 43% after 10 years, and 52% after 15 years of antipsychotic drug exposure. The cumulative incidence of *persistent* TD lasting for at least 3 months is 3% after 1 year, 20% after 5 years, and 34% after 10 years. These rates suggest an annual incidence of approximately 5% overall, including transient and persistent TD, and approximately 3% for cases persisting for at least 3 months. Older age is clearly the most robust risk factor for TD. Other factors, such as female gender, brain damage, dementia, major affective disorder, diabetes, longer duration of antipsychotic drug exposure, use of anticholinergic antiparkinson drugs, and a history of previous acute extrapyramidal reactions to dopamine blockers, have been tentatively associated with greater prevalence of TD.

The prognosis is variable, with spontaneous resolution occurring in approximately half of patients. In patients with persistent symptoms, involuntary movements can generally be reduced with symptomatic treatment but are rarely abolished completely.

KEY POINTS

1. In chorea, involuntary movements may be infrequent, of small amplitude, and relatively isolated, giving an appearance difficult to distinguish from fidgetiness, myoclonus, or tics.
2. Huntington's disease is a trinucleotide expansion disease, with an autosomal dominant pattern of inheritance. Dementia, psychosis, depression, and anxiety are common.
3. TD commonly consists of more repetitive, stereotyped movements than other choreiform disorders and do not exclusively involve muscles of the face, mouth, and tongue.
4. TD has been seen with both older and newer generation neuroleptics, with the notable exceptions of quetiapine and clozapine. Treatment is removal of the offending drugs or, in cases of persistent TD, the dopamine-depleter tetrabenazine.

TABLE 13.5 TYPES OF DYSTONIA

NAME	FEATURES
Cervical dystonia	Begins in midlife, various combinations of torticollis (head rotation), laterocollis (lateral tilt), retrocollis (head extension), and antecollis (head flexion); head jerking or tremor are often present.
Blepharospasm	Increased eyeblink frequency, forced closure of the eyelids, and difficulty opening eyes.
Oromandibular dystonia	Jaw-opening, jaw-closing, and jaw deviation, fairly synchronous and repetitive; may cause dental trauma.
Spasmodic dysphonia (not illustrated)	Involuntary adduction or abduction of the vocal cords; adduction dysphonia results in strained speech and staccato voice pattern with frequent voice breaks; abductor type results in intermittent breathy or whispered voice.
Limb dystonia of the foot	Often presents as unilateral plantar flexion and inversion triggered by action; may be an early manifestation of Parkinson's disease.
Writer's cramp or other limb dystonias	Slowness and deterioration of handwriting; excessive squeezing of pen, involuntary extension movements of individual fingers away from the pen, and involuntary flexion or extension movements of the wrist; one of many occupational dystonias that can affect musicians, typists, tailors, and other occupations requiring manual dexterity.

with anticonvulsant medications. Secondary forms of these disorders also occur, as a result of a variety of causes, including multiple sclerosis, supplementary motor area seizures, endocrine or metabolic disorders, cerebral palsy, and psychogenic disorders.

Secondary Dystonia

The vast majority of dystonias are secondary and are due to other underlying neurological disorders. They are therefore nearly always associated with other neurological findings in addition to dystonia. Dystonia may be associated with diseases with known and suspected metabolic defects, such as Wilson's disease, dopa-responsive dystonia, neuroacanthocytosis, gangliosidoses, metachromatic leukodystrophy, and aminoacidurias. Many degenerative diseases of the basal ganglia, such as PD, PSP, Huntington's disease, olivopontocerebellar atrophy, and pallidal degenerations, may produce dystonia together with other extrapyramidal manifestations (Table 13.6). Miscellaneous structural and toxic disorders that produce dystonia, many of which are associated with abnormal brain imaging, include perinatal anoxia or kernicterus, stroke, head trauma, multiple sclerosis, neoplasm, vascular malformations, neuroleptic and antiparkinson drugs, manganese toxicity, and peripheral trauma (Table 13.7). As with TD, both older and newer generation neuroleptics have been associated with tardive dystonia, with onset often delayed until after years of exposure to dopamine antagonists. Tardive dystonia can resemble idiopathic dystonia, but there are some clinical features that can be used to distinguish the two. Dystonia of the neck and trunk may include retrocollis, torticollis, axial dystonia, shoulder shrugging, rocking and swaying movements, and rotatory or thrusting hip movements. Extremity involvement is often more severe in younger individuals, in whom dystonic postures and ballistic movements may occur.

Childhood forms usually become generalized, regardless of whether primary or secondary. Delayed onset of dystonia may occur in adolescence following perinatal brain injury resulting from kernicterus, anoxia, or trauma. Adult forms of primary dystonia are usually nonprogressive and remain focal or segmental. Generalized or lower extremity dystonia in an adult should therefore raise the possibility of an identifiable underlying cause. Hemidystonia in a child or

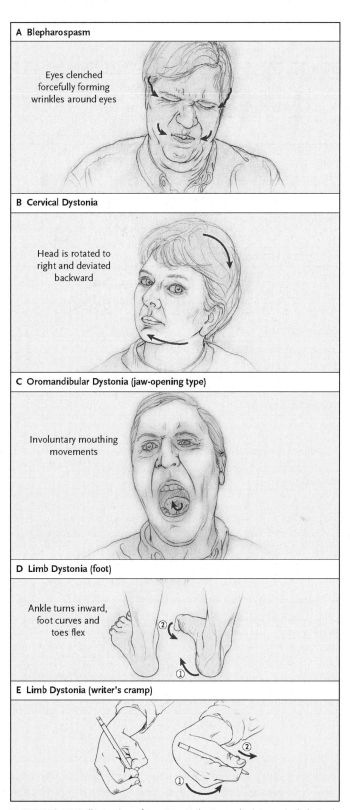

A Blepharospasm

Eyes clenched forcefully forming wrinkles around eyes

B Cervical Dystonia

Head is rotated to right and deviated backward

C Oromandibular Dystonia (jaw-opening type)

Involuntary mouthing movements

D Limb Dystonia (foot)

Ankle turns inward, foot curves and toes flex

E Limb Dystonia (writer's cramp)

■ **FIGURE 13.2** Illustrations from top to bottom depict cervical dystonia with rotation to the right and backward head deviation, blepharospasm with excessive eye blinking and closure, oromandibular dystonia with involuntary jaw opening, focal limb dystonia of the foot demonstrating toe flexion and foot inversion, and writer's cramp causing flexion dystonia of the wrists and fingers during writing. (Reprinted with permission from Tarsy D, Simon DK. Dystonia. *N Engl J Med* 2006;355:818–829. Copyright © 2006 Massachusetts Medical Society. All rights reserved.)

TABLE 13.6 INHERITED CAUSES OF DYSTONIA OR DYSTONIA-PLUS SYNDROMES

Primary torsion dystonia (DYT1)
Autosomal recessive primary torsion dystonia (DYT2)
Lubag's, or X-linked, dystonia-parkinsonism (DYT3)
Non-DYT1 primary torsion dystonia (DYT4)
Dopa-responsive dystonia (GCH1)
Adolescent primary torsion dystonia of mixed type (DYT6)
Adult-onset focal primary torsion dystonia (DYT7)
Paroxysmal nonkinesigenic choreoathetosis (DYT8)
Paroxysmal dystonia choreoathetosis with episodic ataxia (DYT9)
Paroxysmal kinesigenic choreoathetosis (DYT10)
Myoclonus-dystonia (DYT11)
Rapid-onset dystonia-parkinsonism (DYT12)
Focal dystonia with craniocervical features (DYT13)
Deafness-dystonia syndrome 1 (DYT14)
Leber's hereditary optic neuropathy plus dystonia (mitochondrial DNA)
Huntington's disease
Spinocerebellar ataxia (SCA3)
Dentatorubropallidoluysian atrophy
Familial basal ganglia calcifications
Wilson's disease
Gangliosidoses
Metachromatic leukodystrophy
Homocystinuria
Hartnup's disease
Glutaric acidemia
Methylmalonic aciduria
Pantothenate kinase-associated neurodegeneration
Dystonic lipidosis
Ceroid-lipofuscinosis
Ataxia-telangiectasia
Neuroacanthocytosis
Juvenile parkinsonism
Lesch-Nyhan syndrome
Other mitochondrial syndromes (e.g., MERRF/MELAS)

adult is strongly indicative of a contralateral structural basal ganglia abnormality. Action dystonia is more commonly a feature of primary dystonia, whereas the early appearance of a fixed dystonic posture is usually indicative of secondary dystonia. Birth, developmental, medication, toxin, trauma, and family history are all important in identifying secondary dystonia.

Certain clues may help narrow the diagnosis of a secondary dystonia. For example, the combination of tremor and akinesia should suggest Wilson's disease; cerebellar ataxia should suggest olivopontocerebellar atrophy, ataxia telangiectasia, or storage disorders; abnormal eye

TABLE 13.7 SECONDARY CAUSES OF DYSTONIA

Perinatal cerebral injury, including hypoxia or kernicterus

Encephalitis

Head trauma

Pontine myelinolysis

Antiphospholipid antibody syndrome

Stroke

Tumor

Multiple sclerosis

Cervical cord injury or lesion

Peripheral injury

movements should suggest olivopontocerebellar atrophy, dystonic lipidosis, Huntington's disease, or Leigh's disease; and anterior horn cell or peripheral nerve findings should raise the question of metachromatic leukodystrophy, neuroacanthocytosis, ataxia telangiectasia, or olivopontocerebellar atrophy.

KEY POINTS

1. Dystonic movements may be slow or rapid and are typically repetitive and patterned, by contrast with chorea, which is random and unpredictable.
2. Dystonia is classified into primary generalized, focal and segmental, paroxysmal, or secondary dystonia.
3. Common manifestations of focal and segmental dystonias include torticollis, writer's cramp, blepharospasm, and oromandibular dystonia.
4. Dystonia commonly is due to another cause, usually metabolic, structural, or neurodegenerative. Accompanying signs and symptoms can help narrow the diagnosis.
5. Treatment of most dystonias consists of anticholinergics, botulinum toxin administration, and in some cases levodopa or tetrabenazine.

Myoclonus

The term *myoclonus* refers to quick, shocklike muscle contractions that produce brief and sudden movements of a limb or body part. Frequency of muscle jerks may be individual and infrequent or constant and repetitive. Amplitude of movements may range from barely detectable movements within a limb to large jerks of the entire body. In most cases, the pattern of myoclonus is irregular, but it can be rhythmic. The distribution may be focal in one part of the body, segmental involving adjacent body regions, multifocal involving multiple body regions, or generalized involving the entire body. Myoclonus occurring in more than one body part may be asynchronous or synchronous. Muscle jerks may occur spontaneously, as a reflex response to inputs from sudden visual, auditory, or tactile stimuli or as a result of active or passive voluntary movements.

Myoclonus occurs in a very large variety of neurological disorders (Table 13.8). The vast majority of these are central nervous system in origin, but myoclonus occasionally also occurs in peripheral neurological disorders, such as hemifacial spasm, and rarely as an unusual manifestation of nerve or nerve root injuries. Unfortunately, the clinical features of various types of myoclonus usually do not allow reliable classification by etiology or neuroanatomical origin. More common etiologies include physiological myoclonus, such as sleep startles, nocturnal

TABLE 13.8 COMMON CAUSES OF MYOCLONUS

Physiological myoclonus (normal subjects)
Nocturnal
Anxiety
Hiccough

Essential myoclonus (no known cause; no other manifestations)
Hereditary
Sporadic
Benign neonatal sleep myoclonus

Epileptic myoclonus (seizures predominate; no encephalopathy)
Fragments of epilepsy
Isolated epileptic myoclonic jerks
Epilepsia partialis continua
Idiopathic stimulus-sensitive myoclonus
Photosensitive myoclonus
Myoclonic absences
Childhood myoclonic epilepsies
Infantile spasms
Myoclonic astatic epilepsy
Cryptogenic myoclonus epilepsy
Juvenile myoclonus epilepsy
Benign familial myoclonus epilepsy
Baltic myoclonus

Symptomatic myoclonus (encephalopathy predominates)
Storage disease
Lafora body disease
Lipidoses
Ceroid-lipofuscinosis
Sialidosis (cherry-red spot myoclonus)
Spinocerebellar degeneration
Ramsay Hunt syndrome
Friedreich's ataxia
Ataxia telangiectasia
Basal ganglia degeneration
Corticobasal ganglionic degeneration
Wilson's disease
Torsion dystonia
Hallervorden-Spatz disease
Huntington's disease

Dementias
Creutzfeldt-Jakob disease
Alzheimer's disease
Viral encephalopathies
Subacute sclerosing panencephalitis
Encephalitis lethargica
Herpes simplex virus encephalitis
Other viral encephalitides
Postinfectious encephalitis
Metabolic
Hepatic or renal failure
Dialysis encephalopathy
Hyponatremia
Hyperglycemia and hypoglycemia
Infantile myoclonic encephalopathy with polymyoclonus
Toxic encephalopathies
Bismuth
Heavy metals
Methyl bromide
DDT
Drugs (e.g., levodopa, tricyclic antidepressants)
Physical encephalopathies
Hypoxia
Head trauma
Heat stroke
Electric shock
Decompression injury
Focal central nervous system
Stroke
Tumor
Trauma
Olivodentate lesions (palatal myoclonus)
Spinal cord lesions (segmental myoclonus)
Psychogenic

myoclonus, and hiccough; epileptic myoclonus associated with idiopathic seizure disorders, benign or progressive myoclonic epilepsies of childhood, and epilepsy partialis continua; essential myoclonus, an early-onset hereditary or sporadic benign disorder that is usually action-induced and may overlap with essential tremor and myoclonic dystonia; and symptomatic myoclonus caused by a wide variety of structural and metabolic disorders, such as storage diseases, cerebellar and basal ganglia degeneration, mitochondrial encephalopathies, Alzheimer's disease, Creutzfeldt-Jakob disease, encephalitis, systemic metabolic disorders usually associated with asterixis hypoxic and toxic encephalopathies; and focal damage to the brain or spinal cord from a variety of causes.

A history of toxin exposure or drug use is important. Precipitants and circumstances under which the myoclonus appears should be elicited. Asterixis or negative myoclonus often presents as dropping of objects or sudden falls resulting from sudden lapses in extensor muscle tone. Action myoclonus is characteristic of essential myoclonus, for which there may be a family history, but it is also the hallmark of postanoxic myoclonus, for which there should be an obvious history of major acute cerebral anoxia. Myoclonus not uncommonly accompanies idiopathic epilepsy. This myoclonus may be stimulus-sensitive and often occurs at times of reduced seizure control. The presence of myoclonus in a child either with or without epilepsy should prompt assessment of cognitive function and school performance. Symptomatic forms of myoclonus will usually be accompanied by other manifestations of what is usually a significant underlying neurological disorder.

Focal myoclonus limited to distal portions of one extremity suggests a cortical origin, whereas segmental involvement, especially if bilateral, may indicate a brainstem or spinal origin. Multifocal myoclonus is characteristic of systemic metabolic disorders, such as uremia or hepatic failure. When multiple body regions are involved, electromyographic study of synchrony and order of activation of muscle groups may be useful in identifying cortical and subcortical forms of myoclonus. Action myoclonus should be searched for in muscles of the limbs, face, and trunk. Action myoclonus of the upper extremities should be distinguished from severe postural-action or intention tremor, with which it sometimes coexists. Myoclonus is usually lower in frequency and more quick and jerky in its appearance than tremor. Myoclonus present at rest must be distinguished from chorea, which is usually more random, unpredictable, and multifocal in character. Tics usually produce more complex movements and postures, are more suppressible, and are often associated with inner tension and other subjective sensations. Because myoclonus is often accompanied by other manifestations of an underlying neurological disorder, careful examination for associated cerebellar, extrapyramidal, and cognitive abnormalities is necessary for differential diagnosis.

Treatment depends on the underlying cause of myoclonus. If epileptic, anticonvulsants are the main strategy, and valproic acid, levetiracetam, and topiramate are commonly used. In cases in which systemic metabolic disease is involved, such as uremic or hepatic encephalopathy, improving organ dysfunction may reduce the myoclonus. Commonly, the same anticonvulsants are also helpful in myoclonus related to anoxic or metabolic encephalopathy. When essential myoclonus is suspected, clonazepam, propranolol, or primidone can be useful.

KEY POINTS

1. Myoclonus refers to quick, shocklike muscle contractions that produce brief and sudden movements of a limb or body part. They are commonly classified into focal, segmental, multifocal, or generalized.
2. There are many causes of myoclonus; commonly it results from toxic exposure. Important other causes include focal epilepsy, metabolic disorders, and postanoxic brain injury.

Tics

Tics occur as a relatively common phenomenon at one time or another in many neurologically normal individuals, predominantly in children or adolescents. They may also occur as a primary tic disorder or as a part of Tourette's syndrome.

Tic Disorder

Motor tics most commonly appear as brief, high-velocity jerking movements of individual muscles, groups of muscles, or parts of the body. They are random and variable in pattern and frequency and can usually be voluntarily suppressed for limited periods of time. An infinite variety of motor tics may occur and may be classified as simple or complex and clonic or dystonic in type. Common examples of simple motor tics include eye blinking, blepharospasm, facial grimacing, platysma contractions, head jerking, shoulder shrugging, abdominal or pelvic contractions, and arm or leg jerking. Complex motor tics produce patterned and coordinated movements that involve one or more regional groups of muscles and may sometimes appear purposeful, such as repetitive neck or limb shaking or stretching, hitting or touching movements, and whole-body movements such as turning, squatting, or jumping. Complex motor tics are often characterized by ritualistic, obsessive, and compulsive features and in severe tic disorders, such as Tourette's syndrome, may include echopraxia and copropraxia. Clonic tics are brief and jerky, and are characteristic of simple tics, whereas dystonic tics are slower and more protracted movements that usually occur as part of complex tics.

Vocal tics may also be simple or complex in type. Simple vocal tics include nonverbal noisemaking such as sniffing, coughing, throat clearing, humming, grunting, hooting, squealing, or barking. Complex vocal tics are less common and include verbal utterances, such as coprolalia, echolalia, cheers, and oaths, as well as nonverbal tics, such as belching, hiccoughing, and panting.

Tics often occur as an effort to relieve an internal urge and are at least temporarily suppressible. This is especially characteristic of dystonic tics, in which uncomfortable internal sensations, sometimes referred to as "sensory" tics, are experienced in localized body regions, leading to repeated efforts at relief by movements, postures, or other muscle contractions. A period of tic suppression is typically followed by a temporary flurry of increased tic frequency, which the individual will sometimes seek to carry out in private. Although ability to suppress movements is characteristic of tics, this feature may also be found in chorea, dystonia, or athetosis. Most dystonic tics and many simple tics are differentiated from dystonia or chorea by the inner urge and release that characterize tics and the historical features of the disorder. Transient tics are common in children and adolescents, may closely resemble Tourette's syndrome but usually last less than a year or two, and are not usually accompanied by vocal tics. Chronic motor tic disorder appears in childhood or adult life but is usually limited to a single motor tic that remains constant in severity over an extended period. Secondary tic disorders may occur in a wide variety of neurological disorders, as outlined in Table 13.9.

Tourette's Syndrome

Clinical criteria for the diagnosis of Tourette's syndrome include childhood or adolescent onset, multiplicity of tics, presence of vocal tics, a historical pattern of variation in type and severity of tics over time, and suppressibility. Tourette's syndrome must be differentiated from transient

TABLE 13.9 SECONDARY TIC DISORDERS

Chronic neuroleptic exposure or treatment

Amphetamine

Levodopa treatment

Mental retardation

Postencephalitic syndromes

Head trauma

Stroke

Carbon monoxide poisoning

Neuroacanthocytosis

TABLE 13.10 PHARMACOLOGICAL TREATMENT OF TICS AND TOURETTE'S SYNDROME

Tics
　　Alpha-agonists: clonidine (oral, transdermal), guanfacine
　　Atypical antipsychotics: olanzapine, ziprasidone, aripiprazole
　　Classical neuroleptic antipsychotics: haloperidol, pimozide, fluphenazine, others
　　Dopamine-depleters: tetrabenazine
　　Clonazepam
　　Calcium channel antagonists
　　Botulinum toxin (for dystonic tics localized to small muscle groups)

Attention-deficit hyperactivity disorder
　　Alpha agonists: clonidine (oral, transdermal), guanfacine
　　Stimulants: methylphenidate, amphetamine/dextroamphetamine

Obsessive-compulsive behavior
　　Serotonin reuptake inhibitors: clomipramine, fluoxetine, fluvoxamine, paroxetine, clomipramine, and others

and chronic motor tic disorder. A history of fluctuating and changing tics over months or years is typical of Tourette's syndrome and may be absent in patients with transient or chronic motor tic disorder. Tourette's syndrome is often accompanied by obsessive-compulsive disorder, learning disabilities, and attention-deficit disorder, but not by abnormalities in the general neurological examination. The presence of other neurological findings should suggest a secondary tic disorder. Management of tic disorder and Tourette's syndrome is largely aimed at suppressing tics, treating comorbid attention-deficit hyperactivity disorder and obsessive-compulsive disorder. Several of the most effective drugs are listed in Table 13.10. Tics characteristically wax and wane and generally remit as adolescents approach adulthood.

The pathophysiology of tic disorder and Tourette's syndrome is not known. Dopamine-receptor supersensitivity is postulated to contribute to tics mainly based on evidence that dopamine-receptor blockers in relatively small doses are often the most effective drugs for suppressing tics. No gross pathological findings are present on postmortem examination, and no genes have been identified as causative. Numerous functional imaging studies have pointed toward various mechanisms in humans, including observations of increased activity of the dopamine transporter, increased innervation of the ventral striatum, and increased presence of postsynaptic D2 dopamine receptors. Also, several paralimbic regions have been identified as important for tic generation, including the anterior cingulate cortex and insula, followed by activation of superior parietal lobule and cerebellum at the onset of tic action. These data indicate that, as in many other hyperkinetic movement disorders, an overactive corticostriatal-thalamic-cortical circuit is involved in the pathogenesis of Tourette's syndrome.

KEY POINTS

1. Motor and vocal tics often occur as an effort to relieve an internal urge and are at least temporarily suppressible.
2. Clinical criteria for the diagnosis of Tourette's syndrome include childhood or adolescent onset, multiplicity of tics, presence of vocal tics, a historical pattern of variation in type and severity of tics over time, and suppressibility.
3. Treatment of Tourette's syndrome consists of alpha agonists, dopamine-receptor blockers, benzodiazepines, tetrabenazine, and pharmacological treatment for comorbid attention-deficit hyperactivity disorder and obsessive-compulsive disorder.

■ PSYCHOGENIC MOVEMENT DISORDERS

As in other neurological disorders, psychogenic etiologies will sometimes merit consideration in the evaluation of a movement disorder. Movement disorder specialty clinics are currently seeing increasing numbers of patients with movement disorders resulting from psychological causes. These include psychogenic dystonia, tremor, and gait disorder, which are the most common of the group, as well as psychogenic myoclonus, paroxysmal syndromes, and startle disorders. Unfortunately, the diagnosis of many movement disorders is based primarily on an observed pattern of symptoms and signs, with few or no available methods of laboratory confirmation. This is especially true for hyperkinetic syndromes, in which the incidence of psychogenic disorders is higher than for hypokinetic disorders.

Criteria have been recommended for the diagnosis of psychogenic movement disorders. By definition, a documented psychogenic disorder is one in which the manifestations are rapidly and completely eliminated by psychological treatment such as psychotherapy, suggestion therapy, or placebo or the patient is documented to be free of signs when unknowingly observed. With the exception of tics, acute drug-induced dyskinesias, and rare cases of cervical dystonia, organic movement disorders almost never remit suddenly and spontaneously; this serves to document psychogenic movement disorder. A clinically established psychogenic disorder is one in which the disorder is inconsistent over time or is incongruent with the established pattern of a known movement disorder and is accompanied by obvious psychiatric disturbance, other psychosomatic disorders, and other neurological signs that are definitely psychogenic. A probable psychogenic disorder is one in which (a) the movements appear inconsistent or incongruent, but there are no other findings to indicate a psychogenic cause, or (b) the movements appear consistent and congruent, but other psychogenic findings or somatizations are present. One should at least be suspicious of a possible psychogenic disorder in cases in which the movement disorder appears consistent and congruent with an organic disorder but occurs in the setting of an obvious emotional disturbance.

Certain clues in the history and examination may suggest the possibility of a psychogenic disorder. These include sudden onset, a multiplicity of abnormal movements, inconsistency from one examination to another, abnormal movements and postures that do not fit with recognized patterns, large-amplitude shaking movements, bizarre gait without loss of balance or falls, excessive startle responses to a variety of stimuli, overly slow and deliberate voluntary movements, variable tremor frequency, marked relief of involuntary movements with distraction, dystonia beginning as a fixed posture, and false weakness or sensory signs. Although these clues, together with an obvious psychiatric disorder, other previous somatizations, and identifiable secondary gain, may suggest a psychogenic etiology, it is important to view these signs in the context of the diagnostic criteria outlined previously. This is especially true because one is sometimes dealing with rare, unique, or highly unusual movement disorders with variable manifestations, some of which may also be associated with psychiatric disturbance. Finally, as with any apparently psychogenic disorder, one has to be alert to the possibility that psychogenic abnormal movements may occur in patients who also have an underlying organic movement disorder. Inpatient or extended outpatient evaluation, necessary and reasonable laboratory tests, observed and unobserved video recording, psychiatric evaluation, and physical medicine evaluation and treatment should all be considered in the evaluation of such patients.

KEY POINTS

1. A documented psychogenic disorder is one in which the manifestations are rapidly and completely eliminated by psychological treatment such as psychotherapy, suggestion therapy, or placebo, or the patient is documented to be free of signs when unknowingly observed.

2. Clues to a psychogenic movement disorder include sudden onset, a multiplicity of abnormal movements, inconsistency from one examination to another, abnormal movements and postures that do not fit with recognized patterns, large-amplitude shaking movements, bizarre gait, excessive startle responses, overly slow and deliberate voluntary movements, variable tremor frequency, marked relief of involuntary movements with distraction, a dystonia beginning as a fixed posture, and false weakness or sensory signs.

■ SUGGESTED READINGS

de Lau LM, Breteler MM. Epidemiology of Parkinson's disease. *Lancet Neurol* 2006;5;525–535.

Tarsy D. Movement disorders. In: Samuels M, Feske S, eds. *Office Practice of Neurology*, 2nd ed. Philadelphia: Churchill Livingstone, 2003.

Tarsy D. Diagnostic criteria for Parkinson's disease. In: Ebadi M, Pfeiffer R, translator and eds. *Parkinson's Disease*. Boca Raton, Fla: CRC Press, 2005;569–578.

Tarsy D, Baldessarini, RJ. Epidemiology of Tardive dyskinesia: is risk declining with modern antipsychotics? *Mov Disord* 2006;21:589–598.

Tarsy D, Simon DK. Dystonia. *N Engl J Med* 2006;355:818–829.

CHAPTER 14

Epilepsy

Laura C. Miller

■ INTRODUCTION

An *epileptic seizure* is defined as a transient disturbance of cerebral function caused by paroxysmal abnormal and excessive neuronal discharges. The clinical manifestations are varied, depending on the areas of cerebral cortex involved, but can consist of sudden and transitory abnormal phenomena that may include alterations of consciousness, or motor, sensory, autonomic, or psychic events. Clinical manifestations may be perceived by the patient or witnessed by an observer. Seizures are usually self-limited but are often followed by a postictal period of cortical depression that can manifest itself clinically as localized or diffuse neurological deficits. *Epilepsy* is defined as recurrent (two or more) epileptic seizures, unprovoked by any immediate cause.

KEY POINTS

1. Clinical manifestations of seizure are widely varied depending of the area of cerebral cortex involved.
2. In epilepsy, seizures are recurrent and unprovoked by any immediate stimulus.

■ SEIZURE TYPES

Seizures are divided based on clinical manifestations into *partial* seizures, which originate in a part of one cerebral hemisphere, and *generalized* seizures, wherein seizure activity begins in both cerebral hemispheres simultaneously (Table 14.1).

Partial Seizures

Partial seizures that do not alter or impair consciousness are called simple partial seizures. When consciousness is altered or impaired, the seizure is complex partial. The clinical manifestations of partial-onset seizures are often determined by the area of cerebral cortex involved and are further subdivided into motor, somatosensory or special sensory, autonomic, or psychic subtypes (Table 14.2). Motor manifestations in simple partial seizures include versive movements, posturing, or clonic movements of a muscle group. In complex partial seizures, motor signs are usually typified by purposeless and repetitive involuntary muscle movements called automatisms. Examples include lip smacking or chewing, upper extremity gesturing or fidgeting, and lower extremity ambulatory movements. Approximately 70% of complex partial seizures arise from the temporal lobe.

The abnormal cortical discharges in a partial-onset seizure can spread to adjacent cortical areas over time. Consequently, the clinical manifestations of a seizure can evolve. For example, the clonic movements of a partial-onset motor seizure may spread to other body parts as discharges involve adjacent areas of the motor cortex (i.e., Jacksonian march). The discharges can

TABLE 14.1 CLASSIFICATION OF EPILEPTIC SEIZURES

SEIZURE TYPE	KEY FEATURES
Partial Seizures	
Simple partial	May have motor, somatosensory, special sensory, autonomic, or psychic manifestations Consciousness is preserved
Complex partial	May have motor, somatosensory, special sensory, autonomic, or psychic manifestations Consciousness is altered or impaired
Generalized Seizures	
Tonic-clonic	Tonic rigidity followed by synchronous jerking movements of the extremities May be accompanied by incontinence, tongue biting Followed by period of postictal confusion
Absence	Brief (usually <10 seconds) lapse in consciousness with arrest of ongoing activity Rapid onset and offset May be accompanied by automatisms like blinking, orobuccal movements Characteristic 3-Hz spike-and-wave electroencephalogram pattern
Myoclonic	Characterized by single or multiple muscle jerks Consciousness is preserved Usually bilateral and symmetrical but can be regional
Atonic	Brief synchronous loss of muscle tone
Tonic	Prolonged muscle contraction
Clonic	Repetitive alternating jerking and relaxation of an extremity

TABLE 14.2 CLINICAL MANIFESTATIONS OF PARTIAL SEIZURES

SUBTYPE	CLINICAL MANIFESTATIONS
Motor	Versive movements (turning of head or eyes in one direction) Posturing Clonic movements of a muscle group Automatisms (coordinated, repetitive involuntary movements)
Somatosensory	Abnormal tastes Abnormal smells Abnormal visual phenomena
Sensory	Paresthesias (pins-and-needles sensations)
Autonomic	Pupillary changes Diaphoresis Epigastric rising sensation Piloerection Heart rate change Heart rhythm change Blood pressure change
Psychic	Dysphasia Fear Anxiety Depression Distortions of memory (déjà vu or jamais vu) Autoscopy Derealization Depersonalization

also propagate so that a simple partial seizure evolves into a complex partial seizure. Often, patients will refer to the simple partial portion of the seizure as an *aura,* which is the portion of the seizure that occurs before consciousness is altered or lost. Either a simple partial seizure or a complex partial seizure can evolve, or secondarily generalize, into a generalized convulsive seizure.

Generalized Seizures

Generalized seizures are subdivided into several types (Table 14.1). In tonic-clonic seizures there is loss of consciousness, with a tonic phase characterized by rigidity and contraction of body musculature followed by a clonic phase characterized by alternating muscle contraction and relaxation with resultant synchronous jerking limb movements for several minutes. Associated signs include loss of bowel or bladder continence, tongue biting, and postictal confusion or lethargy. Absence seizures consist of a brief (usually less than 10 seconds) lapse in consciousness with arrest of ongoing activity. The impairment in consciousness can be so brief that the patient may be unaware of it. Typical absence seizures have a rapid onset and offset and a characteristic 3-Hz generalized spike-and-wave electroencephalogram (EEG) pattern. Other generalized seizures include the myoclonic, atonic, tonic, and clonic seizure subtypes.

KEY POINTS

1. All seizures can be classified as originating either from part of one hemisphere (partial) or from both hemispheres simultaneously (generalized).
2. *Complex* partial seizures involve an alteration in consciousness.
3. Partial seizure manifestations are focal and depend on the area of cortex involved, but may evolve to become generalized seizures.
4. Generalized seizure types include tonic-clonic, absence, myoclonic, atonic, tonic or clonic.

■ ETIOLOGY

Seizures of new onset can occur as the result of a primary neurological disorder or as the symptomatic result of an underlying systemic dysfunction, such as a metabolic derangement or organ dysfunction (Table 14.3). The International League Against Epilepsy (ILAE) further classifies seizure etiology based on whether there is an identifiable precipitating cause. *Symptomatic* seizures are the consequence of a known or suspected cerebral dysfunction. *Acute symptomatic* (provoked) seizures are those occurring in close association with an acute toxic or metabolic insult or with an acute central nervous system (CNS) insult such as infection, tumor, trauma, ischemic stroke, or hemorrhage. Acute symptomatic seizures usually remit with resolution of the underlying illness. *Remote symptomatic* seizures are those that occur in relation to a well-demonstrated antecedent condition such as earlier head injury, stroke, or infection that causes a static lesion. Such remote symptomatic causes are not likely to resolve and may explain ongoing epilepsy. The term *idiopathic* is reserved for partial or generalized epileptic seizures occurring with particular clinical characteristics and EEG findings that define clear individual syndromes; most are genetic in origin. *Cryptogenic* seizures are those for which no cause can be identified. Identification of symptoms and signs consistent with an epileptic syndrome can help clarify appropriate treatments as well as prognosis.

KEY POINT

New-onset seizures should be classified as being the result of a particular CNS or systemic insult (symptomatic) or as part of an epileptic syndrome.

TABLE 14.3 COMMON CAUSES OF NEW ONSET SEIZURES

Primary CNS disorder
    Stroke or vascular insult
    CNS infection (e.g., meningitis, encephalitis, cysticercosis)
    Head injury or trauma
    Mass lesion
    Idiopathic epilepsy

Systemic disorder
    Hypoglycemia or hyperglycemia
    Hyperosmolar state
    Hyponatremia
    Hypocalcemia
    Hepatic encephalopathy
    Uremic encephalopathy
    Diffuse cerebral ischemia
    Hypertensive encephalopathy
    Eclampsia
    Drug intoxication
    Drug withdrawal

CNS, central nervous system.

■ PATHOPHYSIOLOGY

Current evidence suggests the likelihood that partial and generalized epilepsies originate from different pathophysiological mechanisms. Partial epilepsies presumably arise from a focal lesion, with spread resulting from recruitment of other brain areas. Clinically, there may be an interval between the neurological insult causing the lesion and the development of recurrent seizures. Generalized epilepsies, on the other hand, have been found to arise from abnormalities in the neurons themselves or within an aggregate of neurons fashioned into a network.

■ DIAGNOSTIC APPROACH

History

After an episode of altered consciousness or behavior, the first step is to determine whether the event was truly an epileptic seizure. Paroxysmal disorders that may mimic seizures include syncope, transient ischemic attack, breath-holding spells, hyperventilation syndrome, episodic dyscontrol syndrome, migraine, movement disorders, sleep disorders, and psychogenic nonepileptic seizures (Table 14.4). Misdiagnosis can have adverse effects. There may be delays in initiating the appropriate medical care for underlying medical or psychiatric conditions. In many states, there are restrictions placed on driving after a seizure episode.

    Definitive diagnosis can be made only if a seizure occurs during a period of EEG recording and if the electrographic discharges can be correlated with the patient's signs and symptoms. Therefore the diagnosis of seizure remains primarily a clinical one. The history, both from the patient and from witnesses, is paramount. It is also important to ensure that this was, indeed, the patient's first seizure. Sometimes, the first reported seizure is actually the latest in a series of events such as staring spells or myoclonic jerks that were not previously recognized as seizures. History should be obtained about prior possible neurological insults, such as head trauma, birth injury, history of meningitis or intracranial infection, and stroke, because these can lead to static lesions from which acquired seizures can develop.

TABLE 14.4 DIFFERENTIAL DIAGNOSIS OF SEIZURE

DIAGNOSIS	KEY FEATURES
Partial seizure	Often preceded by positive symptoms Symptoms evolve over seconds Recurrent events stereotyped
Generalized seizure	Onset in any position Loss of consciousness of minutes Tonic phase with increased tone Can be associated with incontinence, tongue biting Minutes in duration Postictal confusion or lethargy Recurrent events stereotyped
Syncope	Onset while standing or during postural change, straining Loss of consciousness is brief Preceded by pallor, nausea, sweating, visual changes such as dimming Flaccid tone typical, but can have brief convulsive activity Recovery usually rapid if recumbent
Transient ischemic attack	Seconds to hours in duration Negative symptoms (loss of motor function or sensation)
Breath-holding spell	Common in children Frequently provoked by frustration or anger Associated with pallor and/or cyanosis, bradycardia If prolonged, may result in loss of consciousness
Hyperventilation syndrome	More common in females More common in patients with underlying anxiety disorder Associated with dyspnea, tachycardia, lightheadedness, circumoral paresthesias
Episodic dyscontrol (rage attack)	More common in males Often situational Goal-directed aggressive behaviors predominate May be amnestic for event
Migraine	Often preceded by positive symptoms Symptoms evolve over minutes Rarely progress to loss of consciousness
Psychogenic nonepileptic seizure	May be precipitated by emotional stressors Recurrent events often not stereotyped May exhibit goal-directed behaviors Can be prolonged (>5 minutes)

The other important historical piece of information is whether the seizure was generalized or partial in onset. This information is garnered from both patient and witness reports. Was there an aura, such as an abnormal taste, smell, vision, déjà vu, jamais vu, or other psychic sensation? The aura is actually the result of simple partial seizure activity, implying a partial onset. Was there head or eye version or limb shaking first on one side of the body? Partial-onset seizures suggest an underlying focal structural abnormality and portend a higher rate of seizure recurrence. Therapy can differ depending on the type of seizure; thus it is important to identify the type of seizure.

Seizures can occur unpredictably, but in some cases may be precipitated by sleep deprivation, alcohol intake or withdrawal, hormonal changes, or stress. Concomitant infection or missed medications are common precipitants for breakthrough seizures in patients with known epilepsy. In a few seizure types, seizures can be provoked by hyperventilation or photic stimulation.

Physical Examination

After determining, based on clinical history, that a seizure likely occurred, the next step in the evaluation is looking for an underlying symptomatic cause. Initial workup should include a general physical examination to look for signs of infection, such as fever, ear infection, meningeal signs, or evidence of head trauma. Detailed and complete neurological examination is essential, looking particularly for focal or lateralizing signs or deficits.

Laboratory Studies

Blood tests should be performed to screen for toxic or metabolic disturbances, such as hyperglycemia or hypoglycemia, hyponatremia, hypocalcemia, renal or hepatic dysfunction, and alcohol or drug intoxication. Lumbar puncture should be performed if fever, meningismus, or infectious prodrome are present.

Neuroimaging

Computed tomography (CT) or magnetic resonance imaging (MRI) of the head should be performed immediately in patients with suspected structural lesions. Specifically, it should be performed in those with focal deficits on examination, altered mental status, history of trauma, fever or other infection, and headache and in those with a history of malignancy, immunosuppression, or anticoagulation. In most other cases, neuroimaging should be considered urgent. Most providers prefer MRI over contrast-enhanced CT given the superior resolution and resultant structural detail provided by MRI.

Electroencephalography

Electroencephalogram is helpful in that approximately 50% of people who have epilepsy have epileptiform EEG discharges between seizures (interictally). Epileptiform discharges include abnormal spikes, polyspike discharges, sharp waves, and spike-and-wave complexes. Because the other 50% do not have an abnormal interictal EEG, a single normal EEG does not rule out seizure. If a routine EEG is normal but suspicion of epilepsy is high, the EEG can be repeated under stress conditions, such as sleep deprivation or by employing additional electrode arrays. Other options include prolonged or long-term EEG monitoring to capture and record the clinical events in question. This can take the form of outpatient ambulatory EEG or inpatient video-EEG monitoring. In addition to confirming the presence of paroxysmal abnormal discharges, long-term EEG can provide information on whether discharges are focal or generalized, help determine the focus of seizure activity, can help quantify frequency of events, and allow for characterization of specific epilepsy syndromes (Table 14.5). Ultimately, though, the EEG is not failsafe; the diagnosis of seizure remains a clinical one, combining and interpreting the information gathered via history, physical examination, and the EEG findings.

KEY POINTS

1. New-onset seizure must first be distinguished from other mimicking conditions to avoid delays in appropriate treatment.
2. Seizure is primarily a clinical diagnosis based on careful history from both patient and observers.
3. Physical examination should focus on possible signs of infection, trauma, or lateralizing deficits.
4. Urgent MRI or head CT is indicated when a CNS insult is suspected from examination or history.
5. EEG may be helpful in characterizing seizure or capturing epileptiform discharge between seizures, but does not rule out a seizure disorder if negative.

TABLE 14.5 INDICATIONS FOR LONG-TERM EEG MONITORING

Characterize paroxysmal events as epileptic or nonepileptic
Quantify seizure frequency
Presurgical localization of epileptic focus
Diagnose epilepsy syndrome

■ MANAGEMENT

The decision to initiate antiepileptic drug (AED) therapy after a single seizure is based on several factors, including the validity of the diagnosis, risk of recurrence, and patient preference. For most patients with unprovoked seizures, the risk of recurrence is under 50% over 2 years, and immediate AED therapy to prevent seizure recurrence does not alter the development of epilepsy or its natural history. Thus AEDs are usually not recommended after a single unprovoked seizure. On the other hand, patients with substantial risks for recurrence, such as focal deficits, presence of an underlying incorrectable cause, or EEG abnormalities, warrant treatment after a single seizure because risk of recurrence is increased in these groups. Patient preferences on risk may affect these recommendations. If a second seizure occurs, the 2-year risk of recurrence increases to approximately 75% and AEDs should be started.

Antiepileptic Medications

Goals of pharmacotherapy include reduction or elimination of seizures while minimizing adverse effects of treatment. Monotherapy is the preferred goal, with the choice of AED based on seizure type or underlying epilepsy syndrome (Table 14.6). In general, carbamazepine, oxcarbazepine, and phenytoin are the preferred first-line medications in cases of partial-onset seizures. Valproic acid and phenytoin are the preferred first-line medications for generalized-onset seizures. Lamotrigine, topiramate, zonisamide, and levetiracetam are effective against both partial-onset and generalized seizures. Side effects, cost, and dosing schedule can play a role in medication selection as well. An adequate trial of antiepileptic medication involves increasing the medication until seizures are controlled or until adverse effects occur. Although serum drug levels are available for most medications, published therapeutic ranges are based on a broad population of patients. Treatment efficacy or toxicity should be used for endpoints in place of a desired therapeutic serum level. Seizure control is achieved at different serum drug levels in different patients. If seizures are not well controlled on the first-choice AED, a second AED is started, followed by gradual taper and discontinuation of the first agent. If seizures are not well controlled after adequate trials of two antiepileptic medications, it is highly likely that seizures will remain refractory to medical therapy. At this point, referral to an epilepsy specialist is warranted.

Side Effects of Antiepileptic Drugs

Commonly reported adverse effects for all of the AEDs include sedation, concentration and memory difficulties, dizziness, and dyspepsia. Adverse effects may be dose related, noted when a drug is first initiated or after dosage increases. Dose-related effects can be minimized by lowering the dosage or by discontinuing the medication. Idiosyncratic reactions are not dose related, but instead may be immune mediated or based on individual factors specific to the patient. Idiosyncratic reactions tend to be more serious and at times even life threatening (Table 14.7). Skin rash can occur with all of the AEDs. Rarely, this can result in severe Stevens-Johnson syndrome, particularly with phenobarbital, phenytoin, carbamazepine, and lamotrigine. Psychiatric side effects are common and will be discussed in a later section.

TABLE 14.6 ANTIEPILEPTIC DRUGS AND TREATED SEIZURE TYPES[a]

MEDICATION	PARTIAL ONSET	SECONDARILY GENERALIZED	GENERALIZED TONIC-CLONIC	ABSENCE	MYOCLONIC	TONIC
Phenobarbital	✓	✓	✓			
Primidone	✓	✓	✓			
Tiagabine	✓	✓				
Vigabatrin[b]	✓	✓				
Phenytoin	✓	✓	✓			
Valproic acid	✓	✓	✓	✓	✓	✓
Carbamazepine	✓	✓	✓			
Oxcarbazepine	✓	✓				
Lamotrigine	✓	✓	✓	✓		
Topiramate	✓	✓	✓			✓
Zonisamide	✓	✓	✓	✓		
Ethosuximide				✓		
Levetiracetam	✓	✓			✓	
Gabapentin	✓	✓				
Felbamate						✓

[a]Recommendations based on literature review.
[b]Vigabatrin not approved by U.S. Food and Drug Administration.

Surgery

Surgery is an effective and safe treatment option for some patients with medically refractory partial seizures. Before surgery, video-EEG monitoring is performed to better localize the focus of epileptic activity. An ideal surgical candidate has seizures that begin in one area of the cortex. Data from invasive EEG and neuroimaging are used to determine the focus. Neuropsychological testing is used to delineate possible deficits after surgery and to determine psychological "readiness" for surgery and its possible outcomes. Excision is planned to remove the epileptogenic cortex while minimizing resection in areas in which neurological impairment could occur. The most common surgical procedure currently is anterior temporal lobectomy, with approximately 50% of patients becoming seizure free after the resection. Psychiatric complications have been reported after temporal lobectomy. Depressive disorders are the most frequent during the first year after surgery. Temporal lobectomy has been associated with *de novo* postoperative psychosis as well. However, depression and anxiety have been shown to improve significantly over the long term after epilepsy surgery, particularly in those patients who become seizure free.

Vagal Nerve Stimulation

Vagal nerve stimulation has been shown to reduce seizure frequency in adults and children with medically refractory epilepsy. It is a pacemaker-like device that is implanted surgically into the chest wall with a lead stimulating the left vagus nerve in the neck. The exact mechanism of action is unknown, but the device has been shown to decrease mean seizure frequency.

TABLE 14.7 ANTIEPILEPTIC DRUG ADVERSE EFFECTS

MEDICATION	DOSE-RELATED ADVERSE EFFECT	IDIOSYNCRATIC ADVERSE EFFECT
Phenobarbital	LFT abnormalities Sedation Behavioral disturbance Osteoporosis Diplopia Ataxia	Hepatotoxicity Rash Stevens-Johnson syndrome
Primidone	Sedation Behavioral disturbance Diplopia Ataxia	Rash
Tiagabine	Sedation	Rash
Vigabatrin	Sedation	
Phenytoin	LFT abnormalities Gingival hyperplasia Hirsutism Coarsened facies Osteoporosis Diplopia Ataxia Polyneuropathy	Hepatotoxicity Rash Stevens-Johnson syndrome Blood dyscrasia Lymphadenopathy
Valproic acid	Dyspepsia LFT abnormalities Sedation Weight gain Hair loss Hirsutism Osteoporosis Tremor	Hepatotoxicity Pancreatitis Thrombocytopenia
Carbamazepine	LFT abnormalities Leukopenia Hyponatremia Osteoporosis Diplopia Ataxia Dizziness Headache	Hepatotoxicity Agranulocytosis Aplastic anemia Rash Stevens-Johnson syndrome
Oxcarbazepine	LFT abnormalities Hyponatremia	Rash
Lamotrigine	Insomnia	Rash Stevens-Johnson syndrome
Topiramate	Weight loss Word finding difficulties	Renal stones Glaucoma
Zonisamide	Dyspepsia Weight loss	Renal stones
Ethosuximide	Dyspepsia Sedation Ataxia Dizziness Headache	Rash Blood dyscrasia
Levetiracetam	Behavioral disturbance	
Gabapentin	Sedation Weight gain	
Felbamate	Anorexia Insomnia	Hepatic failure Aplastic anemia

LFTs, liver function tests.

Discontinuation of Antiepileptic Medication

Patients with epilepsy who are seizure free may eventually wish to discontinue antiepileptic medications. When patients have been seizure free for more than 2 years, this can be considered. Seizure recurrence is more likely in those patients who failed initial AED therapy, those who required multiple AEDs to achieve seizure control, those with abnormalities on neurological examination or neuroimaging, and those with persistent EEG abnormalities. Medication withdrawal should be gradual, over the course of weeks to months. Should seizures recur, previous medications can be reinstituted.

KEY POINTS

1. AEDs are usually not recommended after a single unprovoked seizure without epileptiform EEG findings.
2. An adequate trial of antiepileptic medication involves increasing the dose until seizures are controlled or until adverse effects occur and is not based entirely on drug serum levels.
3. All AEDs have the potential for dose-related or idiosyncratic adverse effects.
4. Surgery is an effective and safe treatment option in some partial seizure patients, with 50% becoming seizure free after resection.
5. Gradual medication withdrawal can be considered after a seizure-free period of more than 2 years.

■ SELECTED EPILEPSY SYNDROMES

Temporal Lobe Epilepsy

The most common adult epilepsy syndrome is complex partial seizures originating in the medial/mesial temporal lobe (Table 14.8). Onset is usually in late childhood or young adulthood. Ictal discharges can be recorded from the hippocampus, amygdala, or other parahippocampal structures. Frequently, there is a history of febrile seizures or a family history of seizures. Seizures often begin with an aura. Abnormal epigastric rising sensations; psychic symptoms; illusions; and olfactory, visual, and gustatory hallucinations are common. Seizures then evolve to loss or alteration in consciousness, with behavioral arrest followed by automatisms. Some seizures secondarily generalize. Hippocampal sclerosis is the most commonly identified pathological condition found in patients with clinical temporal lobe epilepsy syndrome after surgical resection, but it is debated whether hippocampal sclerosis is causative or the effect of the seizures themselves.

TABLE 14.8 CHARACTERISTICS OF TEMPORAL LOBE SEIZURES

Onset in late childhood or young adulthood
Involve mesial temporal lobe structures
May have history of febrile seizures during infancy
Aura with autonomic, sensory, or somatosensory symptoms
Consciousness is impaired or altered
May exhibit automatisms
Stereotyped between attacks

TABLE 14.9 CHARACTERISTICS OF FRONTAL LOBE SEIZURES
Onset during childhood and adolescence
Abrupt onset and offset
Brief duration, usually less than 1 minute
Can occur in clusters
Show a nocturnal preponderance, often out of sleep
May exhibit little to no postictal confusion
Motor manifestations are complex or bizarre
May have gestural and/or sexual automatisms
Vocalizations common
Consciousness may be preserved
Stereotyped between attacks

Frontal Lobe Epilepsy

Frontal lobe seizures can be mistaken for psychogenic seizures. Frontal lobe seizures can have different clinical manifestations, depending on the area of frontal cortex involved (Table 14.9).

Frontal lobe seizures typically have onset during childhood and adolescence. Seizures tend to have an abrupt onset and offset, with little to no postictal confusion. Motor manifestations may be bizarre and complex, such as bicycling leg movements, gestural and sexual automatisms, pelvic thrusting, and asynchronous flailing movements of the extremities. Vocalizations documented include shouting obscenities, singing, and humming. Frontal seizures arising from the supplemental motor areas may manifest as bilateral motor activity but with retained level of consciousness. Surface EEG recordings in frontal lobe seizures may be unrevealing. The features that help differentiate frontal lobe seizures from psychogenic nonepileptic seizures include their length (usually less than 60 seconds), nocturnal preponderance, and stereotyped nature.

KEY POINTS

1. Temporal lobe epilepsy is a complex partial seizure syndrome and is the most common epilepsy syndrome in adults.
2. Frontal lobe seizures may manifest as bizarre and complex automatisms, with little or no postictal confusion.

■ STATUS EPILEPTICUS

Convulsive Status Epilepticus

The operational definition of generalized convulsive status epilepticus (GLSE) varies. It is typically diagnosed when bilateral convulsive seizures last longer than 5 minutes or if multiple seizures occur without return to lucid consciousness in between. Prolonged convulsions lead to the development of physiological stressors in the form of lactic acidosis, hyperthermia, hypoxia, and hypoglycemia. There is significant morbidity and mortality associated with these stressors, and GLSE is treated as a medical emergency. Status epilepticus can be the initial presentation of a seizure disorder and can be precipitated by toxic or metabolic insult, trauma, infection, or acute

TABLE 14.10 CRITERIA FOR DIAGNOSIS OF NONCONVULSIVE STATUS EPILEPTICUS

- Altered mental status, ranging from confusion to impairment of consciousness
- Epileptiform EEG with frequent discrete seizures or continuous discharges
- Response to antiepileptic medications

EEG, electroencephalogram.

neurological insult. In patients with previously diagnosed epilepsy, it is commonly precipitated by medication noncompliance, intercurrent illness, alcohol use, or sleep deprivation.

Emergency treatment to ensure adequate airway, respiration, and circulation is necessary. Identification and treatment of underlying medical conditions is also crucial because outcome is strongly tied to etiology. Treatment is aimed at cessation of seizure activity. Several AED regimens can be used to treat status epilepticus and typically consist of immediate administration of a benzodiazepine agent along with a loading dose of a longer-acting medication, such as phenytoin or its equivalent. EEG monitoring should be utilized in patients with persistent alteration in consciousness and in those with refractory status epilepticus.

Nonconvulsive Status Epilepticus

Nonconvulsive status epilepticus (NCSE) is status epilepticus without obvious generalized tonic-clonic activity. Instead, it manifests mainly with altered mental status ranging from mild confusion to impairment of consciousness (Table 14.10). It can result from intermittent or continued complex partial or absence seizures. It often goes undiagnosed or misdiagnosed. NCSE should be considered on the differential diagnosis in all patients with altered mental status, affective changes, and/or bizarre behavior (Table 14.11). Patients may be intermittently responsive between events with waxing and waning degrees of impairment. Diagnosis is confirmed via demonstration of epileptic discharges on EEG during the periods of confusion. Resolution of epileptiform discharges and improvement in mental status after injection of intravenous benzodiazepines confirms the diagnosis. Prognosis is strongly dependent on etiology. Treatment includes identification and treatment of any precipitating factors, such as underlying medical disorders, toxic or metabolic insults, or infection. Pharmacotherapy involves use of intravenous benzodiazepines in combination with longer-acting antiepileptics.

TABLE 14.11 CLINICAL MANIFESTATIONS OF NONCONVULSIVE STATUS EPILEPTICUS

Cognitive disturbance of impairment (e.g., impaired attention, difficulty in planning)

Emotional lability or mood disturbance

Speech disturbance

Uncharacteristic or bizarre behavior (e.g., laughing inappropriately, agitation)

Psychosis

Autonomic phenomena (e.g., flatulence, belching)

Motor activity (e.g., nystagmoid eye movements, focal jerks, twitching of facial muscles, repetitive motor activity)

Automatisms

KEY POINTS

1. Generalized GLSE is a condition of prolonged or successive convulsions lasting longer than 5 minutes or without a return to baseline between seizures.
2. Status epilepticus is a medical emergency that is associated with significant morbidity and mortality.
3. NCSE manifests without obvious generalized tonic-clonic activity and must be considered in all cases of altered mental status.

■ PSYCHOGENIC NONEPILEPTIC SEIZURES

Definition

Nonepileptic seizures are involuntary episodes of movement, sensation, or behaviors that may resemble seizures but are not the result of abnormal neuronal discharges. They can be physiological in origin (e.g., the physical disorders that are confused with epilepsy, such as syncope, breath-holding spells, hyperventilation syndrome) or psychogenic. The majority of nonepileptic seizures are psychogenic. Psychogenic nonepileptic seizure (PNES), also referred to as psychogenic seizure or pseudoseizure, results from an underlying conversion disorder, somatization disorder, or factitious disorder or from malingering.

Key Features

PNES can occur at all ages, but usually manifests between ages 15 and 35, with a female predominance of 3:1. Notably, PNES is common in patients with epileptic seizures, usually in those with a previous or comorbid psychiatric history. PNES is frequently associated with a history of past sexual or physical abuse or with current significant psychosocial stressors. However, PNES can occur in the absence of a previously diagnosed psychiatric disorder.

PNES can often be distinguished from epileptic seizures on the basis of a few clinically distinguishing features (Table 14.12). Key historical points are whether the patient's eyes are open or closed during the event, the evolution and duration of the event, the characteristics of the limb movements, and whether recurrent events are stereotyped. Typically, eye closure is more common during a PNES, whereas eye opening at onset is seen in epileptic seizures. Motor manifestations in PNES typically lack a tonic phase and are more often flailing, thrashing, asynchronous movements and can include side-to-side head movements, opisthotonic posturing, or pelvic thrusting. Behaviors may be goal directed. If vocalization is present, it is more often weeping or screaming rather than the epileptic cry or moan that results from contraction of respiratory musculature. The duration of the event is often prolonged, lasting more than 2 to 3 minutes. There can be an atypical resolution or lack of a clear postictal state. Recurrent events are rarely stereotyped. Bowel or bladder incontinence is rare, and injury is uncommon. Suggestion or emotional stimuli can sometimes provoke PNES. No one clinical feature reliably distinguishes psychogenic from epileptic seizures, however.

Evaluation and Confirmation

Video-EEG monitoring is the gold standard for confirming a clinical suspicion of PNES. The EEG recording during a PNES does not show abnormal cortical discharges or organized seizure activity. The background rhythm may be preserved, or there may be a lack of expected postictal EEG changes, such as slowing. It is important to record a "typical" seizure event. Again, the EEG is not failsafe and the diagnosis of seizure remains a clinical one. Frontal lobe seizures, for example, can have bizarre clinical manifestations and may not be associated with ictal EEG abnormalities. Subsequently, frontal lobe seizures can be misdiagnosed as psychogenic events.

TABLE 14.12 KEY FEATURES OF EPILEPTIC SEIZURES VERSUS PSYCHOGENIC NONEPILEPTIC SEIZURES

	EPILEPTIC SEIZURES	PSYCHOGENIC NONEPILEPTIC SEIZURES
Age at onset	Onset at all ages	More common between ages 15 and 35
Gender	Male to female ratio equal	3:1 female predominance
Comorbid psychiatric disease	Occasional	Common
Eyelids	Open at onset	Closed at onset, often with resistance to opening during event
Motor manifestations	Synchronous, tonic-clonic movements As seizure evolves, clonic jerks progressively slow in frequency	Asynchronous, commonly with flailing movements, pelvic thrusting, opisthotonic movements, side-to-side head shaking; may wax and wane
Vocalization	Cry or moan during tonic contraction phase with grunting during clonic phase	Screaming, weeping, or shouting obscenities may occur
Consciousness	Rare	Occasional consciousness during event; may be distractible
Goal-directed behaviors	Rare	May exhibit semi-purposeful movements
Duration of attack	Rarely >2–3 minutes	Often >2–3 minutes
Postictal state	Usually lethargic, confused	May be weeping, emotionally distressed
Incontinence	Common	Rare or unwitnessed
Nature of recurrent events	Stereotyped	Usually nonstereotyped

Establishing the diagnosis is important, because early diagnosis has been correlated with improved overall outcome.

Management

Once the diagnosis of PNES has been made, the patient should be informed and educated (Table 14.13). When discussing PNES with a patient, it is important to explain that the symptoms are real and that the patient is not consciously "faking it." It is also important to emphasize reversibility and the chance for recovery. Although the patient does not require treatment with antiepileptic medications, it is important that a therapeutic relationship with the diagnosing physicians be maintained because this has been associated with better outcomes. A multidisciplinary approach

TABLE 14.13 MANAGEMENT OF PSYCHOGENIC NONEPILEPTIC SEIZURES

Presentation of the diagnosis positively, emphasizing reversibility and potential for recovery
Referral to a mental health professional
Continued follow-up with the diagnosing neurologist
Avoidance of unnecessary medications
Maintenance of a treatment alliance
Avoidance of adversarial relationship between the patient and providers

involving patient educators and mental health staff is warranted. Individualized treatment may involve psychotherapy and/or use of psychotropic medication. Although some patients may not readily accept the diagnosis, one should avoid becoming adversarial.

Prognosis

Only approximately one-third of patients with psychogenic seizures completely stop having seizures. Long-term outcome is more related to the underlying psychosocial problems than to the seizures. A treatment plan must be initiated early and focused on identification and management of comorbid conditions.

KEY POINTS

1. PNES usually manifests between ages 15 and 35, with a female predominance, and is common in patients with genuine epilepsy and psychiatric comorbidity.
2. PNES may be distinguished from epileptic seizures based on clinical features, such as closed eyes during the seizure episode, lack of a tonic phase, or atypical resolution.
3. Video-EEG can confirm lack of abnormal cortical discharge during a psychogenic seizure, but lack of findings may not distinguish PNES from frontal lobe seizures.
4. Maintenance of the therapeutic relationship between physician and patient and emphasis on reversibility is paramount in management of psychogenic seizures.

■ PSYCHIATRIC DISORDERS IN PATIENTS WITH EPILEPSY

Up to 30% of patients with epilepsy also have comorbid psychiatric disorders, including depression, anxiety, and psychosis. Increased rates of psychiatric disorders are observed in patients with epilepsy relative to the general population, patients with other neurological disorders, and patients with other chronic nonneurological disorders. Patients with temporal lobe epilepsy have the highest prevalence of psychiatric symptoms. The auras of temporal lobe epilepsy reflect the functions of the limbic and cortical structures within the temporal lobe and manifest as odors, abdominal sensations, formed visual or auditory perceptions, memory distortions, and affective changes such as fear, sadness, or anxiety. Given the similarity of these symptoms to those of primary psychiatric disorders, misdiagnosis is common. When psychiatric symptoms are noted in patients with epilepsy, distinction should be made between symptoms that occur at the time of seizure (during the ictal period), symptoms that occur closely after a seizure (postictal), and those behaviors that manifest between seizure episodes (interictal). More difficult to ascertain is whether symptoms are related to epilepsy, underlying structural brain lesions, or medications or are due to a primary psychiatric disorder.

Depression and Epilepsy

Depression is the most frequent psychiatric disorder in patients with epilepsy, reported in 50% of patients admitted to tertiary-care epilepsy centers. Depression, not seizure frequency, has been shown to predict quality of life in patients with intractable epilepsy. Depression in patients with epilepsy can be multifactorial. Contributing factors include seizure type and focus, adverse effects of antiepileptic medications, reaction to a chronic disorder, and psychosocial factors. Depression is more common in patients with complex partial seizures, with temporal or frontal lobe foci, with left-sided seizure foci, and in those patients with intractable seizures. Preictal symptoms of depression can present as mood dysphoria or irritability hours to days before a seizure. Ictal depression results from a simple partial seizure in which depressive symptoms such as anhedonia, guilt, or suicidality are the predominant clinical feature of the seizure. Depression is the second most common ictal affective complaint, after fear/anxiety. Often, ictal symptoms of depression are followed by alteration of consciousness as a seizure evolves from a simple partial to a complex partial seizure. Interictal forms of depression in patients with epilepsy may be atypical, with intermittent anergia, anhedonia, and irritability predominating, mimicking a dysthymic disorder. This form of atypical depression has been labeled interictal dysphoric disorder. The symptoms of depression have a chronic course but can be interrupted by symptom-free periods of hours to days in duration. Clinical presentations meeting current *Diagnostic and Statistical Manual of Mental Disorders,* fourth edition (DSM-IV), criteria for major depressive disorder are less common.

Management of Depression in Patients with Epilepsy

Depression in patients with epilepsy is underdiagnosed and undertreated. An increased risk of seizure occurrence with antidepressants has been found with high serum concentrations, in the presence of other proconvulsant drugs, with rapid dose escalations, and in the presence of other CNS pathology. The risk of worsening seizures can by minimized by starting antidepressants at low doses, with small dose escalations until desired clinical effects are achieved. The selective serotonin reuptake inhibitors (SSRIs), multireceptor antidepressants (nefazodone and venlafaxine), tricyclic antidepressants, and monoamine oxidase inhibitors have a low risk at low doses for exacerbating seizures in patients with epilepsy. The SSRIs and multireceptor antidepressants are considered first-line agents because of their side effect profile, decreased likelihood to result in death after overdose, and efficacy in treating atypical forms of depression. Drug-drug interactions should be considered as well, because many AEDs and antidepressants use the hepatic cytochrome P450 enzymes for metabolism. Psychotherapy is a worthwhile adjunct to pharmacotherapy in depressed patients with epilepsy. Electroconvulsive therapy (ECT) is not contraindicated in patients with epilepsy and has been shown to be well tolerated in patients refractory to antidepressant treatment.

Anxiety and Epilepsy

After depression, anxiety is the second most common psychiatric disorder in patients with epilepsy. Interictally, the different anxiety disorders present with similar clinical signs and symptoms as in the general population. Ictal anxiety, fear, or panic is the most common ictal psychiatric symptom and usually occurs in simple or complex partial seizures with a mesial temporal lobe focus. Ictal anxiety can be distinguished from anxiety and panic disorders by history and examination (Table 14.14).

TABLE 14.14 KEY FEATURES OF ICTAL ANXIETY VERSUS PANIC DISORDER

KEY FEATURES	ICTAL ANXIETY/PARTIAL SEIZURE	PANIC DISORDER
Duration	Brief episodes (<30 seconds)	Longer episodes (minutes to hours)
Family history	No family history of panic disorder	Family history of panic disorder common
Examination	Neurological examination may reveal temporal lobe dysfunction	Neurological examination normal
Associated symptoms	Odors, auditory or visual hallucinations, psychic symptoms	Tachycardia, dyspnea, diaphoresis
EEG	May have epileptiform EEG	Normal EEG
Consciousness	May progress to loss of consciousness, automatisms	Consciousness preserved
Medication response	Responds to antiepileptic drugs	Responds to antidepressant drugs

EEG, electroencephalogram.

Management of Anxiety in Patients with Epilepsy

Interictal anxiety symptoms are reported in up to two-thirds of epileptics. The rate of generalized anxiety and panic disorders is increased in patients with epilepsy compared to the general population. Treatment with SSRIs or the multireceptor medication venlafaxine may be warranted.

Psychosis of Epilepsy

The frequency of psychosis in patients with epilepsy is greater than in the general population. Ictal, postical, and interictal psychosis have been described as three separate and distinct clinical entities and should be considered in the differential diagnosis in patients presenting with psychosis. In ictal psychosis, symptoms are a direct clinical manifestation of ongoing seizure activity, are episodic, and tend to be stereotyped. In postical psychosis, symptoms follow seizures and are predominantly hallucinations, delusions, affective changes, and paranoia occurring 24 to 72 hours after a lucid interval after prolonged or clustered seizure activity. Although the exact cause is not known, the psychosis is usually self-limited, lasting 1 to 2 weeks. Postical psychosis responds to treatment with low-dose neuroleptic medications or benzodiazepines. Interictal psychosis manifests as psychotic symptoms occurring without a clear temporal relationship to seizures. In most patients, interictal psychosis manifests after more than 10 years of seizure activity. Compared to patients without epilepsy, patients with epilepsy with interictal psychosis tend to show an absence of negative symptoms, have a better premorbid history, and demonstrate rare personality deterioration. Symptoms also tend to be less severe and respond well to treatment. It is postulated that there may be a single underlying pathology to explain both the psychosis and the seizures, likely involving the temporal lobe. When attempting to distinguish from a primary psychosis, psychosis related to underlying seizure activity should be considered in patients with a history of seizures, those with stereotyped events, and in those in whom psychosis is episodic and abrupt in onset. Treatment with antipsychotic medication, both prophylactically and acutely, may be necessary.

Alternative Psychosis

Alternative psychosis or "forced normalization" is the controversial concept of an inverse relationship between seizure control and occurrence of psychotic symptoms. Specifically, with "normalization" of EEG recordings, psychiatric symptoms are noted to appear. This phenomenon has been reported in patients with generalized and temporal lobe epilepsies. A paranoid psychosis without clouding of consciousness is the most frequently reported clinical manifestation. The frequency, relevance, and underlying pathogenesis of this concept are yet to be fully determined.

Management of Psychosis in Patients with Epilepsy

Despite their reported proconvulsant properties, antipsychotic medications can be necessary in the treatment of psychotic disorders in patients with epilepsy. The risk of worsening seizure control is increased with higher doses of antipsychotics, with rapid dose escalations, in the presence of other proconvulsant drugs, and in those patients with abnormal EEGs or history of a CNS disorder. Antipsychotics should be started at lower doses and should undergo slower and smaller dose escalation to minimize the risk of seizures in patients with epilepsy. Clozapine, chlorpromazine, and loxapine are considered the antipsychotics with the highest risk of seizure occurrence and should be avoided in patients with epilepsy unless absolutely necessary.

Medication-Related Psychiatric Symptoms

AED use can result in psychiatric side effects, both positive and negative (Table 14.15). Toxicity should be suspected in the presence of other clinical manifestations of toxicity, such as diplopia, ataxia, or tremor. In some patients, psychiatric symptoms occur in patients on discontinuation of

TABLE 14.15 MEDICATION-RELATED PSYCHOTROPIC EFFECTS

ANTIEPILEPTIC MEDICATION	EFFECT
Phenobarbital	Depression, hyperactivity, psychosis
Primidone	Depression, psychosis
Tiagabine	Depression
Vigabatrin	Depression, psychosis
Phenytoin	Encephalopathy
Valproic acid	Encephalopathy, mood stabilization, antimanic
Carbamazepine	Mood stabilization, antimanic
Oxcarbazepine	Mood stabilization, antimanic
Gabapentin	Mood stabilization, anxiolytic
Topiramate	Depression, psychomotor retardation, psychosis, mood stabilization
Lamotrigine	Antidepressant, mood stabilization
Ethosuximide	Psychosis
Zonisamide	Psychosis
Levetiracetam	Psychosis, irritability

AED therapy because the AEDs may have been helping to treat depressive or psychotic symptoms. This phenomenon has been termed "withdrawal-emergent psychopathology." If the onset of a new psychiatric symptom or worsening of a preexisting psychiatric disorder coincides with a change in AED regimen, the new regimen should be considered as a possible causative factor.

Suicide and Epilepsy

Suicide is more frequent among patients with epilepsy than in the general population, with a lifetime prevalence rate for suicide and suicide attempts of 5% to 14.3% compared to a rate of 1.1% to 4.6% in the general population. Risk factors include interictal depression or other psychiatric comorbidity, history of temporal lobe epilepsy, family history, general health issues, and acute life stressors. Patients with epilepsy should be periodically screened for presence of these risk factors and appropriate interventions undertaken.

KEY POINTS

1. Patients with epilepsy, especially temporal lobe epilepsy, have an increased rate of psychiatric disorders, including depression, anxiety, and psychosis.
2. When evaluating psychiatric conditions in patients with epilepsy, care should be taken to distinguish symptoms associated with seizures from those resulting from a primary psychiatric disorder.
3. Depression is the most common psychiatric comorbidity in patients with epilepsy and is a better predictor of quality of life than seizure frequency.
4. SSRIs and multireceptor antidepressants are considered first-line therapy in treating patients with epilepsy with depression or anxiety, although care should be taken to avoid drug-drug interactions.
5. Psychosis in epilepsy has been described as several distinct clinical entities depending on when the episodes occur. Psychosis may require treatment with antipsychotic medications.
6. Patients with epilepsy have a suicide rate 3 to 4 times higher than the general population and require periodic screening for suicidal risk factors.

TABLE 14.16 PERSONALITY TRAITS ASSOCIATED WITH THE INTERICTAL BEHAVIORAL SYNDROME

Emotionality	Viscosity
Circumstantiality	Paranoia
Hypergraphia	Depression
Religiosity	Aggression
Increased philosophical and moral concerns	Anger
Altered sexual interests or behaviors	Dependence
Obsessiveness	Humorlessness

■ INTERICTAL BEHAVIORAL SYNDROME (GESCHWIND SYNDROME)

An interictal behavioral syndrome, Geschwind syndrome, was first described in patients with temporal lobe epilepsy (Table 14.16). Although use of these traits as an inventory has failed to distinguish temporal lobe epilepsy specifically, the inventory has been found to consistently distinguish patients with epilepsy (regardless of focus or seizure type) from patients with nonepileptic neurological disorders and from normal controls. Because one or more of these traits are noted frequently in patients with epilepsy, the presence of these traits should increase the suspicion for underlying epilepsy. They are, however, by no means sensitive or specific.

KEY POINT

The interictal behavioral syndrome, or Geschwind syndrome, has been developed as an inventory that may help distinguish patients with epilepsy from those with nonepileptic disorders.

■ SUGGESTED READINGS

Barry JJ. The recognition and management of mood disorders as a comorbidity of epilepsy. *Epilepsia* 2003;44(suppl 4):30–40.

Bear DM, Fedio P. Quantitative analysis of interictal behavior in temporal lobe epilepsy. *Arch Neurol* 1977;34:454–467.

Benbadis SR. Epileptic seizures and syndromes. *Neurol Clin* 2001;19:251–270.

Berg AT, Shinnar S. The risk of seizure recurrence following a first unprovoked seizure: a quantitative review. *Neurology* 1991;41:965–972.

Boylan LS, Flint LA, Labovitz DL, et al. Depression but not seizure frequency predicts quality of life in treatment-resistant epilepsy. *Neurology* 2004;62:258–261.

Brodie MJ, Dichter MA. Antiepileptic drugs. *N Engl J Med* 1996;334:168–175.

Brodtkorb E, Mula M. Optimizing therapy of seizures in adult patients with psychiatric comorbidity. *Neurology* 2006;67(suppl 4):S39–S44.

Browne TR, Holmes GL. Epilepsy. *N Engl J Med* 2001;344:1145–1151.

Chang BS, Lowenstein DH. Epilepsy. *N Engl J Med* 2003;349:1257–1266.

Chung SS, Gerber P, Kirlin KA. Ictal eye closure is a reliable indicator for psychogenic nonepileptic seizures. *Neurology* 2006;66:1730–1731.

Commission on Classification and Terminology of the International League Against Epilepsy. Proposal for revised clinical and electroencephalographic classification of epileptic seizures. *Epilepsia* 1981;22:489–501.

Commission on Classification and Terminology of the International League Against Epilepsy. Proposal for revised classification of epilepsies and epileptic syndromes. *Epilepsia* 1989;30:389–399.

Delanty N, Vaughan CJ, French JA. Medical causes of seizures. *Lancet* 1998;352:383–390.

Devinsky O, Vazquez B. Behavioral changes associated with epilepsy. *Neurol Clin* 1993;11:127–149.

Devinsky O, Barr WB, Vickrey BG, et al. Changes in depression and anxiety after resective surgery for epilepsy. *Neurology* 2005;5:1744–1749.

Drislane FW. Presentation, evaluation, and treatment of nonconvulsive status epilepticus. *Epilepsy Behav* 2000;1:301–314.

Engel J Jr, Pedley TA, eds. *Epilepsy: A Comprehensive Textbook*. Philadelphia: Lippincott-Raven, 1998.

Ettinger AB. Psychotropic effects of antiepileptic drugs. *Neurology* 2006;67:1916–1925.

Gates JR, Ramani V, Whalen S, et al. Ictal characteristics of pseudoseizures. *Arch Neurol* 1985;42:1183–1187.

Harden CL. The co-morbidity of depression and epilepsy: epidemiology, etiology, and treatment. *Neurology* 2002;59:S48–S55.

Hauser WA, Hesdorffer DC. *Epilepsy: Frequency, Causes and Consequences.* New York: Demos Press, 1990.

Husain AM, Horn GJ, Jacobson MP. Non-convulsive status epilepticus: usefulness of clinical features in selecting patients for urgent EEG. *J Neurol Neurosurg Psychiatry* 2003;74:189–191.

Jobst BC, Williamson PD. Frontal lobe seizures. *Psychiatr Clin North Am* 2005;28:635–651.

Jones JE, Hermann BP, Barry JJ, et al. Rates and risk factors for suicide, suicidal ideation, and suicide attempts in chronic epilepsy. *Epilepsy Behav* 2003;4:S31–S38.

Lancman M. Psychosis and peri-ictal confusional states. *Neurology* 1999;53(suppl 2):S33–S38.

Kanner AM, Morris HH, Lüders H, et al. Supplementary motor seizures mimicking pseudoseizures: some clinical differences. *Neurology* 1990;40:1404–1407.

Kanner AM, Nieto JCR. Depressive disorders in epilepsy. *Neurology* 1999;53(suppl 2):S26–S32.

Kaplan PW. Clinical presentations of nonconvulsive status epilepticus. In: Drislane FW, ed. *Status Epilepticus: A Clinical Perspective.* Totowa, NJ: Humana Press; 2005:197–220.

Krumholz A. Nonepileptic seizures: diagnosis and management. *Neurology* 1999;53(suppl 2):S76–S83.

LaFrance WC Jr, Kanner AM. Epilepsy. In: Jeste DV, Friedman JH, eds. *Psychiatry for Neurologists.* Totowa, NJ: Humana Press; 2006:191–208.

Leone MA, Solari A, Beghi E for the First Seizure Trial Group (FIRST Group). Treatment of the first tonic-clonic seizure does not affect long-term remission of epilepsy. *Neurology* 2006;67:2227–2229.

Lesser RP. Psychogenic seizures. *Neurology* 1996;46:1499–1507.

Lowenstein CH, Alldredge BK. Status epilepticus. *N Engl J Med* 1998;338:970–976.

Marson A, Jacoby A, Johnson A, et al. Immediate versus deferred antiepileptic drug treatment for early epilepsy and single seizures: a randomized controlled trial. *Lancet* 2005;365:2007–2013.

Miller LC, Drislane FW. Treatment strategies after a single seizure: rationale for immediate versus deferred treatment. *CNS Drugs* 2007;21:89–99.

Morrell MJ. Differential diagnosis of seizures. *Neurol Clin* 1993;11:737–754.

Nadkarni S, LaJoie J, Devinsky O. Current treatments of epilepsy. *Neurology* 2005;64(suppl 3):S2–S11.

Practice parameter: neuroimaging in the emergency patient presenting with seizure. *Neurology* 1996;47:288–291.

Riggio S. Nonconvulsive status epilepticus: clinical features and diagnostic challenges. *Psychiatr Clin North Am* 2005;28:653–664.

Salinsky M, Kanter R, Dasheiff RM. Effectiveness of multiple EEGs in supporting the diagnosis of epilepsy: an operational curve. *Epilepsia.* 1987;28:331–334.

Schmitz B. Psychiatric syndromes related to antiepileptic drugs. *Epilepsia* 1999;40(suppl 10):S65–S70.

Schomer DL, O'Connor M, Spiers P, et al. Temporolimbic epilepsy and behavior. In: Mesulam M-M, ed. *Principles of Behavioral and Cognitive Neurology.* New York: Oxford University Press; 2000:373–405.

Shen W, Bowman ES, Markand ON. Presenting the diagnosis of pseudoseizure. *Neurology* 1990;40:756–759.

Trimble MR. *Psychosis of Epilepsy.* New York: Raven Press, 1991.

van Donselaar CA, Stroink H, Arts W. How confident are we of the diagnosis of epilepsy? *Epilepsia* 2006;47(suppl 1):S9–S13.

Waxman SG, Geschwind N. The interictal behavior syndrome of temporal lobe epilepsy. *Arch Gen Psychiatry* 1975;32:1580–1586.

Williamson PD, Spencer DD, Spencer SS, Novelly RA, Mattson RH. Complex partial seizures of frontal lobe origin. *Ann Neurol* 1985;18:497–504.

CHAPTER 15

Headache

Michael Ronthal

■ INTRODUCTION

Headache is common—approximately 20% of the adult, female childbearing population have migraine; tension-type headache has been estimated to be as prevalent as 80%. In most cases the diagnosis is made by history and the examination is frequently negative; hence an accurate and comprehensive history is mandatory. A distinction must be made between the primary headache syndromes and secondary headaches, in which an underlying, sometimes ominous cause is present and for which further investigation must be undertaken.

■ HEADACHE HISTORY QUESTIONNAIRE

The following questions require specific answers:

- When did the headaches start? (i.e., lifelong, chronic, recent?)
- Frequency?
- Duration?
- Warning or aura?
- Onset gradual or abrupt?
- Site of pain?
- Character of pain (constant or throbbing/pulsatile?)
- Aggravating factors?
- Relieving factors?
- Associated symptoms?
- Precipitants?
- Family history?
- Any history of head or neck trauma?
- Medications tried (failures/successes?)
- Psychiatric history?

Having completed the headache questionnaire, a general medical history should be obtained and the patient is then examined.

■ CLASSIFICATION

The International Classification of Headache Disorders (ICDH-2), published in January 2004, is a comprehensive overview of all headache types, both primary and secondary. The definitions used in this chapter are taken from this classification. Primary headaches are those for which no anatomical pathologic condition can be determined. Secondary headaches, by definition, are secondary to some definable neurological abnormality and perforce carry a higher morbidity and even mortality depending on the underlying pathology.

■ PRIMARY HEADACHES

Migraine

Migraine is an intermittent and recurrent, usually familial headache. Migraine may be subclassified as migraine without aura or migraine with aura. The clinical features of migraine without aura are listed in Table 15.1.

The aura may come before, during, or after the headache or may not be associated with headache at all. The aura is regarded as a reversible neurological deficit, lasting less than 60 minutes. The deficit is cortically based and may include visual, motor, somatosensory, or language symptoms, and the diagnosis of migraine is made because the symptoms progress, or march, in an extremity over time. Thus "pins and needles" or numbness in an arm could start in the hand and march up the limb to the shoulder over approximately 10 to 15 minutes. The visual aura (shimmering or scintillating light, scotomas, fortification spectra) will gradually spread across the visual field; the language deficit will change over minutes. Weakness will spread in a fashion similar to a sensory march.

Before or simultaneously with the aura, regional cortical cerebral blood flow is decreased in the somatic cortical area corresponding to the body part involved (e.g., occipital area for a visual aura). The spread of dysfunction is currently usually equated with the experimentally induced spreading depression of Leão. If potassium is dripped onto the cortex, it causes local depolarization, which leads to further potassium egress from the depolarized cell that in turn depolarizes its neighbor, setting up a chain reaction that spreads over the cortex at a rate of approximately 3 mm per minute. This spread correlates with the migraine march. The aura is distinct from the headache and has a different pathophysiology.

The headache of migraine is typically throbbing; aggravated by coughing, straining, and stooping; and relieved by lying still in a dark room. It is regarded as a neurovascular phenomenon associated with neurally mediated inflammation and activation of deep pain pathways. The periaqueductal gray in the brainstem is activated during the headache.

Triggers for migraine attacks include emotional upsets or stress, irregular sleep habits, missing meals, and hormonal changes. Curiously, patients will cope well during a stressful episode, but have a migraine once the stress passes. Migraine related to the menstrual period is called catamenial migraine—the trigger is estrogen withdrawal. Some patients report that specific foods may trigger an attack—common foods are red wine, chocolate, and Chinese food. The basic pathophysiological connection between any particular trigger and an attack of migraine remains obscure. During pregnancy, migraine usually improves, only to return after delivery.

Hemiplegia as part of migraine is rare but may be familial or sporadic. Familial hemiplegic migraine (FHM) has been tracked to mutations in the *CACNA1A* gene on chromosome 19

TABLE 15.1 ICDH-2 DIAGNOSTIC CRITERIA FOR MIGRAINE WITHOUT AURA

A. At least five attacks fulfilling criteria B–D
B. Headache attacks lasting 4 to 72 hours

C. Headache has at least two of the following characteristics:
  1. Unilateral
  2. Pulsating
  3. Moderate or severe pain
  4. Aggravation by or causing avoidance of routine physical activity (e.g., walking or climbing stairs).

D. During the headache at least one of the following:
  1. Nausea and/or vomiting
  2. Photophobia and phonophobia

E. Not attributed to another disorder

(FHM1) and to mutations in the *ATP1A2* gene on chromosome 1 (FHM2). In FHM1, basilar symptoms are common, headache is almost always present, and disturbances of consciousness, fever, and cerebrospinal fluid (CSF) pleocytosis can occur. In approximately 50% of families with FHM1, chronic progressive cerebellar ataxia occurs.

If a migraine headache is very severe and lasts without remission for more than 72 hours, the label status migrainosus is warranted.

Psychopathology of Migraine

The prodrome of an attack of migraine may include depression, euphoria, irritability, anxiety, hyperactivity, poor concentration, anorexia, or increased appetite. There is a significant association of migraine with affective disorders and anxiety disorders.

Anxiety disorder generally precedes the onset of migraine, and major depression usually occurs after the onset of migraine. Odds ratios for psychiatric disorders in migraineurs versus nonmigraineurs have been reported as 2.2 for major depressive disorder, 2.9 for bipolar spectrum disorders, 5.3 for generalized anxiety disorders, 3.3 for panic disorder, 2.4 for simple phobia disorder, and 2 for social phobia. Dysregulation of serotonergic transmission has been postulated as a common cause.

Patients with comorbid migraine and psychiatric disorder experience a more severe or complex clinical course, with greater impairment of health-related quality of life measures. The odds ratio for suicide attempts is 3.0. The odds ratio for suicide attempts in major depression is 7.8, but in those with migraine as a comorbidity the rate is 23.2.

Red Flags: The finding of a focal deficit, papilledema, cranial bruit, recent onset, fever, meningismus, are indications for imaging and CSF analysis.

Treatment

The patient should be counseled about "daily life" precipitants of migraine. Some alteration in lifestyle often goes a long way. Medication is indicated for *prophylaxis* and for *symptomatic* treatment of an attack.

Prophylaxis: One or two headaches a week is sufficient to warrant prophylaxis. The response to placebo is approximately 30% to 50%, so the response of an effective prophylactic agent must exceed these numbers.

Antidepressants: Tricyclic antidepressants have stood the test of time and are probably the first choice. Selective serotonin reuptake inhibitors (SSRIs) are the next choice. Calcium blockers, such as verapamil, have few side effects and are worth a trial. Beta-blockers should not be used if the patient is depressed, but are generally good anxiolytics. Anticonvulsants are next in line. Valproate works quite well (80%), but it is contraindicated in women in the childbearing years for fear of congenital malformations in the fetus. Topiramate is somewhat sedating in some patients but often works well, as does lamotrigine. There are reports that riboflavin is effective, and because migraineurs are sometimes magnesium-depleted, magnesium supplements have been suggested and occasionally help.

When using prophylactic medications the rule is to start with a small dose and gradually escalate, to tolerance if necessary, before declaring any particular drug a failure.

Symptomatic Treatment: Ibuprofen is a good starting point. If it fails, a triptan should be used. For a rapid effect a nasal triptan spray is worth trying. About 60% of patients may rebound, when a longer-acting preparation such as frovatriptan is worth considering. If a triptan fails, analgesics of varying strength, ranging from tramadol through narcotics, are used, but in general it is best to avoid narcotics.

Tension-Type Headache

Tension-type headache (TTH), also known as tension headache, muscle contraction headache, psychomyogenic headache, stress headache, and psychogenic headache is classified as:

- Infrequent episodic tension-type headache
- Frequent episodic tension-type headache
- Chronic tension-type headache

These classifications are further subdivided in the International Classification Impairments, Disabilities, and Handicaps (ICDH-2) into those with and those without pericranial tenderness.

The prevalence of TTH in the general population ranges from 30% to 78%, but, as in migraine, the figures quoted are likely on the low side.

Diagnostic criteria for infrequent episodic TTH are listed in Table 15.2.

Infrequent headaches by definition occur less frequently than 1 day per month, frequent headaches occur on more than 1 but fewer than 15 days per month for at least 3 months, and chronic headache implies that the occurrence of headache occurs on more than 15 days per month.

These patients describe their headaches variously as pressure, a band around the head, a bursting sensation, or tight scalp. The posterior cervical muscles are usually tight and tender, and there may be tenderness to pressure over the temporalis and masseter. Likely the headache is pain referred from extracranial muscle in spasm. In young patients the social background is almost always of stress, and in older individuals the root cause is likely to be cervical spondylosis diagnosed by restricted neck movement, cervical root signs, or long tract signs.

Treatment

Often, reassurance is all that is necessary, but relaxation exercises and biofeedback offer a non-medication route of therapy.

Mechanical help by way of firm to hard pillows for sleep, local heat to the neck, or gentle massage may be of value. In patients with cervical spondylosis, a soft cervical collar is usually of benefit.

Prophylactic medication includes muscle relaxant drugs such as cyclobenzaprine, methocarbamol, metaxalone, tizanidine, and orphenadrine, but all of these have a potential for sedation and may not be tolerated. Diazepam is a good muscle relaxant, especially when anxiety is part of the syndrome. A muscle relaxant combined with a tricyclic antidepressant usually works for prophylaxis.

TABLE 15.2 ICDH-2 DIAGNOSTIC CRITERIA FOR INFREQUENT EPISODIC TENSION-TYPE HEADACHE

A. At least 10 episodes occurring on fewer than 1 day per month on average (<12 days per year) and fulfilling criteria B through D

B. Headache lasting from 30 minutes to 7 days

C. Headache has at least two of the following characteristics:
  1. Bilateral location
  2. Pressing/tightening (nonpulsatile) quality
  3. Mild or moderate intensity
  4. Not aggravated by routine physical activity such as walking or climbing stairs

D. Both of the following:
  1. No nausea or vomiting (anorexia may occur)
  2. No more than one of photophobia or phonophobia

E. Not attributed to another disorder

Symptomatic treatment should begin with ibuprofen or acetaminophen, which is often combined with a muscle relaxant, but a stronger analgesic may be required.

Red Flags: Sudden onset, worsening headache pattern without response to treatment, fever and meningismus, focal signs, papilledema, aggravation by cough or exertion, history of cancer, or human immunodeficiency virus (HIV) infection.

Trigeminal Autonomic Cephalgias

The primary short-lasting headaches with prominent autonomic features include cluster headache, chronic paroxysmal hemicrania, episodic paroxysmal hemicrania, short-lasting unilateral neuralgiaform headache attacks with conjunctival injection and tearing (SUNCT) syndrome, and hemicrania continua.

Common to all of these is the presence of short-lived unilateral pain and ipsilateral autonomic features—*trigeminal* because the headache is in the distribution of the trigeminal nerve (V1) and *autonomic* because of activation of cranial parasympathetic efferents. This does not imply a common underlying pathogenesis for all of the varieties but does suggest activation of similar structures.

Cluster Headache

The prevalence is less than 1%, and it affects almost entirely men.

The term "cluster" refers to the fact that there are periods of recurrent headache or "clusters" of headache, and a cluster may recur at the same patient-specific time of the year. Each cluster lasts from 7 days to 12 months, and during it there may be from one to eight attacks per day. If a remission lasts less than 30 days, or there is no remission after a year, the label is chronic cluster headache.

A familial history is present in 11% of patients, but no clear molecular genetic predisposition has yet been established.

The diagnostic criteria for cluster headache are described in Table 15.3.

Cluster headaches tend to be time-locked or circadian, occurring at the same time every day or night, suggesting that a biological clock (hypothalamus) must be involved. They may be precipitated by alcohol. The Horner may become permanent.

Current theories of pathophysiology suggest that autonomic dysregulation might originate centrally in the hypothalamus and that parasympathetic overactivity may result in vasodilatation or perivascular edema affecting sympathetic pathways in the carotid wall and that autonomic symptoms are secondary to trigeminal discharge.

TABLE 15.3 ICDH-2 DIAGNOSTIC CRITERIA FOR CLUSTER HEADACHE

A. At least five attacks fulfilling criteria B through D

B. Severe or very severe unilateral orbital, supraorbital, and/or temporal pain lasting 15 to 180 minutes if untreated

C. Headache is accompanied by at least one of the following:
 1. Ipsilateral conjunctival injection and/or lacrimation
 2. Ipsilateral nasal congestion and/or rhinorrhea
 3. Ipsilateral eyelid edema
 4. Ipsilateral forehead and facial sweating
 5. Ipsilateral miosis and/or ptosis
 6. A sense of restlessness or agitation

D. Attacks have a frequency from one every other day to eight per day

E. Not attributed to another disorder

Functional imaging with positron emission tomography (PET) confirms activation of the hypothalamus, and functional magnetic resonance imaging (MRI) supports that notion.

Treatment

Prophylaxis: Verapamil in an initial dose of 80 mg three times daily is usually the key to success, but the dose may have to be increased, and a total daily dose of 480 to 720 mg is recommended before the treatment is regarded as unsuccessful. Nimodipine may also be effective. Prednisone 30 to 100 mg daily may abort the cluster. Lithium has been shown to be effective (78%), with a rate of effectiveness similar to that of verapamil.

In 10% to 20% of patients the first-line drugs fail; pizotifen, valproate, or topiramate may then be tried. Intranasal capsaicin has shown some efficacy.

Ergotamine was the mainstay of treatment in the past. A trial of ergotamine suppositories at night as a preventive for night headaches is worth considering.

Occipital nerve block may help, although the mechanism of action is unknown, but deep brain stimulation of the posterior inferior hypothalamus has been shown to be effective in patients with refractory cluster headache.

Symptomatic: Inhalation of pure oxygen with a nonrebreathing mask at a flow rate of 7 liters per minute is effective in 60% of patients. Intranasal 4% lidocaine drops sometimes works, presumably by anesthetizing the sphenopalatine ganglion. Dihydroergotamine intravenous or sumatriptan subcutaneous injections are effective in more than 75% of patients. Sumatriptan or zolmitriptan nasal spray into the contralateral nasal passage is effective.

Chronic Paroxysmal Hemicrania

The distribution and autonomic accompaniments of chronic paroxysmal hemicrania (CPH) are as in cluster headache. Onset is usually in the 20- to 30-year age range. The headache lasts 2 to 45 minutes and recurs more than 5 times per day, but case reports document a frequency of 1 to 40 attacks per day. The distinction from cluster headaches is that the headaches are shorter, are more frequent, are female predominant (3:1), and respond to indomethacin. Whereas patients with cluster headaches are restless during an attack, patients with CPH may take to their beds.

MRI has shown narrowing of ophthalmic veins on orbital phlebography, but this is nonspecific.

Treatment

Indomethacin 25 mg three times daily, increasing to 50 mg three times daily, can be administered if there is no response. A proton pump inhibitor may protect the stomach from gastrointestinal side effects and should be combined with the indomethacin. Verapamil is preventive.

Episodic Paroxysmal Hemicrania

Episodic paroxysmal hemicrania (EPH) is a rare headache syndrome characterized by frequent daily attacks of short-lived, very severe headache with ipsilateral autonomic features. It may be a variant of CPH, but it is cluster-like, occurring in bursts lasting 7 days to 1 year, separated by pain-free periods lasting a month or longer. It also responds to indomethacin and calcium blockers. CPH and EPH may be headaches at opposite ends of a spectrum, and some reported patients transition from one to the other.

Short-Lasting Unilateral Neuralgiform Headache with Conjunctival Injection and Tearing

Short-lasting unilateral neuralgiform headache with conjunctival injection and tearing (SUNCT) is a disorder of male individuals (17:2 male to female ratio), with paroxysms of pain lasting 5 to 250 seconds, rarely longer. Attacks recur at approximately 5 to 6 times per hour,

TABLE 15.4 ICDH-2 DIAGNOSTIC CRITERIA FOR SUNCT

A. At least 30 attacks fulfilling B through E

B. Attacks of unilateral, moderately severe orbital or temporal stabbing or throbbing pain lasting 15 to 120 seconds.

C. Attack frequency from 3 to 100 per day

D. Pain is associated with at least one of the following signs or symptoms on the affected side, with conjunctival injection being most often present and very prominent.
   1. Conjunctival injection
   2. Lacrimation
   3. Nasal congestion
   4. Rhinorrhea
   5. Ptosis
   6. Eyelid edema

E. At least one of the following:
   1. There is no suggestion of other diagnosis (i.e., a secondary headache)
   2. Such a diagnosis is suggested but excluded by appropriate investigations

Clinical note: The literature suggests that the most common secondary cause of SUNCT would be a lesion in the posterior fossa.

occasionally as frequently as 30 episodes in an hour. One study showed a range of frequency of 6 to 77 attacks per day, with a mean of 28 attacks per day. Conjunctival injection is the most prominent autonomic feature (Table 15.4). Occasionally this turns out to be a secondary headache with pathology in the cerebellar pontine angle or brainstem. Orbital phlebography may demonstrate narrowing of the superior ophthalmic vein.

Treatment

Whereas CPH and EPH respond to indomethacin, SUNCT is refractory to virtually all treatment suggested so far.

Hemicrania Continua

Hemicrania continua (HC) is characterized by a continuous unilateral pain of moderate severity punctuated by superimposed intense episodes that are associated with autonomic features. This headache responds to indomethacin.

HC is differentiated from the other headaches in this group by its continuous moderate pain without autonomic features between the painful exacerbations.

Escalating requirements for indomethacin or lack of response should indicate imaging (a case of a sphenoid bone tumor with HC features has been described), but imaging in this condition is generally negative.

There remains a group of rare and unusual headache types, all poorly understood and treated. These include thunderclap headache, primary stabbing headache, primary exertional headache, primary cough headache, primary headache associated with sexual intercourse, and hypnic headache. Their names describe the headaches fairly.

Chronic Daily Headache

Chronic daily headache (CDH) by definition is headache lasting for more than 15 days per month, for longer than 3 months. CDH is a syndrome, not a diagnosis, and the syndrome may be part of primary or secondary headache, and secondary headache must be excluded.

The prevalence of CDH is 3% to 5%, worldwide, and it is a cause of considerable disability and diminished quality of life. Depression and anxiety are present in more than half of the patients.

The two common causes of CDH are transformed migraine and medication overuse headache.

Transformed Migraine

Most patients are women with a history of episodic migraine that gradually escalates until a pattern of daily or near-daily headache emerges that, by history, suggests a combination of migraine and tension type headache.

Medication Overuse Headache

Medication overuse headache (MOH) or analgesic rebound headache is prevalent in 1.4% of the population. Patients with transformed migraine are part of this pool. By definition, this is a CDH that resolves within 2 months of discontinuing the analgesics. There should be a history of regular use of headache medication for more than 3 months. Drugs include ergotamine, triptans, opioids, and combination analgesics used for more than 10 days per month or of simple analgesics used for more than 15 days per month.

There has been some debate about cause and consequence of using analgesics to excess. If the headache remits within 2 months of analgesic withdrawal, MOH is diagnosed; if the headaches continue, transformed migraine is diagnosed.

Treatment

No controlled studies are available to assess withdrawal of medication, but simple analgesics, ergotamine, triptans, and most combination analgesics can be abruptly withdrawn on an outpatient basis. Opioids and barbiturates should be tapered over weeks. A short course of phenobarbital or clonidine may cushion narcotic or barbiturate withdrawal. Occasionally, inpatient management is required.

Prednisone 100 mg for 5 days has been shown in some studies to reduce withdrawal headache in MOH, and tizanidine 2 to 16 mg at bedtime has also been helpful.

Repeated migraine or analgesic overuse may lead to central sensitization of pain pathways. PET scanning has shown hypometabolism in pain-processing areas of the brain: bilateral thalami, orbitofrontal cortex, anterior cingulated gyrus, insula and ventral striatum, and right inferior parietal lobule. The cerebellar vermis was hyperactive with analgesic withdrawal, except the orbitofrontal cortex. These structures are involved in other chronic pain disorders.

■ SECONDARY HEADACHES

The diagnosis of secondary headache implies that there is significant neurological pathology as the underlying cause. That pathology irritates or deforms pain-sensitive structures, including the dura, arterial and venous vessels, sensory cranial nerves, and cervical structures. Given this, the causes are legion and some may be associated with a high morbidity and mortality risk, so a precise diagnosis is imperative and prompt and appropriate treatment a requisite.

The ICDH-2 recognizes the following broad categories:

- Headache attributed to head and neck trauma
- Headache attributed to cranial or cervical vascular disorder
- Headache attributed to a vascular intracranial disorder
- Headache attributed to a substance or its withdrawal
- Headache attributed to infection
- Headache attributed to a disturbance of homeostasis
- Headache or facial pain attributed to a disorder of cranium, neck, eyes, ears, nose, sinuses, teeth, mouth, or other facial or cranial structures
- Headache attributed to psychiatric disorder

TABLE 15.5 SECONDARY HEADACHE

SUDDEN ONSET	CONSIDER SUBARACHNOID HEMORRHAGE
Fever/meningismus	Infective meningitis, acute or chronic, carcinomatous meningitis, chemical meningitis
Worse with coughing/straining/papilledema	Raised intracranial pressure—mass lesion, hydrocephalus, pseudotumor
Focal features	Mass lesion, tumor, abscess
Throbbing, lateralized, jaw claudication, elevated sedimentation rate or C-reactive protein	Temporal arteritis
Worse in upright posture	Spinal fluid leak
Background human immunodeficiency syndrome	Opportunistic infection, lymphoma

This brief discussion pretty much includes a whole textbook of internal medicine!

Features that should prompt consideration of secondary headaches and therefore continued investigation are presented in Table 15.5.

Consider the following factors:

- A new headache not conforming to the syndromes described in the preceding section on primary headache.
- A headache of sudden onset suggests some form of mechanical trigger, the most important of which is a vascular event such as a subarachnoid hemorrhage (SAH). The "worst headache of my life" does not necessarily carry the same ominous portent in each individual—everyone at some point has the "worst" headache! Arterial strokes of all types may present with sudden headache, as can venous occlusions.
- Fever or meningismus may indicate meningitis.
- Patients with a background illness that might spread to the nervous system should be treated with caution; thus a history of malignancy or HIV infection will prompt further study.
- The characteristic features of a headache secondary to raised intracranial pressure are coughing, straining, or stooping. This type of headache often wakes the patient in the early hours of the morning.
- The finding of papilledema.
- The finding of focal features on clinical examination.
- Patients over the age of 50 with temporal or facial pain, jaw claudication, or visual symptoms may have temporal arteritis, which requires immediate treatment if vision is to be preserved. Emergency sedimentation rate and C-reactive protein values should be requested.
- A headache that is worse in the upright posture and settles on recumbency suggests a low-pressure state that may be due to spinal fluid leak—itself a portal of entry for infection.

These scenarios represent red flags in headache diagnosis and will always suggest further imaging, CSF studies, and blood studies as appropriate.

Sudden-Onset Headache

Sudden-onset headache as a syndrome deserves more attention here and also in practice.

By "sudden," we mean onset over seconds; this is often referred to as a thunderclap headache, suggesting a mechanical cause of some sort. Of all of the many causes, the most important one and the one potentially having lethal implications is SAH.

The CT scan is sensitive for blood and will detect approximately 95% of cases. When the CT is bland but the history persuasive, it is mandatory to perform a spinal tap and examine the CSF for blood or blood products. The spinal tap should be performed by an experienced operator. A traumatic tap with bleeding at the site of puncture makes for uncertainty and results in a host of further investigations that might not really be necessary.

The fluid should be spun down and the supernatant examined for a yellow tinge, or xanthochromia; the collecting tube is held up against a pure white background. In SAH the red cells will be crenated when examined with a microscope. The protein is elevated, and the elevation depends on the degree of bleeding. The spinal fluid glucose is often decreased as it is in meningitis.

SAH requires extensive imaging and angiography to determine the source of bleeding.

Other causes of sudden headache include stroke of any type, cerebral venous thrombosis, pituitary apoplexy, benign thunderclap headache, cranioverterbral subluxation, and sometimes just cervical spondylosis. Intermittent hydrocephalus, such as might be produced by a third-ventricle colloid cyst, is always mentioned in this differential diagnosis but is very rare.

Headache Attributed to Psychiatric Disorders

The headache attributed to psychiatric disorders must be manifest only during times when the symptoms of the psychiatric disorder also manifest.

In this category the ICDH-2 recognizes the following:

- Headache attributed to major depressive disorder
- Headache attributed to panic disorder
- Headache attributed to generalized anxiety disorder
- Headache attributed to undifferentiated somatoform disorder
- Headache attributed to social phobia
- Headache attributed to separation anxiety disorder
- Headache attributed to posttraumatic stress disorder

In all of these the caveat is that other causes of headache must be excluded and any of the headache types can coincide with a psychiatric condition.

KEY POINTS

1. The history is paramount in headache diagnosis and must be meticulous.
2. Unusual features such as sudden onset, fever, history of HIV or malignancy, or an abnormal physical examination may be regarded as red flags and suggest a secondary rather than a primary headache.
3. The physician should be familiar with the patterns of headache, which are now well delineated.
4. Treatment may be prophylactic or symptomatic and should be individualized for each patient.

■ SUGGESTED READINGS

Breslau N, Schultz LR, Stewart WF, et al. Headache and major depression: Is the association specific to migraine. *Neurology* 2000;54:308–313.

Cahill CM, Murphy KC. Migraine: Another headache for the psychiatrists? *BMJ* 2004;185:191–193.

Dodick DW. Chronic daily headache. *N Engl J Med* 2006;354:158–165.

Fumal A, Laureys S, Di Clemente L, et al. Orbitofrontal cortex involvement in chronic analgesic-overuse headache evolving from episodic migraine. *Brain* 2006;129:543–550.

Goadsby PJ, Lipton RB. A review of paroxysmal hemicranias, SUNCT syndrome and other short-lasting headaches with autonomic features, including new cases. *Brain* 1997;120:193–209.

Kumar KL, Reuler JB. Uncommon headaches: Diagnosis and treatment. *J Gen Int Med* 1993;8:333–341.

Lake AE, Saper JR. Chronic headache: New advances in treatment strategies. *Neurology* 2002;59:S8–S13.

Lake AE, Rains JC, Penzion DB, et al. Headache and psychiatric comorbidity: Historical context, clinical implication, and research relevance. *Headache* 2005;45:493–506.

Lipton RB, Bigal ME. Chronic daily headache: Is analgesic overuse a cause or a consequence? *Neurology* 2003;61: 154–155.

Lipton RB, Bigal ME, Steiner TJ, et al. Classification of primary headaches. *Neurology* 2004;63:427–435.

May A. Cluster headache: Pathogenesis, diagnosis, and management. *Lancet* 2005;366:843–855.

Merikangas KR, Angst J, Isler H. Migraine and psychopathology: Results of the Zurich cohort study of young adulta. *Arch Gen Psychiatry* 1990;47:849–853.

CHAPTER 16

Spinal Cord Disorders

Michael Ronthal

■ MYELOPATHY

Introduction

The term "myelopathy" implies dysfunction of the spinal cord, which extends from the craniocervical junction to the level of the L1/2 interspace. The salient feature to suggest cord dysfunction is the presence of bilateral signs or symptoms in the lower limbs, but occasionally a localized intramedullary cervical cord lesion will present with signs or symptoms referable only to the upper limbs, again, usually bilaterally. The clinical diagnosis will depend on a combination of symptoms and signs that suggest root or tract dysfunction (Fig. 16.1). The following discussion excludes acute traumatic spinal cord injury.

Symptoms

Root Related

Motor: Each motor root supplies a group of muscles labeled a myotome. The motor deficit, or weakness, is related to the particular root or myotome involved. Thus weakness in the distribution of C5 may result in the complaint of difficulty lifting objects when the movement requires elbow flexion or difficulty brushing the hair, which requires deltoid action. Weakness in the distribution of C6–7 may result in the complaint of difficulty with pushups when the triceps is weak. Lower cervical root dysfunction results in weak hands.

Sensory: Root pain is typically superficial, sharp, lancinating, shooting down the arm to the hand, or in the thoracic area around the trunk in a girdle distribution. At times the complaint may be of numbness or loss of sensation down the arms or in the hands, but patients rarely report trunk numbness.

Tract Related

Motor: Weakness in the lower limbs results in the complaint of "I can't walk." Because of weakness of toe (and also foot) extension the patient may catch the toes and trip, especially when walking on thick rugs. The distal soles of the shoes wear out from constant scraping on the ground with each step, and the patient may be aware of shuffling. Weakness of hip flexion impairs walking up stairs or getting in and out of an automobile.

Sensory: Sensory symptoms depend on which ascending fiber tract is dysfunctional. Posterior column dysfunction may result in deep aching or boring pain caudally. There may be bizarre sensations such as tight garter or stocking sensation in the legs. The fingers may feel "like blown-up sausages." An occasional complaint is of "water trickling down the leg." Spinothalamic tract dysfunction may, rarely, result in superficial sharp, root-like pain in the legs. Itching is a pain equivalent. On occasion a pseudo-radicular girdle pain, tight sensation, or sensory loss is due to tract dysfunction in the cervical cord.

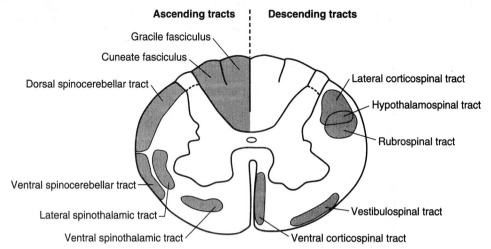

Ascending tracts | **Descending tracts**

Gracile fasciculus
Cuneate fasciculus
Dorsal spinocerebellar tract
Lateral corticospinal tract
Hypothalamospinal tract
Rubrospinal tract
Ventral spinocerebellar tract
Lateral spinothalamic tract
Vestibulospinal tract
Ventral spinothalamic tract
Ventral corticospinal tract

■ **FIGURE 16.1** Horizontal section through the cervical spinal cord depicting the ascending and descending tracts. (Reprinted with permission from Fix JD. *High-Yield Neuroanatomy*, 3rd ed. Baltimore: Lippincott Williams & Wilkins; 2005:62.)

Bladder Related

Motor: In upper motor neuron (UMN) bladder dysfunction the bladder is small and contracted. This results in the complaint of frequency of small amounts of urine, nocturia, and, because the bladder is hyperexcitable, urgency and urgency incontinence. Lesions of the thoracic cord may result in bladder dyssynergia—the detrusor contracts on a tight sphincter, with the result of hesitancy.

Sensory: Deafferentation of the bladder leads to a large-volume "sack" with no desire to void and no bladder pain. Ultimately, overflow incontinence occurs. This is termed a tabetic bladder.

Signs

Root Related

Motor: It is fairly easy to detect myotomal weakness in the upper limbs, and the distribution of weakness discloses the root involved. There is considerable overlap; the main muscles involved in particular myotomes are indicated in Table 16.1. With weakness, given time, there is myotomal wasting and sometimes fasciculations, so it is often possible to localize the root level simply by inspection.

Weakness of the abductor digiti minimus (ADM), which abducts the little finger, can be problematic. It may be part of an ulnar neuropathy, but absent a peripheral cause, centrally

TABLE 16.1 MAIN MUSCLES INVOLVED IN PARTICULAR MYOTOMES

SEGMENTAL LEVEL	MUSCLE	ACTION
C4	Infraspinatus	External rotation of the shoulder
C5	Deltoid, biceps/brachialis	Shoulder abduction
C6	Extensor carpi radialis	Radial wrist extension
C6/7	Triceps	Elbow extension
C7	Extensor digitorum	Finger extension
C8	Flexor digitorum	Finger flexion
T1	Interossei, abductor digiti minimi	Finger abduction

mediated ADM weakness is often labeled pseudo-ulnar syndrome generated at cord level, but not at a definite segmental level, and can be seen with lesions as high as C1. This falls into the rubric of false localizing signs.

Weakness in myotome distribution localizes the segmental level of the pathology.

Sensory: The sensory component of root dysfunction is dermatomal, and the dermatomes are illustrated in Figure 16.2. Pinprick, temperature sensation, and light touch sensation are variously involved in an unpredictable manner.

In the upper limbs, dissociated loss of pinprick and temperature sensation, but with retained light touch, suggests central cord dysfunction that could be due to primary pathology in the cord itself or secondary to extramedullary cord compression.

As with hypothenar weakness, dissociated pinprick loss over the hypothenar eminence could be ulnar nerve in origin or it may be a part of the pseudo-ulnar syndrome. If the pinprick level is exactly at the wrist crease, it is more likely to be ulnar nerve in origin, whereas a level above the wrist crease supports root or cord origin.

On the trunk, the finding of a band of sensory loss is referred to as suspended sensory loss and may be secondary to thoracic radiculopathy or is occasionally tract related.

Sensory dysfunction secondary to radicular pathology localizes the segmental level of pathology.

Tract Related

Motor: The lower limbs may be spastic, and clonus at the patella or Achilles tendon is part of the UMN syndrome. The distribution of weakness in the UMN syndrome is all-important in diagnosis. In the upper limbs there is preferential weakness of deltoid, triceps, wrist, and finger extension and finger abduction. In the lower limbs there is preferential weakness of hip flexion, foot and toe dorsiflexion, and hamstring and thigh abduction.

Sensory: Spinothalamic tract (pinprick) sensory loss secondary to cord dysfunction is variable but will result in a "level" either in the legs or on the trunk. As the dysfunction progresses, the level will rise until the radicular segmental level is reached. The normal segment between the tract level and the root level is called a "skip area." As the level rises, it ultimately reaches the root level of pathology and the skip disappears. The lesson is to never accept trunk or leg level as indicative of the segmental level of pathology until one is sure that there is no more cephalad (radicular) sensory loss. The rising level or skip area is usually attributed to the somatic layering of fiber tracts in the cord, such that, in the spinothalamic tract, the lateral or external part of the tract contains the more sacral or caudal segments and the medial part contains the upper or cervical segments.

Posterior column dysfunction results in loss of position sense in the toes and a characteristic gait—with each step the anterior foot is slapped down, which exaggerates sensory feedback. The Romberg test will usually be positive. Loss of position sense in the fingers indicates a very high cervical cord lesion.

Central cord dysfunction interferes with spinothalamic sensation as the fibers cross over to the contralateral ascending tract, having entered the cord via the dorsal root. Light touch is spared in that a good deal of touch sensory information ascends in the ipsilateral posterior column, thus causing dissociation. Central cord dysfunction is usually seen in the cervical region and affects the cape area, but can occur at any segmental cord level.

Loss of vibration sense at the ankles is common in cord lesions, and if the vibration level is at the costal margin, a cervical pathology is likely. The precise ascending tract for vibratory sense has not yet been established.

Reflexes

In UMN lesions the reflexes are exaggerated below the level of pathology. The plantar reflex can be extensor, but a flexor response in the presence of a multitude of cord signs, as described

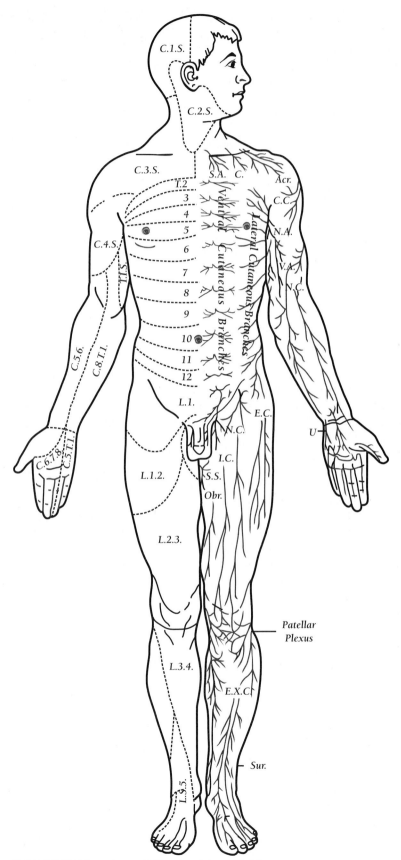

■ **FIGURE 16.2** Dermatomes (*left*) and peripheral (*right*) nerves.

earlier, should be recorded but does not detract from the diagnosis. An extensor plantar response or Babinski sign indicates a pyramidal tract lesion, but the UMN syndrome is pyramidal and also includes other descending nonpyramidal tracts.

An absent tendon reflex in the upper limbs points to a specific segmental level and may be localizing. An absent biceps reflex in the presence of cord dysfunction, which promotes hyperreflexia, may lead to spread of the reflex to other segments, such as triceps or finger flexors, which contract when the biceps tendon is struck. This sign is known as an "inverted biceps reflex" and localizes with precision to C5.

Anatomical Diagnosis

The objectives of the physical examination are to first establish the presence of spinal cord dysfunction and then to diagnose the segmental level of pathology. *Only if a clear root lesion is established, can one be sure of a segmental level.* Other signs related to tract dysfunction do not localize the level of pathology. The root level is diagnosed by the finding of a lower motor neuron myotomal level, dermatomal sensory loss, or absent tendon reflex.

Pathology

A useful approach to the pathology of spinal cord disease or myelopathy is to divide the various causes into medical or surgical categories. Surgical disease implies a structural pathology that is amenable to operation or perhaps radiotherapy.

Surgical Myelopathy

Intramedullary: Intramedullary tumors include primary gliomas, ependymomas, and lymphoma, which may be isolated or part of a more generalized disease. Occasionally, infection may result in an abscess or granuloma. Syringomyelia is a cystic cavity within the cord, usually cervical, and results in the dissociated sensory loss syndrome, sometimes with pain, and also long tract dysfunction.

Extramedullary: The cord may be compressed by a variety of pathologies, both benign and malignant. Herniated disc, spondylotic spurs, and pathological vertebral fractures should be considered. Primary tumors such as meningiomas and schwannomas can compress the cord. Metastatic malignancy usually spreads in the epidural space and destroys bone early, whereas epidural abscess or granuloma often seeds the disc and then in time may spread to bone. Arteriovenous anomalies cause cord dysfunction by increasing venous pressure with resulting cord edema. Occasional rarities such as herniation of the cord through a dural window may cause myelopathy.

Medical Myelopathy

Demyelinating myelitis may be part of multiple sclerosis or of the neuromyelitis optica syndrome. Although metastatic malignant cord compression is more common, carcinomatous meningitis can cause myelopathy and, occasionally, paraneoplastic necrotizing myelitis is seen. Infective myelitis secondary to herpes zoster or simplex or *Mycoplasma* infection should be considered in the absence of overt cord compression, and tuberculosis should always be in the differential diagnosis of myelopathy. Syphilis can affect the cord in the secondary stage or in the tertiary stage by way of meningovascular disease, tabes dorsalis, or even a gumma. Other granulomatous disease, such as sarcoidosis, can cause cord dysfunction. Human immunodeficiency virus (HIV) myelopathy is a diagnosis of exclusion in patients with that disease. In patients who have resided in the tropics, consider infestations with parasitic cysts, schistosomiasis, and human T-cell lymphotropic virus (HTLV1)-related tropical spastic paraplegia. Sudden-onset myelopathy may be due to cord infarction, either atheromatous or vasculitic.

Metabolic myelopathy may be seen in, for example, adrenoleukodystrophy. If skeletal markers such as scoliosis and pes cavus are present, consider a hereditary spinocerebellar degenerative disease.

In motor neuron disease there is usually evidence of anterior horn loss, but in primary lateral sclerosis only a motor UMN syndrome is present.

Approach to Diagnosis

It behooves the clinician to make a diagnosis of the cause of new myelopathy with haste. If there is any sign or symptom of bladder dysfunction, the situation is a true emergency. The best prognostic sign is that of "still walking"—once paraplegia ensues the prognosis for recovery is poor, whatever the treatment. Time is of the essence!

The clinical level is suspected by way of the examination. Fever may suggest an infection. Localized bone tenderness to percussion may suggest metastatic disease or other surgical zathology.

The emergency investigation of choice is magnetic resonance imaging (MRI). In the case of known malignancy the whole cord should be scanned because the deposits may be multiple. If multiple sclerosis is a possibility, the brain should also be scanned, but all patients should in any case have routine blood work for inflammatory disease and chest radiography for a primary source of pathology.

If epidural abscess is suspected, the radiologist should be especially alert because the MRI signs may be subtle.

If the MRI results are negative, the spinal fluid should be examined and cultured, and, if indicated, polymerase chain reaction for specific organisms should be requested. Serology and cytological evaluation should be done in all cases.

If an arteriovenous anomaly is suspected, spinal angiography may be required.

Approach to Management

Treatment depends on the cause of the myelopathy and is specific for each entity.

It is worth recording the emergency management of acute or subacute cord compression in metastatic disease. High-dose dexamethasone 100 mg intravenously is administered, followed by a dose of 16 mg daily. More specific treatment by radiotherapy or surgical decompression will be determined for each individual patient.

- Infections indicate appropriate antibiotics.
- Demyelinating disease is treated with high-dose intravenous steroids in the hope of shortening the duration of the episode.
- Extramedullary tumors indicate surgical decompression.
- Occasionally a syrinx is so large that it warrants drainage.
- Arteriovenous anomalies may be treated surgically or via embolization.
- There may be no adequate treatment for some conditions, and rehabilitation in a spinal cord unit is appropriate.

Prognosis and Counseling

Paraplegia is a devastating disability, and a good deal of psychological support is required. Depression is present in approximately 60% of patients, and sleep disturbances, suicidal ideation, and guilt occur with the same frequency. Suicide rates in patients with spinal cord injury are about five times higher than in the general population. Effective coping mechanisms result in higher quality of life scores. Although there may be reduced interest in sexual activity and less frequency after spinal cord injury, even in patients with what appear to be complete cord lesions, sexual activity and even orgasm are possible. A spinal cord injury in a female patient does not preclude the possibility of having a family and caring for children adequately. Sporting activities play a large role in rehabilitation and are associated with a better psychological status in patients with spinal cord injury.

KEY POINTS

1. In patients with acute or subacute myelopathy, time is of the essence. These patients should be evaluated and treated on an emergency basis.
2. Bladder dysfunction increases the sense of urgency.
3. At the bedside the level of pathology is related to the root signs and symptoms.
4. Cord compression can cause dysfunction in any tract at the level of compression and is usually treatable.
5. MRI is the investigation method of choice, but if the results are negative, a spinal tap should follow immediately

---

■ CERVICAL SPONDYLOSIS

Introduction

Cervical spondylosis is a degenerative disorder of the cervical spine characterized by softening of the discs, which results in narrowing of the disc spaces, secondary bone overgrowth to produces spurs and ridges, and hypertrophy of the facet joints, which may contribute to nerve root compression. There may be hypertrophy and sometimes calcification of the anterior and posterior longitudinal ligaments and of the ligamentum flava; the latter can compress the spinal cord in neck extension. The risk of mechanical cord compression is related to the anteroposterior diameter of the neural canal. If the canal diameter is approximately 12 to 13 mm, the chance of cord compression by ridges, spurs, or hypertrophied ligaments is accordingly increased. Torn or lax ligaments may predispose to subluxation, which causes dynamic and intermittent cord compression when the neck is flexed or extended.

Symptoms and Signs

Pain

The most common symptom is pain. If one considers the various pain-sensitive structures in the neck, it is possible to deduce the source. These are the cervical muscles, annulus of discs, bone, facet joints, ligaments, and sensory portions of the nerve roots.

A "stiff" neck or just posterior neck pain aggravated by head movement is likely to be on the basis of muscle spasm. Because of the confluence of sensory input (ascending spinothalamic tracts converge with trigeminal afferents) the pain may be referred to virtually any part of trigeminal territory, for example, the orbit. Headache secondary to posterior cervical muscle spasm has the signature of a simple muscle contraction headache—diffuse or circumferential, aching tightness, pressure, but not throbbing, which would imply a vascular component.

If the pain radiates down the upper limb, root irritation is present. Root pain may be sudden, shooting, electrical in type (neuralgic), or it can be deep, dull, and boring. If the pain is aggravated or precipitated by head and neck movement, the diagnosis of radiculopathic pain is clinched. Diagnosis by history of which particular root is involved in the process can be difficult because of overlap of dermatomes; on occasion, anterior upper chest wall pain, often misdiagnosed as cardiogenic, points to the fourth cervical root (C4).

Occasionally, tract dysfunction in the cord can refer pain as a girdle sensation in the trunk and even rarer as pseudo-sciatic pain.

Numbness and tingling in the arm or hand is also a referred symptom from nerve root pathology.

Sensory Loss

Dermatomal sensory loss in the upper limbs signifies which particular cervical nerve *root* is dysfunctional. Pinprick loss on the trunk or in the legs signifies *tract* dysfunction and, accordingly, myelopathy.

Loss of pinprick sensation with sparing of light touch in the arms (dissociated sensory loss) suggests central cord dysfunction secondary to extramedullary cord compression.

Vibration sense is frequently a casualty of spondylotic myelopathy, often extending from the rib margin and below that level to the feet.

Loss of position sense in the toes signifies a significant myelopathy, and loss of proprioception, if severe, can be as great a handicap as a motor deficit. Loss of proprioception in the fingers indicates a very high cervical cord lesion.

Weakness

Weakness, like sensory loss, may be root related or tract related. Diagnosis depends on the pattern of weakness.

Root Dysfunction: Because there is overlap in myotomal (root) innervation it may be difficult to pinpoint a specific segmental level, but if the main points of anatomy are remembered, despite some minor inaccuracies, a reasonable degree of clinical certainty is possible (Table 16.1).

Myelopathy is signaled by hypertonia in the lower limbs, or, if there is a UMN pattern of weakness, hip flexion, toe or even foot dorsiflexion, hamstring and thigh abduction weakness.

Bladder Dysfunction: The symptoms of UMN bladder dysfunction are frequency of small amounts of urine, urgency, and urgency incontinence. The bladder is small, spastic, and hyperreflexic. Bladder symptoms indicate fairly urgent imaging of the cord.

The Neck: The best clinical test of spondylosis is limitation of active or passive neck movement, and the most sensitive indicator is restriction of neck rotation. Normal rotation implies the ability to twist the neck so that the chin approximates the point of the shoulder; anything less is abnormal.

Reactive posterior muscle spasm is palpable and tender.

Investigations

Radiography

Regular radiographic examination will demonstrate reduction in disc spaces and reactive bone change by way of spurring.

It is important to measure the anteroposterior diameter of the neural canal. A canal diameter of less than 12 to 13 mm sets the scene for myelopathy because of cord compression.

If more sophisticated imaging does not demonstrate cord compression in patients with myelopathy, flexion and extension lateral films may show subluxation of the vertebral bodies. More than 3 mm of movement is considered pathological.

Magnetic Resonance Imaging

MRI is the method of choice to make the diagnosis of cervical spondylosis and, more particularly, spondylotic myelopathy. It is used to demonstrate the neural canal and the exit foramina; both may be impinged by osteophytes, discs, or hypertrophied or sometimes calcified ligaments. The cord may be deformed, or, on T2 images, can show an area of high attenuation (whiteness) in its substance, indicating either edema or gliosis.

Computed Tomography

Computed tomography (CT) is used when MRI is, for whatever reason, not available. It is excellent at displaying the bony anatomy. When combined with contrast myelography the cord is well outlined.

Pathophysiology

Nerve root compression by disc or osteophyte may be accompanied by a local inflammatory reaction and results in the appropriate motor or sensory signs and symptoms. Nerve root irritation triggers cervical muscle spasm, which causes local pain and referred headache.

Myelopathy may be on the basis of simple cord compression, but, despite adequate decompression, some patients continue to progress so that simple compression may not be the only mechanism. Various hypotheses to explain cord damage have been advanced. Ischemia, edema, and progressive gliosis are candidates. With flexion or extension movements of the neck the cord rides up and down one or two segments and may be subject to rubbing or friction anteriorly (by osteophytes and occasionally an enlarged or calcified posterior longitudinal ligament) and posteriorly (by a thickened ligamentum flava). Furthermore, in flexion and particularly in extension the degree of spinal stenosis is increased. The fact that patients do improve when treated with a cervical collar, which limits flexion and extension, but does very little else, supports this hypothesis.

Treatment

The vast majority of patients can be treated conservatively, which will produce symptomatic improvement, but with the likelihood of relapses in the future. There are no adequate trials of the various recommended conservative therapies, so best practice is described in the following sections. There is very little evidence to support surgery, but progressive myelopathy, severe cord compression, or an unstable subluxation are usually taken to indicate a more invasive approach.

Neck Pain and Headache

Muscle relaxants, such as metaxolone 800 mg three times daily combined with over-the-counter analgesics, are worth a trial. Application of local heat helps relieve pain.

Many patients aggravate the underlying pathology when sleeping, because of poor posture or abnormal movement. Two inexpensive, firm feather pillows provide good support for the neck. A buckwheat husk pillow may also help. If this fails, the patient should sleep in a soft cervical collar at night.

Chronic headache often responds to an antidepressant, either a small dose of a tricyclic antidepressant (e.g., desipramine 25 mg at night) or any of the selective serotonin reuptake inhibitor (SSRI) drugs. If there is a problem with falling asleep, trazodone 50 mg at night is usually beneficial.

Gentle massage of the posterior cervical muscle feels good and helps ease the pain at least temporarily. Manipulation of the neck by physical therapists or chiropractors is to be avoided. Vigorous manipulation carries a risk for vertebral artery dissection.

Root Pain

If root pain is severe, an analgesic will be required. One uses "what it takes to control the pain," and at times narcotics in small doses are required. Gabapentin or pregabalin may help to control neuropathic root pain, but the response is unpredictable. The linchpin of treatment is a soft cervical collar used around the clock for a few weeks.

If there is no adequate pain control within a week or two, an epidural steroid injection administered by anesthesia in the pain clinic is often of symptomatic benefit.

When root pain is secondary to an acute disc rupture and a trial of conservative treatment, including a short burst of corticosteroid treatment fails, anterior discectomy usually provides dramatic symptomatic relief.

Myelopathy

Although surgery, either laminectomy or anterior fusion, is the most commonly performed neurosurgical operation in the United States, and is accepted as standard of care for cervical stenosis and cord compression, the evidence for its efficacy is sparse. Most reported trials of surgery are retrospective. A single prospective controlled trial concluded that surgical decompression was of no benefit for mild stenosis.

If the patient does not improve in a cervical collar, has significant gait problems, or is experiencing bladder dysfunction, a surgical opinion is certainly warranted. If significant subluxation is present, surgical fusion may be the only therapeutic option.

KEY POINTS

1. Approximately 50% of people older than 50 years and 75% of people older than 65 years have radiological evidence of spondylosis.
2. Cervical spondylosis should not be equated with an acute disc rupture or herniation, rather it is a gradually evolving condition with fluctuation in symptomatology at irregular and unpredictable intervals.
3. The natural history is variable, but in general the symptoms are likely to fluctuate and recur.

■ SUGGESTED READINGS

Alexander CJ, Sipski ML, Findley TW. Sexual activities, desire and satisfaction in males pre- and post-spinal cord injury. *Arch Sex Behav* 1993;22:217–228.

Ahn NU, Ahn UM, Ipsen B, et al. Mechanical neck pain and cervicogenic headache. *Neurosurgery* 2007;60:S1–S21.

Assendelft WJ, Bouter LM, Knipschild PG, et al. Complications of spinal manipulation: a comprehensive review of the literature. *J Fam Pract* 1996;42:475–480.

Baker JH, Silver JR. Hysterical paraplegia. *J Neurol Neurosurg Psychiatry* 1987;50:375–382.

Baron EM, Young WF. Cervical spondylotic myelopathy: a brief review of its pathophysiology, clinical course, and diagnosis. *Neurosurgery* 2007;60:S1–S35.

Conway R, Graham J, Kidd J, et al. What happens to people after malignant cord compression? Survival, function, quality of life, emotional well-being and place of care 1 month after diagnosis. *Clin Oncol (R Coll Radiol)* 2007;19:56–62.

De Carvalho SA, Andrade MJ, Tavares MA, et al. Spinal cord injury and psychological response. *Gen Hosp Psychiatry* 1998;20:353–359.

Delattre JY, Arbit E, Thaler HT, et al. A dose-response study of dexamethasone in a model of spinal cord compression caused by epidural tumor. *J Neurosurg* 1989;70:920–925.

Gioia MC, Cerasa A, Di Lucente L, et al. Psychological impact of sports activity in spinal cord injury patients. *Scand J Med Sci Sports* 2006;16:412–416.

Hartkopp A, Bronnum-Hansen H, Seidenschnur AM, et al. Suicide in a spinal injured population: its relation to functional status. *Arch Phys Med Rehabil* 1998;79:1356–1361.

Kadanka Z, Mares M, Bednarik J, et al. Predictive factors for spondylotic cervical myelopathy treated conservatively or surgically. *Eur J Neurol* 2005;12:55–63.

King JT, McGinnis KA, Roberts MS. Quality of life assessment with the medical outcomes study short form-36 among patients with cervical spondylotic myelopathy. *Neurosurgery* 2003;52:113–120.

Loblaw DA, Perry J, Chambers A, et al. Systematic review of the diagnosis and management of malignant extradural spinal cord compression: the Cancer Care Ontario Practice Guidelines Initiative's Neuro-Oncology Disease Site Group. *J Clin Oncol* 2005;23:2028–2037.

Mazanec D, Reddy A. Medical management of cervical spondylosis. *Neurosurgery* 2007;60:S1–S43.

Parkinson J. *An Essay on the Shaking Palsy*. London: Sherwood, Neely and Jones, 1817.

Patchell RA, Tibbs PA, Regine F, et al. Direct decompressive surgical resection in the treatment of spinal cord compression caused by metastatic cancer: a randomized trial. *Lancet* 2005;366:643–648.

Ronthal M. *Neck Complaints*. Boston: Butterworth Heinemann; 2000.

Shedid D, Benzel EC. Cervical spondylosis anatomy: pathophysiology and biomechanics. *Neurosurgery* 2007;60:S1–S7.

Thomas KC, Nosyk B, Fisher CG, et al. Cost-effectiveness of surgery plus radiotherapy versus radiotherapy alone for metastatic epidural spinal cord compression. *Int J Radiat Oncol Biol Phys* 2006;66:1212–1218.

Transverse Myelitis Consortium Group. Proposed diagnostic criteria and nosology of acute transverse myelitis. *Neurology* 2002;59:499–505.

Westgren N, Levi R. Motherhood after traumatic spinal injury. *Paraplegia* 1994;32:517–523.

Wieser ES, Wang JC. Surgery for neck pain. *Neurosurgery* 2007;60:S1–S51.

CHAPTER 17

Neuromuscular Disorders

Andrew W. Tarulli

■ INTRODUCTION

The evaluation of a suspected neuromuscular disorder begins, like the evaluation of all other neurological disorders, with an attempt to localize the problem to a specific level of the neuraxis. The peripheral nervous system encompasses a variety of structures (Fig. 17.1), and dysfunction at each level produces a characteristic pattern of neurological signs and symptoms.

Motor Neuron and Motor Unit

A motor neuron is a nerve cell with its cell body in the anterior horn of the spinal cord. A motor unit consists of a motor neuron and all the muscles it innervates. The features that suggest a motor neuron disorder include painless weakness, muscle cramps, fasciculations, and muscle atrophy.

Nerve Root

Sensory fibers from the peripheral nervous system have their cell bodies in dorsal root ganglia and enter the spinal cord as dorsal nerve roots. The sensory distribution supplied by a sensory nerve root is known as a dermatome. Motor fibers emerge from anterior horn cells and exit from the spinal cord as ventral nerve roots. The motor territory supplied by a motor nerve is called a myotome. In clinical neurology, the structure that is referred to as the "nerve root" is actually a mixed spinal nerve consisting of the fused dorsal and ventral nerve roots. Characteristics of nerve root dysfunction, or radiculopathy, include pain, paresthesias, and numbness radiating in a dermatomal distribution and weakness in a myotomal distribution.

Plexus

The most anatomically complex structures of the peripheral nervous system are the collections of peripheral nerves known as the brachial and lumbosacral plexuses. The brachial plexus provides sensory and motor innervation to the upper extremity, and the lumbosacral plexus provides sensory and motor innervation to the lower extremity. The identification of plexus disorders can be challenging and relies on demonstrating sensory and motor deficits in the distribution of multiple nerves and nerve roots.

Nerve

Characteristics of nerve dysfunction include pain, sensory loss, paresthesias, and weakness in the distribution of a nerve or multiple nerves. Either sensory or motor findings may predominate, or a mixed sensorimotor picture may be observed. Mononeuropathy involves a single named nerve, mononeuropathy multiplex involves multiple nerves, and polyneuropathy is a generalized process involving all nerves, often (but with many exceptions) with a length-dependent distribution. Axonal neuropathies involve injury to the nerve cell itself, and

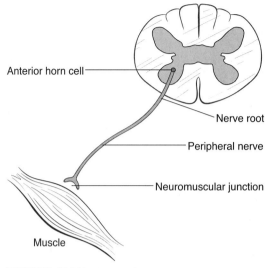

■ **FIGURE 17.1** Neuromuscular anatomy.

demyelinating neuropathies attack the myelin coating of the nerve. This distinction may not be apparent clinically, but axonal and demyelinating neuropathies can be differentiated electrophysiologically, as discussed in the section on neurophysiological testing.

Neuromuscular Junction

The neuromuscular junction is the interface between the nerve and muscle. The nerve releases vesicles containing the neurotransmitter acetylcholine, which binds to postsynaptic acetylcholine receptors on the muscle, resulting in the firing of miniature end-plate potentials. Disorders of the neuromuscular junction produce painless, often fatigable weakness without sensory loss.

Muscle

Muscle disorders produce wasting and weakness without sensory abnormalities, although cramps and myalgias may occur. Most muscle disorders preferentially affect proximal muscles such as neck flexors and extensors, deltoids, iliopsoas, and quadriceps. Distal muscles, extraocular muscles, and respiratory muscles may be involved, however, in specific types of myopathies.

■ NEUROPHYSIOLOGICAL TESTING

After a careful history and physical examination, further diagnostic testing to establish the localization of a suspected peripheral nervous system disorder may not be necessary. If the localization is in doubt, however, electromyography (EMG) and nerve conduction studies (NCS) may be required.

Nerve Conduction Studies

In NCS, nerves are stimulated with surface electrodes and signals produced by the nerves or the muscles that they innervate are recorded. The most commonly measured NCS parameters are the compound muscle action potential (CMAP) amplitude, sensory nerve action potential (SNAP) amplitude, and conduction velocity.

Late Responses

Late responses are used to assess proximal nerve segments and are recorded using the NCS technique. There are two types of late responses. F waves are produced by stimulation of a motor nerve, conduction of the electrical impulse back toward the spinal cord, firing of a select portion of anterior horn cells, and conduction of the signal back toward the muscle. H reflexes are most commonly obtained by stimulating the sensory component of the tibial nerve, conduction of this signal back to the spinal cord, synapse with the anterior horn cell, and conduction back down the motor nerve to cause contraction of the soleus. The H reflex is the neurophysiological equivalent of the ankle jerk, and it should be emphasized that the stimulus is conducted by both sensory and motor nerves, unlike F waves, which are conducted *entirely by motor nerves.*

Needle Electromyography

During EMG, a small electrode embedded in a needle is inserted into a muscle, and muscle electrical potentials are analyzed semi-quantitatively. Spontaneous muscle activity is measured by inserting the needle into the muscle while the patient is completely relaxed. Abnormal spontaneous muscle activity (fibrillations, positive sharp waves, myotonia, fasciculations) can be seen in a variety of neuromuscular pathologies. Motor unit activity is recorded and analyzed by having the patient contract the muscle. In chronic neurogenic lesions (anterior horn cell, nerve root, plexus, and nerve), the characteristic EMG findings are long duration, large amplitude, and polyphasic motor units, reflecting reinnervation of denervated muscles. Myopathic motor units are of short duration, of small amplitude, and polyphasic.

Two important EMG concepts are those of activation and recruitment. There are two ways to increase muscular force. The first is by activating an individual motor unit to increase its firing rate, a process mediated by the central nervous system (CNS). The second way to increase muscular force is by recruiting additional motor units, a process mediated by the peripheral nervous system. In CNS disorders, therefore, activation is poor and recruitment is normal. Nerve root and peripheral nerve disorders produce normal muscle activation but decreased recruitment. In combined disorders of the central and peripheral nervous systems (such as amyotrophic lateral sclerosis), both activation and recruitment are abnormal. Muscle disorders are characterized by normal muscle activation and early recruitment.

A brief summary of the expected findings of EMG and NCS is presented in Tables 17.1 and 17.2.

TABLE 17.1 NERVE CONDUCTION STUDY FINDINGS IN NEUROMUSCULAR DISEASES

LOCALIZATION	CMAP AMPLITUDE	CMAP VELOCITY	SNAP AMPLITUDE	SNAP VELOCITY
Anterior horn cell	May be decreased	Normal	Normal	Normal
Nerve root	May be decreased	Normal	Normal	Normal
Plexus	Decreased	Normal	Decreased	Normal
Nerve: axonal pathology	Decreased	Mildly decreased	Decreased	Mildly decreased
Nerve: demyelinating pathology	Mildly decreased	Markedly decreased	Mildly decreased	Markedly decreased
Neuromuscular junction-presynaptic	Often decreased	Normal	Normal	Normal
Neuromuscular junction-postsynaptic	Normal	Normal	Normal	Normal
Muscle	May be decreased	Normal	Normal	Normal

CMAP, compound motor action potential; SNAP, sensory nerve action potential.

TABLE 17.2 ELECTROMYOGRAPHIC FINDINGS IN NEUROMUSCULAR DISEASES

LOCALIZATION	SPONTANEOUS ACTIVITY	MOTOR UNIT MORPHOLOGY
Anterior horn cell	Fibrillations, positive sharp waves, fasciculations, cramps	Large, polyphasic motor units with decreased activation and recruitment
Nerve root	Fibrillations, positive sharp waves	Large, polyphasic motor units with decreased recruitment
Nerve, plexus	Fibrillations, positive sharp waves	Large, polyphasic motor units with decreased recruitment
Neuromuscular junction	Normal	Normal
Muscle	Fibrillations and positive sharp waves possible in inflammatory myopathies	Small, polyphasic motor units with early recruitment

■ MOTOR NEURON DISEASES

Amyotrophic Lateral Sclerosis

Amyotrophic lateral sclerosis (ALS) is a progressive and uniformly fatal disorder characterized by wasting and weakness that often begins asymmetrically in an arm or leg. Later, involvement of the other limbs, bulbar muscles, and respiratory muscles occurs. A diagnosis of probable ALS is made when muscles of at least three of four different myotomal levels (bulbar, cervical, thoracic, and lumbosacral) are affected. A combination of upper (spasticity, hyperreflexia) and lower (wasting, weakness, fasciculations) motor neuron dysfunction is required to make a diagnosis, and EMG has a confirmatory role. Familial ALS accounts for only 10% of all cases and is associated with mutations in the superoxide dismutase (SOD) gene in 20% of these cases. Variants of ALS include primary lateral sclerosis (PLS), which involves isolated degeneration of upper motor neurons, and progressive muscular atrophy (PMA), which involves lower motor neurons exclusively. Both of these variants have better prognoses than ALS. Treatment of ALS is largely supportive and includes assistive devices, positive pressure ventilation at night, and the glutamate antagonist riluzole. Despite these treatments, the mean survival is approximately 3 to 4 years, with a universally fatal outcome in those patients who are not mechanically ventilated.

Kennedy's Disease

Kennedy's disease is an X-linked bulbospinal neuronopathy caused by a CAG trinucleotide repeat expansion in the androgen receptor gene. The disorder affects men exclusively and is characterized by muscle wasting and weakness, without signs of upper motor neuron dysfunction such as spasticity or hyperreflexia. Fasciculations in the lower face and gynecomastia are often prominent. No specific treatment is available for Kennedy's disease, although the prognosis is better than that for ALS.

Spinal Muscular Atrophy

The three most common types of spinal muscular atrophy (SMA) are caused by deletions in the survival motor neuron gene on chromosome 5 and are inherited in autosomal recessive fashion.

SMA I (Werdnig-Hoffmann disease) begins between birth and 6 months of age, with death usually occurring before age 2. Presenting symptoms include hypotonia, a weak cry, poor suck, and respiratory distress.

SMA II begins between 6 and 18 months, although symptoms may be present at birth. Delayed motor milestones bring these patients to neurological attention. Most children with

SMA II are able to roll over and sit, but do not achieve the ability to walk independently. Death from respiratory failure occurs in childhood or early adulthood.

SMA III (Kugelberg-Welander disease) may not be evident until after age 5. Some patients with SMA III may remain ambulatory well into adulthood, but most require a wheelchair by the time they are in their mid 30s. Treatment of SMA III is supportive, with the goals being maintenance of ambulation, respiratory support, and prevention of contractures.

Polio

Caused by poliovirus infection, acute poliomyelitis is now uncommon in the industrialized world as a result of childhood immunization. Most patients infected by the virus develop a gastrointestinal illness or are asymptomatic. Acute poliomyelitis, however, begins as aseptic meningitis, followed by flaccid, asymmetrical paralysis developing within a week. Spinal fluid analysis shows polymorphonuclear cells in the acute stage. Treatment is supportive. If bulbar and respiratory muscles are involved, intubation may be required. The post-polio syndrome is characterized by progressive wasting, weakness, cramps, fasciculation, pain, and fatigue many years after an episode of acute poliomyelitis. Supportive care with an emphasis on physical therapy is the mainstay of post-polio syndrome treatment.

Benign Fasciculations (Cramp-Fasciculation Syndrome)

Fasciculations are spontaneous discharges of individual motor units. Although frequently prompting investigation for ALS, fasciculations may also be a benign phenomenon as in cramp-fasciculation syndrome. Benign fasciculations can be distinguished from ALS-associated fasciculations by the absence of associated weakness and denervation changes on EMG. Reassurance that the patient does not have ALS is often helpful in relieving symptoms, although recalcitrant fasciculations may require treatment with agents such as quinine or carbamazepine.

KEY POINTS

1. Mutations in the SOD gene can be found in 20% of patients with familial ALS.
2. The most common types of SMA are associated with mutations in the survival motor neuron gene on chromosome 5.
3. Benign fasciculations can be differentiated from the fasciculations of ALS by the lack of denervation changes on EMG.

■ DISORDERS OF THE BRACHIAL PLEXUS

Traumatic Injury

In adults the most common forms of traumatic injury to the brachial plexus are falls and motor vehicle accidents. Violent downward movement of the shoulder results in an upper trunk disorder affecting predominantly the C5–6 nerve roots (Erb's palsy). Hyperabduction causes a lower trunk injury affecting predominantly the C8–T1 nerve roots (Klumpke's palsy). In newborns, Erb's palsy may occur at delivery, with risk factors for the development of the condition including large gestational weight and small pelvic diameter. Brachial plexus injuries in the newborn may require surgery if improvement in muscle strength is not noted within 3 to 6 months.

Neoplastic-Related Brachial Plexopathy

The two main causes of neoplastic-related brachial plexopathy are direct infiltration of the plexus by tumor and radiation-related injury. Infiltrative lesions are usually derived from tumors of the lung or breast, are associated with a higher incidence of pain, tend to affect the lower plexus, and can produce Horner's syndrome. Radiation-related plexopathy occurs months to years after radiation therapy and is generally less painful than plexopathy caused by tumor infiltration. A characteristic EMG finding in patients with radiation-induced brachial plexopathy is myokymia—rhythmic, grouped repetitive discharges of the same motor unit. Radiation therapy is the mainstay of treatment of neoplastic infiltration; the treatment for radiation-related plexopathy is mainly supportive.

Idiopathic Brachial Neuritis

Idiopathic brachial neuritis is known by a variety of names, including Parsonage-Turner syndrome, brachial plexitis, and neuralgic amyotrophy. Typically, a patient who develops idiopathic brachial neuritis has an upper respiratory tract infection several weeks prior and then experiences the sudden onset of pain in the arm and shoulder, and in several days to weeks develops weakness in the affected limb. Recovery is generally spontaneous, but may be prolonged over several months. In cases with poor recovery or severe deficits, corticosteroids or intravenous immunoglobulin (IVIg) may be beneficial.

Neurogenic Thoracic Outlet Syndrome

Neurogenic thoracic outlet syndrome is an uncommon syndrome characterized by a lower trunk brachial plexopathy, predominantly affecting T1 fibers. The causes of neurogenic thoracic outlet syndrome include cervical ribs, fibrous bands, and scalene muscle anomalies. Symptoms include pain in the cervical and suprascapular regions, with pain and weakness in the hand. On physical examination, sensory loss is characteristically confined to the medial hand and forearm and weakness is found in intrinsic hand muscles. The mainstay of treatment is physical therapy, with surgical decompression necessary for refractory cases.

■ DISORDERS OF THE LUMBOSACRAL PLEXUS

Traumatic Injury

Because of the protected location of the lumbosacral plexus, traumatic injury to this structure is less common than traumatic brachial plexopathy. Traumatic lumbosacral plexopathy may occur in women during childbirth, especially in the presence of fetal-pelvic disproportion.

Mass Lesions

Retroperitoneal hematomas, tumors, and abscesses may produce lumbosacral plexopathy. Anticoagulation, pelvic and abdominal surgery, and femoral catheterization may produce hematomas of the lumbosacral plexus. Evaluation should include computed tomography (CT) or magnetic resonance imaging (MRI) of the pelvis to exclude these lesions. Treatment is directed at the underlying source and may involve surgical intervention and reversal of anticoagulation.

Neoplastic Lumbosacral Plexopathy

Like the analogous syndrome affecting the brachial plexus, direct infiltration of the lumbosacral plexus by tumor produces a syndrome of subacute pain and limb weakness. Radiation-induced lumbosacral plexopathy is typically less painful than infiltrative plexopathy and may be associated with myokymia on EMG. Radiation therapy is the treatment of lumbosacral plexopathy related to tumor infiltration, whereas radiation-related plexopathy is poorly responsive to treatment.

Diabetic Amyotrophy

Diabetic amyotrophy occurs in individuals with type 2 diabetes, often with well-controlled diabetes. The subacute development of hip and leg pain that progresses over several weeks precedes proximal leg weakness, which may be severe. The mechanism of diabetic amyotrophy is not entirely clear, with vasculitic insults, inflammatory processes, and autoimmune attacks against the lumbosacral plexus or nerve roots implicated. Although many patients recover from the condition without treatment, patients may benefit from a course of IVIg or corticosteroids. Treatment must also incorporate strict glucose control.

Idiopathic Lumbosacral Plexitis

Less common than its brachial plexus counterpart, idiopathic lumbosacral plexitis is characterized by the subacute development of pain followed by weakness in the lower extremity. Unlike idiopathic brachial neuritis, however, the prognosis of idiopathic lumbosacral plexitis is more guarded, with a larger proportion of patients having a prolonged course or poor recovery. Treatment with IVIg or corticosteroids may improve outcome.

KEY POINTS

1. Radiation-induced plexopathy can be differentiated from neoplastic infiltration of the plexus by the presence of myokymia.
2. Diabetic amyotrophy occurs in patients with type 2 diabetes, often with well-controlled diabetes, and is characterized by pain followed by the subacute development of proximal leg weakness.

■ MONONEUROPATHIES

Any nerve can be involved in isolation by a variety of compressive, ischemic, infiltrative, or inflammatory conditions. Tables 17.3 and 17.4 present examples of the most common mononeuropathies of the upper and lower extremities, but are by no means exhaustive.

■ DEMYELINATING POLYNEUROPATHIES

As noted above, demyelinating neuropathies are characterized by damage to the myelin coating of peripheral nerves. These neuropathies are often indistinguishable from axonal neuropathies on clinical grounds; the neurophysiological features of demyelinating neuropathies

---

TABLE 17.3 COMMON MONONEUROPATHIES OF THE UPPER EXTREMITY

NERVE	MECHANISM OF INJURY	MOST COMMON CLINICAL FINDINGS
Median	Entrapment at the carpal tunnel	Pain and tingling on palmar surface of first three digits; sensory loss in first three digits, sparing the palm; weakness of thumb abduction
Ulnar	Entrapment at the elbow	Pain and tingling in fourth and fifth digits, weakness of intrinsic hand muscles
Radial	Entrapment at spiral groove: "Saturday night palsy" develops when pressure is applied to the humerus during deep sleep/intoxication	Wrist and finger drop, with sparing of arm extension; sensory loss over dorsum of hand
Axillary	Injured during fracture or dislocation of the humerus	Weakness of shoulder abduction, sensory loss over upper arm
Long thoracic	Pressure injuries to shoulder, idiopathic brachial neuritis	Winging of scapula

TABLE 17.4 COMMON MONONEUROPATHIES OF THE LOWER EXTREMITY

NERVE	MECHANISM OF INJURY	MOST COMMON CLINICAL FINDINGS
Femoral	Hip/pelvic fractures, childbirth, retroperitoneal hematomas	Weakness of hip flexion and knee extension, sensory loss over anterior and medial thigh and medial leg
Lateral femoral cutaneous	Entrapment at the inguinal ligament, often in obese patients	Meralgia paresthetica: numbness and pain in lateral thigh and around knee
Common peroneal	Entrapment at the fibular neck	Weakness of foot dorsiflexion and eversion, with sparing of inversion; sensory loss over dorsum of foot and lateral shin
Tibial	Compression at the tarsal tunnel, usually history of foot/ankle trauma	Pain involving the sole of the foot and toes
Sciatic	Hip surgery, hip or femoral fracture	Symptoms in the distribution of peroneal and tibial nerves, usually peroneal nerve symptoms predominate

are marked slowing of conduction velocities (to less than 75% of normal values) with relative preservation of CMAP and SNAP amplitudes. Conduction block is a feature of acquired demyelinating neuropathies: stimulation of a nerve distal to the site of conduction block produces a normal response amplitude and stimulation proximal to that site produces a reduced response amplitude.

Acute Inflammatory Demyelinating Polyradiculoneuropathy

Acute inflammatory demyelinating polyradiculoneuropathy (AIDP) (Guillain-Barré syndrome) is classically characterized by the acute development of ascending symmetrical weakness accompanied by hyporeflexia or areflexia. Many variations on this theme exist, however, and proximal greater than distal weakness or asymmetrical weakness may also occur. Severely affected patients have bulbar and diaphragmatic weakness and autonomic dysfunction. Upper respiratory tract infections and gastrointestinal illnesses are frequent antecedent events, and the illness is often associated with *Campylobacter jejuni* infection. Cerebrospinal fluid (CSF) analysis characteristically shows albuminocytologic dissociation—elevated protein with a normal cell count. Although EMG should demonstrate demyelinating features, if it is performed too early, these features may not be seen. Additionally, axonal variants of Guillain-Barré syndrome have also been described. Other disorders that may produce an AIDP-type picture of rapidly progressive areflexic weakness are human immunodeficiency (HIV) seroconversion, porphyria, and heavy metal intoxication (lead, thallium, arsenic). Although mild cases of AIDP may not require treatment, most patients are treated with IVIg or plasma exchange, both of which are effective in hastening recovery. In patients with severe disease resulting in respiratory dysfunction, negative inspiratory force and forced vital capacity is necessary, and mechanical ventilation may be required. Prognosis in AIDP depends on the severity of the initial deficit, with more severely affected patients having worse long-term outcomes. A small minority of patients relapse despite treatment with IVIg or plasmapheresis.

The Miller-Fisher variant of Guillain-Barré syndrome consists of the triad of ophthalmoplegia, ataxia, and areflexia and is associated with antibodies to the GQ1b ganglioside in 90% of patients. Recovery from Miller-Fisher syndrome typically takes 3 to 6 months, and IVIg or plasma exchange may hasten recovery.

Chronic Inflammatory Demyelinating Polyradiculoneuropathy

Chronic inflammatory demyelinating polyradiculoneuropathy (CIDP) is characterized by the progressive development of motor and sensory dysfunction over the course of 2 months or longer. Similar to AIDP, the symptoms may be predominantly proximal or distal, and hyporeflexia or areflexia is expected. CIDP can be associated with a variety of medical conditions, including HIV and osteosclerotic myeloma. In this setting, a syndrome known by the acronym POEMS may occur: Polyneuropathy, Organomegaly, Endocrinopathy, Myeloma, and Skin changes. Like AIDP, CIDP is characterized by demyelination on NCS and often is associated with albuminocytologic dissociation in the CSF. The mainstay of treatment of CIDP is prednisone. Other treatment options include plasmapheresis, IVIg, and immunosuppressants such as azathioprine, cyclosporine, and cyclophosphamide. Up to 90% of patients can be successfully treated, but on discontinuation of treatment, approximately half will relapse.

Charcot-Marie Tooth

Charcot-Marie Tooth (CMT), or hereditary sensory motor neuropathy, is a group of genetic disorders that share predominantly distal muscle weakness and atrophy, sensory loss, and absent or diminished deep tendon reflexes. There are multiple subtypes of CMT and related disorders, the most important of which are outlined in Table 17.5. With the exception of CMT2, CMT is characterized neurophysiologically by demyelination without conduction block.

Hereditary Neuropathy with Liability to Pressure Palsies

Hereditary neuropathy with liability to pressure palsies (HNPP) usually comes to clinical attention in the second or third decade of life and most typically presents as painless numbness and weakness in the distribution of a single or multiple peripheral nerves, often precipitated by minor trauma or nerve compression. Nerve biopsy shows focal thickening of the myelin sheath, which lends the condition the name tomaculous neuropathy.

Dejerine-Sottas Disease

Dejerine-Sottas disease (DSD) is a polyneuropathy that can present in infancy as generalized weakness and hypotonia or begin in young children as distal sensory loss with ataxia, pes cavus, kyphoscoliosis, weakness, and atrophy in a length-dependent pattern. The peripheral nerves are enlarged and often palpable. Treatment for Dejerine-Sottas is supportive.

TABLE 17.5 CHARCOT-MARIE TOOTH AND RELATED DISORDERS

DISORDER	PHYSIOLOGY	INHERITANCE	CHROMOSOME	GENE DEFECT
CMT1A	Demyelinating	AD	17	PMP duplication
CMT1B	Demyelinating	AD	1	P_o point mutation
CMTX	Demyelinating	X-linked	X	CX32 point mutation
CMT2	Axonal	AD	1	Multiple
HNPP	Demyelinating with conduction block	AD	17	PMP deletion/point mutation
Dejerine-Sottas (CMT3)	Demyelinating	NK	17 or 1	PMP or P_o mutation

AD, autosomal dominant; CMT, Charcot-Marie Tooth; CX32, connexin 32; HNPP, hereditary neuropathy with liability to pressure palsies; NK, not known; PMP, peripheral myelin protein.

Multifocal Motor Neuropathy with Conduction Block

Multifocal motor neuropathy with conduction block (MMNCB) is an immune-mediated demyelinating neuropathy characterized by asymmetrical weakness and atrophy in the distribution of multiple peripheral nerves and conduction block on EMG. Men are affected more often than women, and the arms are involved more often than the legs. Antibodies to the ganglioside GM1 are seen in approximately 50% of patients with MMNCB. The treatment of choice is IVIg.

■ AXONAL POLYNEUROPATHIES

The majority of polyneuropathies are axonal in nature, characterized neurophysiologically by amplitude reduction in SNAPs or CMAPs, with mild slowing of conduction velocity.

Often, a specific etiological diagnosis for an axonal polyneuropathy cannot be made. In that case, the term idiopathic polyneuropathy is used.

Most cases of axonal polyneuropathy are not reversible, and symptomatic treatment includes medications for neuropathic pain (Table 17.6), careful foot examinations to prevent ulcers and infections, and referral for podiatric care and physical therapy.

Discussion of some of the more common varieties of axonal polyneuropathies follows.

Diabetes

The most common form of diabetic neuropathy is a distal, symmetrical sensorimotor polyneuropathy that usually develops in patients with long-standing, often poorly controlled diabetes. Tight blood sugar control may help to improve the condition, but in most cases treatment of the neuropathy is symptomatic (see later discussion).

Alcohol

The pathophysiology of alcoholic polyneuropathy is controversial, with both direct toxic effects and nutritional factors being implicated. Most commonly, alcoholic neuropathy is a distal, symmetrical sensorimotor polyneuropathy. Specific treatments are not available, but adequate nutrition should be maintained. Thiamine supplementation is advocated by some.

TABLE 17.6 MEDICATIONS USED TO TREAT NEUROPATHIC PAIN

MEDICATION	CLASS	COMMON SIDE EFFECTS
Gabapentin	Anticonvulsant	Weight gain, fatigue, peripheral edema
Nortriptyline	Tricyclic antidepressant	Dry mouth, constipation, cardiac conduction defects, fewer sedating effects than amitriptyline
Amitriptyline	Tricyclic antidepressant	Dry mouth, constipation, cardiac conduction defects, sedation
Topiramate	Anticonvulsant	Paresthesias, nephrolithiasis, anomia
Tramadol	Nonopioid analgesic	Dizziness, nausea, constipation
Opioids	Opioids	Sedation, addiction, constipation
Pregabalin	Anticonvulsant	Dizziness, somnolence
Duloxetine	Serotonin/norepinephrine reuptake inhibitor	Nausea, insomnia, constipation

Vitamin B$_{12}$ Deficiency

The neuropathy caused by B$_{12}$ deficiency usually begins with paresthesias and numbness in the feet and is often accompanied by dorsal column degeneration in the spinal cord, resulting in vibratory/proprioceptive deficits. B$_{12}$ deficiency is associated with vegetarianism, pernicious anemia, malabsorption syndrome, and certain parasitic infestations. Laboratory testing demonstrating low B$_{12}$ levels helps establish the diagnosis. In cases in which the B$_{12}$ level is low-normal, elevations of methylmalonic acid and homocysteine are suggestive of early B$_{12}$ deficiency. Supplementation with intramuscular B$_{12}$ injections or high-dose oral B$_{12}$ is the treatments of choice.

Human Immunodeficiency Virus Infection

Painful paresthesias of the feet tend to dominate the clinical picture of HIV polyneuropathy, a disorder that tends to occur in patients with more advanced disease. The pathogenesis of the condition is poorly understood and likely multifactorial. The neuropathy is poorly responsive to treatment, including antiretroviral agents.

Lyme

A tick-borne illness caused by the spirochete *Borrelia burgdorferi,* Lyme disease may produce several different peripheral nervous system manifestations, including facial palsy, polyradiculoneuropathy, mononeuropathy multiplex, and sensorimotor polyneuropathy. Facial palsy can be treated with oral doxycycline; other peripheral nervous system manifestations of Lyme disease require treatment with intravenous ceftriaxone for 2 to 4 weeks.

Amyloidosis

Amyloidosis is heterogeneous group of disorders characterized by the deposition of amyloid in a variety of organs, affecting the peripheral nerves in 15% to 20% of patients with the condition. Usually, small-diameter nerve fibers are affected first, resulting in painful dysesthesias in the limbs and autonomic dysfunction, including orthostatic hypotension, impotence, impaired perspiration, and bowel or bladder dysfunction. Nerve biopsy helps to establish the diagnosis. Unfortunately, there are no effective treatments for amyloidosis and patients usually succumb to cardiovascular or renal complications.

Heavy Metal Intoxication

Lead, thallium, and arsenic intoxication may result in axonal polyneuropathies, sometimes resembling AIDP. Lead intoxication classically produces wrist drop or foot drop, with no sensory disturbances. Basophilic stippling of erythrocytes is a characteristic hematological finding. Thallium intoxication is characterized by painful dysesthesias in the feet and is classically associated with alopecia. Arsenic neuropathy is usually preceded by several days of gastrointestinal distress and is associated with Mees lines, which are linear white discolorations seen at the bases of the fingernails and toenails. In all cases, treatment of heavy metal intoxication involves supportive care. Chelation therapy can be effectively employed for lead intoxication, but does not have a role in the treatment of thallium or arsenic intoxication.

Porphyria

Porphyria refers to a group of disorders of heme biosynthesis inherited in an autosomal dominant fashion. Symptoms are intermittent and precipitated by a variety of drugs, especially barbiturates and sulfonamides. The classic picture involves abdominal pain followed by agitation and a rapidly developing motor neuropathy that resembles AIDP. Porphyria is diagnosed by examining the stool or urine for accumulation of heme precursors. Patients are treated with hematin, glucose, and supportive therapy. Avoidance of medications that may precipitate the clinical syndrome is also necessary to prevent recurrent attacks.

Mononeuropathy Multiplex

Leprosy

The most common cause of neuropathy worldwide, infection with *Mycobacterium leprae* is classically associated with multiple mononeuropathies affecting the cooler regions of the body, such as the ulnar nerve at the elbow and the peroneal nerve at the fibular neck. A distal, symmetrical, sensorimotor polyneuropathy may also occur. Multidrug therapy with dapsone and rifampin is the standard treatment in the United States.

Vasculitis

The classic pattern of peripheral nervous system involvement in vasculitis is mononeuropathy multiplex. A distal, relatively symmetrical polyneuropathy may also occur in vasculitis, as may a hybrid of mononeuropathy multiplex and symmetrical polyneuropathy. Examples of vasculitides that produce peripheral neuropathy and mononeuropathy multiplex are polyarteritis nodosa (also associated with vasculitis of the kidneys and gastrointestinal tract), Churg-Strauss syndrome (associated with respiratory involvement), and Wegener's granulomatosis (associated with upper and lower respiratory tract involvement and glomerulonephritis). Screening laboratory tests, including erythrocyte sedimentation rate and C-reactive protein, are helpful in suggesting a diagnosis of vasculitis. Definitive diagnosis, however, requires biopsy demonstrating transmural inflammation and necrosis of blood vessel walls.

Sarcoidosis

A multisystem granulomatous disorder of unclear etiology, sarcoidosis may produce mononeuropathy multiplex or, less commonly, generalized sensorimotor polyneuropathy. Multiple cranial neuropathies may also occur, with the facial, vestibulocochlear, and optic nerves most commonly involved. Biopsy demonstrating noncaseating granulomas establishes the diagnosis of sarcoidosis. The mainstay of treatment is corticosteroids, with supplementation by other immunosuppressants in patients with refractory disease.

KEY POINTS

1. Conduction block is a feature of acquired demyelinating neuropathies not seen in hereditary demyelinating neuropathies.
2. AIDP is frequently preceded by respiratory or gastrointestinal infections, with *Campylobacter jejuni* being one of the more common precipitating agents.
3. CSF analysis in AIDP shows and elevated protein value and normal cell count.
4. The Miller-Fisher variant of Guillain-Barré syndrome consists of ophthalmoplegia, ataxia, and areflexia and is associated with antibodies to GQ1b.
5. Mononeuropathy multiplex is classically associated with vasculitis.

■ NEUROMUSCULAR JUNCTION DISORDERS

Myasthenia Gravis

Myasthenia gravis is an autoimmune disorder caused by antibodies directed against the postsynaptic neuromuscular junction. There are two peaks of age of onset in myasthenia gravis: one in young women and a second in older men. Although each patient with myasthenia gravis may have a different constellation of symptoms, the broad patterns of disease are generalized fatigable muscle weakness, ocular myasthenia (ptosis and diplopia), and bulbar dysfunction (dysphagia and dysarthria). Myasthenic crisis is a life-threatening condition characterized by weakness of upper airway muscles, leading to obstruction and aspiration, or weakness of respiratory muscles, resulting in decreased air intake. Patients with this condition require intubation and intensive care.

Several bedside and laboratory tests may help to confirm a diagnosis of myasthenia gravis. Tensilon (edrophonium) is a cholinesterase inhibitor that is injected intravenously while monitoring for a clinical response, such as an improvement in ptosis, diplopia, or muscle strength. Because edrophonium may cause bradycardia, the patient's heart rate should be monitored during the test and atropine should be available in the event that bradycardia does occur. Testing for acetylcholine-receptor (AChR) antibodies is positive in 80% of patients with generalized myasthenia gravis but in only 50% of patients with isolated ocular involvement. Antibodies to a muscle-specific tyrosine kinase (MuSK) are seen in approximately half of patients without AChR antibodies. All patients with myasthenia gravis should have a chest CT scan with contrast, because 10% to 15% will have a thymoma requiring surgical removal.

Two electrophysiological tests, repetitive nerve stimulation (RNS) and single-fiber EMG (SFEMG), are frequently employed in the diagnosis of myasthenia gravis. In 60% of patients with myasthenia gravis, RNS performed at 3 Hz results in a U-shaped decremental response. SFEMG involves recording the time interval between the firing of two adjacent muscle fibers from a single motor unit, or jitter. Myasthenia gravis is characterized by increased jitter, because of the prolonged time for the end-plate potential to reach threshold. If this increased neuromuscular transmission time is sufficiently prolonged, the muscle fiber may never reach threshold, a phenomenon known as blocking.

Treatments available for myasthenia gravis are detailed in Table 17.7. Although most patients with myasthenia gravis require lifelong immunosuppression, there is an excellent chance for meaningful improvement with treatment.

TABLE 17.7 MEDICAL TREATMENT OF MYASTHENIA GRAVIS

TREATMENT	USES	POTENTIAL SIDE EFFECTS
Pyridostigmine	Acetylcholinesterase inhibitor that can be effective as a sole treatment for ocular myasthenia or in conjunction with immunosuppression in generalized myasthenia	Nausea, abdominal cramping, diarrhea, increased salivation, rhinorrhea
Prednisone	Corticosteroid that is the mainstay of treatment for generalized myasthenia gravis	Weight gain, glaucoma, osteoporosis, hypertension, diabetes
Mycophenolate mofetil	Steroid-sparing agent that suppresses B and T cell proliferation	Diarrhea, myelosuppression (uncommon)
Azathioprine	Steroid-sparing agent that inhibits T lymphocytes	Leukopenia, hepatotoxicity
Cyclosporine	Steroid-sparing agent that inhibits helper T cells, facilitates suppressor T cells, and blocks production and secretion of IL-2	Tremor, paresthesias, anemia, hepatotoxicity
IVIg	Used in myasthenic crisis: 0.4 g/kg for 5 days	Headache with infusions, nephrotoxicity, thrombotic events, aseptic meningitis
Plasma exchange	Used in myasthenic crisis: five exchanges performed every other day	Risks of central line placement, hypotension

Botulism

Caused by toxins of the bacterium *Clostridium botulinum,* botulism is a life-threatening disorder with several possible routes of acquisition. Food-borne botulism is caused by ingestion of botulinum toxin and begins several hours to days after eating contaminated food, often home canned. The initial symptoms are oculobulbar dysfunction, followed by descending weakness, which may be rapidly progressive, resulting in respiratory paralysis and necessitating mechanical ventilation. In infant botulism, *C. botulinum* spores are ingested and elaborate the toxin while in the intestine. The first symptom is usually constipation, which is followed by a weak cry, difficulty feeding, and muscle weakness, which can progress to complete paralysis. Inadvertent botulism is caused by accidental spread of botulinum toxin from injections used in the treatment of dystonia or for cosmetic purposes. Electrodiagnostic features of botulism include decreased CMAP amplitudes and posttetanic facilitation or an increase in CMAP response amplitude with either sustained exercise or 30- to 50-Hz repetitive nerve stimulation. Treatment for botulism consists of mechanical ventilation and supportive care. Antitoxin administration does not reverse existing paralysis, but it may prevent development of further weakness. Recovery from botulism is usually prolonged, requiring several months of intensive care.

Lambert-Eaton Myasthenic Syndrome

Lambert-Eaton myasthenic syndrome (LEMS) is a syndrome produced by antibodies directed against presynaptic voltage-gated calcium channels. In approximately two thirds of cases, LEMS is associated with cancer, most commonly small cell lung carcinoma. Development of LEMS may precede a cancer diagnosis by up to 2 years. Other autoimmune diseases, such as hypothyroidism and pernicious anemia, may also be associated with LEMS. Like myasthenia gravis, the main clinical feature of LEMS is fatigable proximal weakness. Autonomic dysfunction, including dry mouth, dry eyes, and constipation, is seen in 75% of patients. Unlike in myasthenia gravis and botulism, bulbar and ocular symptoms are less common in LEMS. A characteristic finding on neurological examination is diminished deep tendon reflexes with facilitation of reflexes after sustained muscle exercise. Electrophysiological testing demonstrates baseline reduction in CMAP amplitudes. Similar to myasthenia gravis, low (3 Hz) repetitive nerve stimulation (RNS) produces a decremental response. Unlike in myasthenia, however, either sustained exercise or 30- to 50-Hz RNS produces an incremental response in the CMAP amplitudes. Evaluation of LEMS should include screening for an underlying cancer. Treatment of LEMS should first be directed at treating the underlying cancer, if applicable. 3,4-diaminopyridine, a potassium-channel blocker that facilitates presynaptic calcium entry, is effective in the treatment of LEMS, but is not currently Food and Drug Administration approved. Other treatment options that are employed with varying degrees of success include pyridostigmine, corticosteroids, and IVIg.

KEY POINTS

1. AChR antibodies are present in 80% of patients with myasthenia gravis. Antibodies to MuSK are seen in approximately 50% of patients without AChR antibodies.
2. LEMS is associated with antibodies to presynaptic voltage-gated calcium channels and is frequently seen as a paraneoplastic disorder.

■ MYOPATHIES

Dystrophies

Muscular dystrophies are inherited, progressive diseases affecting muscle that are pathologically characterized by destruction of muscle tissue and replacement by connective and fatty tissue. A discussion of some of the more common dystrophies follows.

Duchenne and Becker Muscular Dystrophy

Duchenne and Becker muscular dystrophy (DMD and BMD) are X-linked re. dystrophies that are caused by deficiency of the muscle membrane prot. Symptoms of DMD, the most common muscular dystrophy, are first seen betw. 6 and include proximal weakness, gait abnormalities, calf pseudohypertrophy, . impairment. Cardiomyopathy and dysrhythmias are seen later in the disease. E presents between ages 5 and 15, has a milder clinical phenotype, and is not associate. .п cognitive impairment. Creatine kinase (CK) enzyme levels at the time of diagnosis are elevated in both conditions. Female carriers of the dystrophin gene mutation may have milder clinical phenotypes and muscle enzyme elevations. Dystrophin immunostaining shows marked reductions in DMD (less than 3% of normal) and milder reductions in BMD (usually 20% to 50% of normal). DNA testing for dystrophin gene mutation is also available. Treatment of DMD and BMD with prednisone increases strength and function and delays progression of the disease. Supportive care, including bracing to prevent contractures, physical therapy, and respiratory therapy, is also essential. Children with DMD are confined to wheelchairs by age 12 and usually die by their early 20s. Patients with BMD have a milder disease course, often maintaining the ability to ambulate into adulthood, occasionally into late adulthood.

Limb-Girdle Muscular Dystrophy

The limb-girdle muscular dystrophies (LGMDs) are a heterogeneous group of disorders characterized, as their name suggests, by slowly progressive weakness in a limb-girdle distribution. The majority of these disorders are inherited in an autosomal recessive fashion, with a smaller minority inherited in an autosomal dominant fashion. Serum CK levels are modestly elevated and tend to be higher in autosomal recessive varieties of LGMD. Muscle biopsy reveals degeneration and regeneration of muscle fibers, fiber splitting, and internalized nuclei. DNA testing is available for several forms of LGMD. Treatment is supportive, with the principal goals being contracture prevention and maintenance of physical activity.

Facioscapulohumeral Muscular Dystrophy

Facioscapulohumeral muscular dystrophy (FSHD) is inherited in an autosomal dominant fashion with high penetrance. Patients are affected at a wide range of ages, from early childhood until well into adulthood. As its name suggests, both facial muscles (resulting in widened palpebral fissures, pouting lips, and decreased facial expression) and scapular stabilizers (producing scapular winging) are affected. Humeral muscles are affected disproportionately compared to the forearm muscles. Foot dorsiflexors are also characteristically weak. Serum CK levels may be normal or mildly elevated. Treatment for FSHD is supportive. In the absence of respiratory, bulbar, or cardiac involvement, the prognosis of FSHD is excellent, with a normal life expectancy.

Emery-Dreifuss Muscular Dystrophy

Emery-Dreifuss muscular dystrophy is characterized by early contractures of the Achilles tendons and elbows, slowly progressive muscular weakness, and cardiac conduction defects. A variety of inheritance patterns have been described, with the most common being X-linked (associated with a defect in the protein emerin) or autosomal dominant (associated with a defect in the protein lamin A/C). Serum CK is usually normal or mildly elevated. Electrocardiogram (ECG) can show several abnormalities, including sinus bradycardia, PR interval prolongation, and conduction block. Monitoring of the patient's ECG on a yearly basis and consideration of pacemaker placement are therefore essential. Physical therapy is necessary to minimize the severity of contractures.

Oculopharyngeal Muscular Dystrophy

Oculopharyngeal muscular dystrophy is inherited in an autosomal dominant fashion and usually becomes clinically manifest between the fourth and sixth decades. It is particularly common in people of French-Canadian descent. The most common clinical features are ptosis and dysphagia, with weakness of extraocular muscles and frank diplopia being less comon. In patients with severe dysphagia, swallowing studies should be performed, with feeding tube placement to prevent aspiration if necessary. Ptosis can be treated with eyelid crutches or surgery.

Myotonic Dystrophy

Myotonic dystrophy is a multisystem, autosomal dominant disorder, caused by a CTG trinucleotide repeat expansion. Because the number of repeats is unstable and increases from generation to generation, the anticipation phenomenon, in which more severe disease affects each subsequent generation, is seen. Ptosis and generalized facial weakness with atrophy of the temporal muscles is characteristic of myotonic dystrophy. Patients also have weakness of sternomastoid and distal limb muscles. Most affected patients will demonstrate myotonia, which can be clinically detected as impaired relaxation of grip or eyelid closure or delayed relaxation of the thenar eminence or deltoid after percussion. EMG shows myotonic potentials. Cardiac conduction defects and involvement of smooth muscles, including the gastrointestinal tract and gallbladder, are also characteristic of myotonic dystrophy. Other features include frontal balding, cataracts, testicular atrophy, apathy, and sometimes mild mental retardation. Genetic testing shows an increased number of CTG repeats in the dystrophia myotonica protein kinase gene on chromosome 19. There are few options for the treatment of muscle weakness in myotonic dystrophy; myotonia can be treated with several agents, including mexiletine, phenytoin, quinine, and procainamide. Some of these agents, however, may potentiate arrhythmias and should be avoided. Cardiac evaluation, including Holter monitoring, is essential to screen for arrhythmias and to plan placement of pacemakers/defibrillators.

Inflammatory Myopathies

Inflammatory myopathies are characterized by muscle weakness, elevated serum CK, and inflammatory infiltrates on muscle biopsy. EMG typically shows increased insertional and spontaneous activity, with small-amplitude, short-duration, polyphasic motor units. The three most common inflammatory myopathies are dermatomyositis, polymyositis, and inclusion body myositis.

Dermatomyositis: Dermatomyositis is an acquired microangiopathy that typically presents with proximal muscle weakness and several characteristic skin findings, including a heliotrope (violet-colored) rash affecting the forehead and malar regions, chest and neck, extensor surfaces of the joints, and Gottron's papules. Interstitial lung disease, myocarditis, and gastrointestinal bleeding may result from involvement of other organ systems. Serum CK is almost always elevated. Characteristic biopsy findings include perifascicular atrophy and perimysial and perivascular inflammation. The mainstay of treatment for dermatomyositis is corticosteroids. For patients with disease refractory to steroids, other agents, including methotrexate, azathioprine, and IVIg, can be added. There is an increased risk for cancer in patients with dermatomyositis, and screening should include chest CT, colonoscopy, mammography, and prostate specific antigen assay.

Polymyositis: Polymyositis is an autoimmune disorder mediated by cytotoxic T cells that target muscle fibers, producing slowly progressive proximal muscle weakness. Muscle biopsy demonstrates endomysial inflammation, consisting of mononuclear cells. Similar to dermatomyositis, the mainstays of treatment are corticosteroids, with medications such as methotrexate and azathioprine being used as steroid-sparing agents.

Inclusion Body Myositis: Inclusion body myositis (IBM) is the most common inflammatory myopathy. It primarily affects patients over age 50 and is characterized by the gradual onset of proximal and distal muscle weakness. Preferential involvement of wrist flexors, finger flexors, and quadriceps distinguishes this disorder from other inflammatory myopathies. Dysphagia occurs in about half of patients with IBM. CK elevations are usually modest compared to those seen in other inflammatory myopathies. Muscle biopsy demonstrates endomysial mononuclear infiltrates and muscle fibers that contain the rimmed vacuoles from which IBM derives its name. Unlike polymyositis and dermatomyositis, IBM is poorly responsive to therapy such as corticosteroids, and the mainstays of treatment are supportive.

Toxic and Iatrogenic Myopathies

Alcohol: Acute necrotizing alcoholic myopathy is a syndrome of severe muscle pain, cramps, weakness, and tenderness. In severe cases, rhabdomyolysis may occur. Supportive treatment is indicated to expedite resolution. Chronic alcoholic myopathy is characterized by the gradual development of proximal muscle weakness and atrophy in the absence of tenderness and pain and follows a history of many years of excessive alcohol use. CK is usually normal or mildly elevated. Other stigmata of chronic alcohol abuse are often present. Improvement in chronic alcoholic myopathy may take place after several months of abstinence from alcohol.

Statins: Statins (HMG-CoA reductase inhibitors) characteristically produce a syndrome of myalgias, cramping, fatigue, and elevation of CK that develops within weeks to months after initiating therapy. Rhabdomyolysis is a rare complication, and syndromes resembling dermatomyositis or polymyositis are even less common. The risk of developing muscle complaints from statins increases with higher drug doses. Lovastatin, simvastatin, and atorvastatin are more likely to produce myopathy than pravastatin or fluvastatin. Treatment for statin-related myopathy depends on the severity of the symptoms: rhabdomyolysis necessitates medication discontinuation, and myositis or myalgias should prompt consideration of switching to an alternative cholesterol-lowering agent. Asymptomatic, mild elevation of CK does not necessitate statin discontinuation and should be followed clinically and with repeat CK assessments.

Steroids and Other Drugs: Corticosteroids may produce myopathy, characteristically as a painless process affecting the legs more than the arms, and often associated with other signs of steroid excess. Serum CK concentration is typically normal. Needle EMG shows normal insertional activity and small-amplitude, short-duration, polyphasic motor units in about half of patients. Muscle biopsy characteristically shows atrophy of type II fibers. Because type II muscle fibers are preferentially involved, EMG motor unit activity may be normal. After discontinuation of therapy, the symptoms of 90% of patients will resolve within 6 months.

Other medications that may produce myopathy include antimalarial drugs (particularly chloroquine and hydroxychloroquine), colchicine, phenothiazines, interferon alpha, vincristine, penicillamine, amiodarone, and perhexiline.

Metabolic Myopathies

Inherited disorders of glycogen and fatty acid metabolism are uncommon causes of myopathies. Although these conditions are mostly seen in children, they may also be diagnosed in adults. Hypotonia and progressive weakness with lethargy, seizures, and hypoglycemia are characteristic of infantile-onset metabolic myopathies. Hepatomegaly, macroglossia, and cardiomyopathy may also occur in infants with metabolic myopathies. Clinical clues to help diagnose an underlying metabolic myopathy in older children and adults include exercise intolerance, muscle cramps, and myoglobinuria. Unfortunately, most of the metabolic myopathies do not have specific treatments. The noteworthy exception is carnitine deficiency, which can be treated by carnitine supplementation. In older children and adults who develop a metabolic myopathy, strenuous exercise, which may precipitate rhabdomyolysis, should be avoided.

Acid Maltase Deficiency

Although a detailed review of the features of all of the metabolic myopathies is beyond the scope of this text, this autosomal recessive deficiency of lysosomal acid maltase produces several characteristic phenotypes. The severe infantile multisystem disorder (Pompe's disease) is associated with cardiomegaly, macroglossia, hepatomegaly, weakness, and hypotonia. Juvenile-onset acid maltase deficiency presents in the first decade of life with proximal greater than distal weakness and respiratory muscle weakness. Adult-onset acid maltase deficiency begins in the third or fourth decade and is characterized by proximal and respiratory muscle weakness. Myotonic discharges in the paraspinal muscles are an EMG feature of acid maltase deficiency in adults. There is no specific treatment for acid maltase deficiency other than supportive care, although enzyme replacement therapy is being actively investigated for infantile-onset disease.

Mitochondrial Myopathies

Mitochondrial myopathies are transmitted via a maternal inheritance pattern. A variety of clinical features, including short stature, ophthalmoparesis, proximal muscle weakness, cardiomyopathy, neuropathy, sensorineural hearing loss, pigmentary retinopathy, myoclonic epilepsy, headaches, stroke-like symptoms, and gastroparesis, suggest the possibility of a mitochondrial disorder. The characteristic biopsy findings in patients with mitochondrial myopathy are ragged red fibers and abnormalities in oxidative enzyme stains. There are no specific therapies for patients with mitochondrial myopathy, although coenzyme Q and creatine monohydrate are often prescribed. Some of the more common mitochondrial myopathies include the following:

- Mitochondrial encephalomyopathy, lactic acidosis, and stroke-like episodes (MELAS)
- Myoclonic epilepsy with ragged red fibers (MERRF)
- Chronic progressive external ophthalmoplegia (CPEO): progressive immobility of extraocular movements and ptosis
- Kearns-Sayre syndrome: CPEO with pigmentary retinopathy and cardiac conduction defects
- Leigh's disease: CPEO; abnormal movements, including ataxia, chorea, and myoclonus; and respiratory disorders, including episodic hyperventilation

Critical Illness Myopathy

Critical illness myopathy usually occurs in intensive care patients with sepsis who have received high doses of intravenous steroids and nondepolarizing neuromuscular blocking agents. Generalized muscle weakness develops over several days and may be profound. Often the first suspicion of critical illness myopathy is failure to wean a patient from a ventilator. Serum CK levels are normal or moderately elevated. Muscle biopsy shows loss of myosin on electron microscopy. Extensive supportive care is required to improve the patient's clinical condition, but no specific therapies are available. The prognosis of patients who develop critical illness myopathy is poor and generally related to the underlying medical process that necessitated intensive care.

Congenital Myopathies

A variety of uncommon myopathies may come to clinical attention at or shortly after birth. Muscle biopsy findings lend these disorders their names, which include central core myopathy, nemaline rod myopathy, and centronuclear myopathy. Central core myopathy is caused by a mutation in the ryanodine receptor (RYR1), and patients with this mutation, even in the absence of the classic congenital myopathy picture, are at risk for later development of malignant hyperthermia. Specific treatments are not available for the congenital myopathies.

KEY POINTS

1. Duchenne and Becker muscular dystrophy are both X-linked disorders produced by mutations in the dystrophin gene.
2. Myotonic dystrophy is a multisystem disorder caused by a CTG trinucleotide repeat expansion. Among the important components of the disorder are distal muscle weakness, myotonia (an impaired ability to relax the muscles), and cardiac conduction defects.
3. Polymyositis and dermatomyositis are steroid responsive; IBM is not.

■ **SUGGESTED READINGS**

Amato AA, Dumitru D. Hereditary myopathies. In: Dumitru D, Amato AA, Zwarts MJ, eds. *Electrodiagnostic Medicine*, 2nd ed. Philadelphia: Hanley & Belfus, Inc., 2002;1265–1370.

Barohn RJ, Kissel JT, Warmolts JR, et al. Chronic inflammatory polyradiculoneuropathy: Clinical characteristics, course, and recommendations for diagnostic criteria. *Arch Neurol* 1989;46:878–884.

Charness ME, Simon RP, Greenberg DA. Ethanol and the nervous system. *N Engl J Med* 1989;321:442–454.

Dalakas MC. Polymyositis, dermatomyositis, and inclusion body myositis. *N Engl J Med* 1991;325:1487–1498.

Dyck PJ, Windebank AJ. Diabetic and nondiabetic lumbosacral radiculoplexus neuropathies: New insights into pathophysiology and treatment. *Muscle Nerve* 2002;25:477–491.

Halperin J, Luft BJ, Volman DJ, et al. Lyme neuroborreliosis: Peripheral nervous system manifestations. *Brain* 1990;113:1207–1221.

Jaeckle KA. Neurological manifestations of neoplastic and radiation-induced plexopathies. *Semin Neurol* 2004;24:385–393.

Pascuzzi RM. Pearls and pitfalls in the diagnosis and management of neuromuscular junction disorders. *Semin Neurol* 2001;21:425–440.

Preston DC, Shapiro BE. *Electromyography and Neuromuscular Disorders*. Boston: Butterworth-Heinemann; 1998.

Ropper AH. The Guillain-Barré syndrome. *N Engl J Med* 1992;326:1130–1136.

Stewart JD. *Focal Peripheral Neuropathies*, 2nd ed. New York: Raven Press; 1993.

CHAPTER 18

Pediatric Neurology for Psychiatrists

Magdi M. Sobeih

■ INTRODUCTION

As the child's brain develops, new developmental abilities arise. Skills in multiple domains are acquired concurrently. These domains include motor, sensory, language, cognitive, attention, social, and self-care skills. Development of any one or multiple domains may go awry in childhood, resulting in patterns of developmental impairments with clinical diagnostic features.

■ BRAIN DEVELOPMENT

The fetal brain develops from the neural tube and prosencephalon. Neuronal precursors proliferate between 12 and 16 weeks of gestation. Neurons migrate to form the six-layered inside-out cortex between 12 and 20 weeks gestational age. Subsequently (in fetal as well as years into postnatal brain development), organization of the multilayered cortex takes place, with dendritic arborization, synaptogenesis, pruning of synapses, and apoptosis. Glial cells proliferate, and the myelin-forming cells, oligodendrocytes, differentiate. Finally, myelination prenatally proceeds first in the brainstem and cerebellum. Myelination continues into young adulthood, with central sensory system pathways becoming myelinated before motor systems. Myelination of central cortical sites occurs, followed by the occipital and then frontotemporal poles. From early development into late adolescence, functional connectivity of neural networks is continuously modified.

■ EXPECTED DEVELOPMENTAL MILESTONES

Evaluation of children relies heavily on comparison of their developmental abilities relative to those of their peers. For this reason, adjustments for conceptual age and knowledge of typical developmental milestones are essential. Children's early development proceeds in an orderly fashion in several areas, first with primitive reflexes and then more complex developmental processes (Tables 18.1 and 18.2). Much like in neurological examination of adults, children's developmental milestones can be organized based on various domains. These include motor skills (both fine motor and gross motor), language abilities (both receptive and expressive), socialization skills, cognitive abilities, and executive function. Significant delays in acquisition of these milestones can occur in any of the domains or a combination of domains. For example, a child may have language delay only, delays in fine or gross motor skills, or a combination of language and motor delay. These delays assume an otherwise normal neurological examination, without evidence of focal or lateralizing neurological signs indicating a possible underlying structural etiology. Regression warrants neurological consultation for metabolic disorder or neurodegenerative disorder, such as leukodystrophy or gray matter disorder.

TABLE 18.1 PRIMITIVE REFLEXES IN FULL-TERM INFANT

REFLEX	DISAPPEARS BY
Moro	3–4 months
Tonic neck	6 months
Babinski	Usually 12 months
	Up to 3 years old is normal if symmetrical
Grasp reflex	4–6 months in hand, 10 months in foot
Suck	4 months
Stepping reflex	6 weeks

TABLE 18.2 TYPICAL DEVELOPMENTAL MILESTONES

AGE	GROSS MOTOR	FINE MOTOR	LANGUAGE	SOCIAL
1 month				Smiles responsively
2 months			Coos	Recognizes mother, tracks 180 degrees
3 months	Head control, rolls over	Reaches for objects	Babbling and cooing	
4 months		Reaches whole hand		Laughs
5 months	Head up on horizontal suspension			
6 months	Sits with support	Transfers objects	Turns to name	
8 months	Sits unsupported	Pincer grasp		
9 months	Stands with support, crawls		"Dadda," "Mamma" specifically	
10 months	Cruises			
11 months				Plays peek-a-boo
12 months	Walks independently	Handedness develops, tower of 2 cubes	One or two words more to identify objects specifically	
15 months			Points for communication to desired objects	
18 months	Walks forward and backward, stoops and recovers, ascends steps	Tower of 3 cubes	10–20-word expressive vocabulary, larger receptive	Imaginative play
2 years	Runs well	Tower of 8 cubes	200-word expressive vocabulary, two-word phrases	Helps around house
3 years	Throw, catch, kick, pedals	Copies circle	Speaks in sentences, follows two-step directions	Toilet trained, Pretend play
4 years	Hops	Copies cross	Begins to write	
5 years	Skips	Copies square	Beginning to read	

■ DISORDERS PRESENTING IN EARLY CHILDHOOD

Motor Delay and Motor Skills Disorder: Developmental Coordination Disorder and Developmental Dyspraxia

Important motor milestones center around handedness and ambulation. Children usually develop hand dominance by 18 months (but may be as early as 12 months) and have started walking independently at 12 months. Motor skills are characterized by progressive development of fine and gross motor skills (Table 18.2). Screening for motor skills is accomplished using the motor quotient, the movement ABC test, and the Bruininks-Oseretsky test.

Developmental dyspraxia is a disorder in the organization, planning, and execution of coordinated movement compared with age-appropriate skilled motor abilities. This is similar to the *Diagnostic and Statistical Manual of Mental Disorders,* fourth edition (DSM-IV), diagnostic category of developmental coordination disorder, which is diagnosed by motor coordination that is substantially below that expected for chronological age and intelligence quotient (IQ); this motor coordination difficulty interferes with academic abilities and socialization.

If there are lateralizing or focal signs on neurological examination, further studies, including neuroimaging and electrophysiological studies, such as electroencephalography, should be considered. Otherwise, neuroimaging is unnecessary. The only proven etiology for any developmental dyspraxia is the dominant mutation of the *FoxP2* gene on 7q31. Other than this rare cause, there is no known cause and thus no standard workup.

Language Impairment

Important language milestones include prelinguistic skills, such as babbling and pointing, before the age of 1 year. The use of first words starts at 12 months plus or minus 3 months. In most cultures, a child first uses words to describe or name objects. At around 18 months children understand actions, and by the age of 2 years they use action words and coincidentally typically begin to speak in two-word phrases. Vocabulary at this time should be at least 50 words; the average is 200 words. By 3 years old, a child's vocabulary should be approximately 1000 words and the child should be speaking in sentences.

Any delay or deviation in achieving these milestones should raise concern. Workup should include a formal hearing evaluation by visual-reinforced audiometry, a behavioral technique of evaluating hearing. If the child is not cooperative or the test cannot be performed, brainstem auditory evoked response (BAER) should be performed.

If a child has gained language through the first few years of life along a typical trajectory but then loses language abilities suddenly, temporal lobe seizures may be the cause, as in Landau-Kleffner syndrome.

Treatment with the antiepileptic medication valproic acid or high-dose valium may allow recovery in about one third of patients. Otherwise, the child should be evaluated by a speech pathologist, and speech and language therapy should be initiated.

Cognitive Impairment: Global Developmental Delay

The definition of mental retardation requires evaluation by standardized IQ testing (see later discussion). This is applicable only after 3 years of age and reliable after 5 years of age. Before that, a child with significant deficits in learning and adaptive skills is diagnosed with global developmental delay (GDD). GDD implies functioning at least 2 standard deviations below the mean in at least 2 of the following developmental skills: motor, language, cognitive, personal-social, and adaptive living skills.

Autism Spectrum Disorder

Autism spectrum disorder is a neurodevelopmental disorder resulting in the impairment of communicative and social development in children (Fig. 18.1). DSM-IV classifies the disorders under pervasive developmental disorder (PDD) with autism, Rett's syndrome, Asperger's syndrome, and PDD not otherwise specified (PDD-NOS). Diagnosis of autism requires symptoms before 3 years of age.

Workup for a diagnosis of autism should include genetic studies for fragile X syndrome (FMR1 triple repeat number analysis), karyotype, and examination of submicroscopic subtelomeric chromosomal microarray analysis. In addition, girls may have MeCP2 mutation testing for Rett syndrome.

Although there is no specific treatment for autism, early identification and therapy assists in socialization and improved language function.

Pervasive Developmental Disorder

Approximately 1 in 150 children may be diagnosed with PDD, which affects individuals across the lifespan. Features of autism include impairment in language development, with both verbal and nonverbal communication affected, diminished age-appropriate social ability, and activities characterized by repetitive or a restricted range of activities or inflexible adherence to routines or rituals.

Asperger's Syndrome

Children with Asperger's syndrome reach typical early language milestones and have an IQ in the average range. However, social abilities, pragmatic language abilities, and comprehension are severely impaired. Those with Asperger's syndrome fail to interpret social cues, gestures, and body language. This results in difficulty forming peer relations, despite a desire to form these relationships, and may lead to depression or mood disorder.

Rett's Syndrome

Rett's syndrome is a genetic disorder characterized by regression of developmental abilities in girls. These patients typically lose functional use of their hands and develop stereotypies involving the hands.

■ DISORDERS PRESENTING IN LATER CHILDHOOD

Learning Disability

There is no universally accepted definition of learning disability. A discrepancy between ability as judged by IQ, and academic achievement as evaluated by standardized measures such as

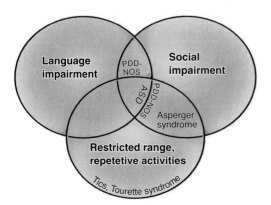

■ **FIGURE 18.1** Venn diagram of autism spectrum disorders showing the intersection of language impairment, social impairment, and repetitive behaviors.

the Wechsler Individual Achievement Test (WIAT II), Wide Range Achievement Test (WRAT-3), and the Woodcock-Johnson Tests of Achievement (WJ-III), is one method of establishing a learning disability. The most common learning disability is impairment in basic reading skills, also known as dyslexia. Children with a language-based learning disability show good visuospatial skills but impaired verbal comprehension and expression. By contrast, children with nonverbal learning disability are able to perform well on repetitive motor skills and have good auditory comprehension.

Workup for a learning disability should include neuropsychological evaluation using standardized measures of IQ and academic ability. Medical evaluation should be considered if there are concerning signs and symptoms on history or physical examination findings.

Mental Retardation

Neuropsychological evaluation using normed, standardized IQ tests has an average set at 100, with a standard deviation of 15. Thus 2 standard deviations below average with impaired self-care abilities under 18 years of age defines mental retardation (MR). Mild MR implies IQ between 50 and 70, moderate MR from 35 to 49, severe MR from 20 to 34, and profound MR lower than 20. This implies administration of IQ tests, which usually are applicable after 5 years of age. Children younger than 5 who have not had IQ tests but nevertheless perform lower than 2 standard deviations below the mean in two areas of development from the following list are considered to have GDD: motor, language, cognitive, personal-social, and activities of daily living.

MR results from perinatal insult, toxic or metabolic exposure, or genetic causes (syndromic or nonsyndromic).

Perinatal causes include preterm delivery with complications, hypoxia or ischemia, infection, hemorrhage, or trauma.

Toxic or metabolic causes include congenital hypothyroidism; TORCH infection (toxoplasmosis, other [congenital syphilis, and viruses], rubella, cytomegalovirus, and herpes simplex virus); malnutrition; plumbism; and fetal alcohol exposure, which may cause specific dysmorphic features (Fig. 18.2), or fetal alcohol effect, which is characterized by behavioral symptoms of hyperactivity and cognitive impairment.

Genetic causes account for up to 15% of neurodevelopmental disorders including MR. The most common syndromes include Down syndrome (trisomy 21), fragile X syndrome (mutation

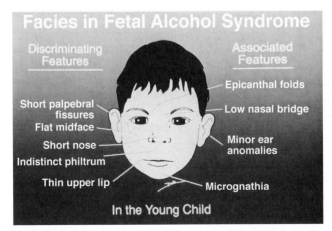

■ **FIGURE 18.2** Facies in fetal alcohol syndrome. (From Streissguth AP, Little RE. *Alcohol, Pregnancy, and the Fetal Alcohol Syndrome,* 2nd ed. Project Cork Institute Medical School Curriculum [slide lecture series] on Biomedical Education: Alcohol Use and Its Medical Consequences. Produced by Dartmouth Medical School, Hanover, NH, 1994.)

of *FMR1* on the X chromosome [expansion of triple-repeat CCG]), Rett's syndrome (mutation of the methyl CpG binding protein 2 *MeCP2* gene on the X chromosome), and chromosomal and submicroscopic subtelomeric chromosomal rearrangements.

The most commonly used tests for IQ in children are the Wechsler Preschool and Primary Scale of Intelligence (WPPSI), used between 3 and 7 years of age, and the Wechsler Intelligence Scales for Children (WISC IV) for 6- to 12-year-old children.

Workup

If there is a history of perinatal difficulties or trauma, or asymmetrical neurological examination, neuroimaging by brain MRI is warranted, otherwise no neuroimaging is required. Genetic screening is recommended to include karyotype, *FMR1* analysis for fragile X syndrome, *MeCP2* analysis for Rett's syndrome in girls, and higher resolution chromosomal testing using subtelomeric FISH or comparative genomic hybridization.

Attention Deficit (Hyperactivity) Disorder

Neural networks for attention serve to guide attention to an activity, sustain that attention, and then disengage when appropriate. Disorders of attention in childhood present after the age of 4 years, persist for at least 6 months, are maladaptive (interfering with academics or social or family interaction), and are inconsistent with age-expected attention ability.

The differential diagnosis includes depression, learning disability, MR, and anxiety disorder.

Workup for a disorder of attention includes objective measures of behavior characterizing attention and motor hyperactivity in multiple settings, such as school and home. This can be accomplished using inventories such as the Achenbach Child Behavior Checklist and the Connors ADHD Index. Testing using continuous performance tasks provide age-appropriate, standardized measures.

Treatment for attentional disorders includes behavioral therapy and school accommodations. Pharmacotherapeutic options include alpha-adrenergic agents, such as clonidine or guanfacine, especially for impulsive type attention-deficit hyperactivity disorder (ADHD). Stimulants such as methylphenidate or amphetamine preparations have an approximately 70% efficacy rate. Nonstimulants, such as atomoxetine, or second-line agents, including selective serotonin reuptake inhibitors (SSRIs) may also be tried. Empiric trials of these different medication classes may be necessary.

Tic Disorders and Tourette's Syndrome

Tic disorders and Tourette's syndrome are clinical diagnoses of neurodevelopmental disorders characterized by sudden, rapid, repeated, stereotyped motor movement. These movements are ultimately sensed by the subject as an uncontrollable urge to perform the movement. This movement may be simple, involving only one muscle or muscle group, or complex, in which sequential muscle movements are made. Tics may also be vocal (phonic), in which grunts, squeaking, chirping, throat clearing, or coughing sounds, among others, may be made. These too may be complex, including echolalia (repeating something heard), pallilalia (repeating what one says), or coprolalia (cursing or vulgarities), which is the least common. If present for 4 weeks to less than 1 year, tics are classified as transient. Presence longer than 1 year constitutes chronic tics, even if the tics disappear for up to 3 months during that time. The presence during that 1 year of multifocal motor tics and a phonic tic in a child under 18 years old defines Tourette's syndrome. Tourette's syndrome is more common in boys than girls. Comorbid conditions with Tourette's syndrome include ADHD and obsessive-compulsive disorder (OCD). These may each be present in approximately one third of patients with Tourette's syndrome.

Functional neuroimaging studies implicate the basal ganglia as the focus of generation of the tics. Regions in the basal ganglia use dopamine as a neurotransmitter. Thus it is not surprising that some medications may trigger tics. Note, however, that the presence of tics in a child does not preclude the use of stimulants to treat AD(H)D.

The differential diagnosis for tics includes other movement disorders, such as dystonias or drug-induced tics (such as with dopaminergic stimulants or antipsychotics).

Tics need only be treated if their presence is interfering with the child's social or academic development. Pharmacotherapy for tics includes alpha-adrenergic agents, atypical antipsychotics, and botulinum toxin injection.

Pediatric Autoimmune Neuropsychiatric Disorders Associated with Streptococcus Infection

There is some evidence that an immune reaction to streptococcus infection leads to an autoimmune reaction giving rise to neuropsychiatric disorders including OCD and tics. This evidence is inconsistent and not universally accepted.

KEY POINTS

1. Comparison of a child's development with known typical developmental milestones is essential in establishing diagnoses.
2. Impairments in development may affect motor, language, social, or cognitive spheres.
3. Evaluation should be based on standardized measures.
4. A combination of behavioral intervention and pharmacotherapy is often most effective.

■ **SUGGESTED READINGS**

American Psychiatric Association. *Diagnostic and Statistical Manual of Mental Disorders.* 4th ed. Washington, DC: American Psychiatric Association; 1994.

Augustyn M. Diagnosis of Autism spectrum disorders. In: Rose BD. *UpToDate.* Wellesley, MA: UpToDate; 2007.

Cohen D, Pichard N, Tordjman S, et al. Specific genetic disorders and autism: clinical contribution towards their identification. *J Autism Dev Disord* 2005;35:103–116.

Dosenbach NU, Visscher KM, Palmer, et al. A core system for the implementation of task sets. *Neuron* 2006;50:799–812.

Fair DA, Dosenbach NU, Church JA, et al. Development of distinct control networks through segregation and integration. *Proc Natl Acad Sci U S A* 2007;104:13507–13512.

Jankovich J. *Tourette Syndrome.* In: Rose BD. *UpToDate.* Wellesley, MA: UpToDate; 2007.

McPartland J, Klin A. Asperger's syndrome. *Adolesc Med Clin* 2006;17:771–788, abstract xiii.

Pliszka S. Practice parameter for the assessment and treatment of children and adolescents with attention-deficit/hyperactivity disorder. *J Am Acad Child Adolesc Psychiatry* 2007;46:894–921.

Sanger TD, Chen D, Delgado MR, et al. Definition and classification of negative motor signs in childhood. *Pediatrics* 2006;118:2159–2167.

Sebat J, Lakshmi B, et al. Strong association of de novo copy number mutations with autism. *Science* 2007;316:445–449.

Volpe J. *Neurology of the Newborn.* Philadelphia: WB Saunders; 2001.

Watkins KE, Dronkers NF, Vargha-Khadem F. Behavioural analysis of an inherited speech and language disorder: comparison with acquired aphasia. *Brain* 2002;125(Pt 3):452–464.

Weiss LA, Shen Y, Korn JM, et al. Association between microdeletion and microduplication at 16p11.2 and autism. *N Engl J Med* 2008;358:667–675.

CHAPTER 19

Multiple Sclerosis

Alexandra Degenhardt

■ INTRODUCTION

Multiple sclerosis (MS) is a chronic autoimmune demyelinating disease of uncertain etiology involving the central nervous system (CNS). In 70% to 85% of cases the initial course is relapsing-remitting (RRMS), in which episodes of subacute neurological deterioration (relapses) are followed by complete or near-complete recovery over weeks to months. Relapses must last for at least 24 hours, be separated in time by at least 1 month, and involve separate lesions in the CNS.

In 15% to 30% of cases, the initial course is predominantly one of progressive neurological deterioration (PPMS) without distinct relapses. Approximately 70% of patients with RRMS transition to a progressive course within 25 years, which is termed secondary progressive multiple sclerosis (SPMS).

KEY POINTS

1. Of MS cases, 80% are relapsing-remitting, 70% of these transition to a progressive course within 25 years termed SPMS.
2. Of MS cases, 20% are primarily progressive.

■ SYMPTOMS AND SIGNS

General

Typical symptoms during relapses may include any of the following: hemiparesis, paraparesis, monoparesis, numbness, paresthesias, ataxia, diplopia, and vertigo. Additional symptoms that are often troublesome and persistent include pain, fatigue, depression, and cognitive and urinary dysfunction. Cognitive impairments usually involve executive functions and short-term memory. Urinary dysfunction often begins with urge incontinence (detrusor hyperreflexia) and later progresses to dyssynergia (in which the bladder contracts against the closed sphincter), or urinary retention secondary to detrusor flaccidity or a hyperactive sphincter.

On examination, there are signs referable to the CNS consistent with the patient's symptoms, such as weakness in an upper motor neuron pattern, ataxia, and sensory loss. Upper motor neuron signs of the CNS include increased tone, hyperreflexia, the extensor plantar response, clonus, and weakness (involving shoulder abduction, elbow, hand and finger extension, flexion of the hip and knee, and dorsiflexion). Characteristic signs include Lhermitte's sign (neck flexion elicits a shooting unpleasant sensation down the spine), Uhthoff's phenomenon (exercise- or heat-induced worsening of symptoms), Marcus Gunn pupil (dilation of the affected pupil during the swinging flashlight test), and internuclear ophthalmoplegia (paresis of the adducting eye on conjugate lateral gaze with nystagmus of the abducting eye). The degree of disability on the neurological examination is quantified by the Expanded Disability Status Scale (Table 19.1).

TABLE 19.1 THE EXPANDED DISABILITY STATUS SCALE (EDSS)

EDSS SCORE	DESCRIPTION
0	Normal neurologic examination
1	No disability, minimal signs in one FS
1.5	No disability, minimal signs in more than one FS
2.0	Minimal disability in one FS
2.5	Minimal disability in two FS
3.0	Moderate disability in one FS
3.5	Fully ambulatory but with moderate disability
4.0	Fully ambulatory without aid, self-sufficient, up and about some 12 hours per day despite relatively severe disability; able to walk without aid or rest some 500 meters
4.5	Fully ambulatory without aid, up and about much of the day, able to work a full day; characterized by relatively severe disability; able to walk without aid or rest for some 300 meters
5.0	Ambulatory without aid or rest for about 200 meters; disability severe enough to impair full daily activities
5.5	Ambulatory without aid or rest for about 100 meters; disability severe enough to preclude full daily activities
6.0	Intermittent or unilateral constant assistance (cane, crutch, or brace) required to walk about 100 meters with or without resting
6.5	Constant bilateral assistance (canes, crutches, or braces) required to walk approximately 20 meters without resting
7.0	Unable to walk beyond about 5 meters even with aid; essentially restricted to wheelchair
7.5	Unable to take more than a few steps; restricted to wheelchair; wheels self but cannot carry on in standard wheelchair a full day
8.0	Essentially restricted to bed or chair or perambulated in wheelchair, but may be out of bed itself much of the day; retains many self-care functions
8.5	Essentially restricted to bed much of the day; has some effective use of arm(s); retains some self-care functions
9.0	Helpless bed patient; can communicate and eat
9.5	Totally helpless bed patient; unable to communicate effectively or eat/swallow
10	Death due to MS

FS, functional system, including pyramidal, cerebellar, brainstem, sensory, bowel and bladder, visual (or optic), and cerebral. (Adapted from Kurtzke J. Rating neurologic impairment in multiple sclerosis: an expanded disability status scale [EDSS]. *Neurology* 1983;33:1444–1452.)

Psychiatric Symptoms

Depression and anxiety are more common in MS than in most chronic diseases, including most neurological disorders. The prevalence of depression in patients with MS is 14%, with a lifetime prevalence of 50%. Anxiety is common, with a prevalence of 34% in patients attending an MS clinic and 40% of partners with anxiety. Anxiety disorders more common in MS than in the general population include panic disorder (10% versus 3.5%), obsessive-compulsive disorder (8.6% versus 2.5%), and generalized anxiety disorder (18.6% versus 5.1%). Patients with anxiety were more likely to be women, abuse alcohol, report higher levels of stress, and have a history of depression.

Patients with both depression and anxiety are at highest risk for attempting suicide. Of note, the incidence and degree of depressive symptoms correlate with greater cognitive impairments and modestly with brain atrophy. Suicide is thought to be the cause of 15% of deaths in MS; 6.4% of patients will attempt to commit suicide during their lifetime. Suicidal intent occurs in 28.6% of patients during their lifetime. The greatest risk factors include depression, alcohol abuse, and living alone.

Medications used to treat MS are associated with a variety of psychiatric symptoms. High-dose steroids can cause mania, increased energy, insomnia, and euphoria. Depressive symptoms can occur with the abrupt tapering of steroids or their chronic use. The interferons used to treat MS are associated with a worsening of preexisting depression, but not clearly with the development of depression.

KEY POINTS

1. On examination, one can find upper motor neuron patterns of weakness, dermatomal and patchy sensory loss, hyperreflexia, Lhermitte's sign, Marcus Gunn pupil, and internuclear ophthalmoplegia.
2. Depression occurs with a prevalence of 14% in MS clinics and a lifetime prevalence of 50%. The prevalence of anxiety is 34%.
3. High-dose steroids can cause mania, increased energy, insomnia, and euphoria.

■ MULTIPLE SCLEROSIS VARIANTS

Clinical variants include progressive-relapsing MS (PRMS) and single-attack progressive MS (SAPMS). PRMS is rare. It is primarily progressive at onset with occasional relapses, and appears to have a similar prognosis to PPMS. Single-attack progressive cases demonstrate progression after one relapse and also have a prognosis similar to that of PPMS.

Other variants of MS include Balo's concentric sclerosis (in which alternating rings of myelination and demyelination are seen on imaging), Marburg's disease (widespread demyelination that is often destructive, with rapid clinical progression), and tumefactive MS (in which a large single lesion with significant edema is seen on imaging). Neuromyelitis optica, otherwise known as Devic's disease, is presently considered a separate demyelinating autoimmune disease that involves primarily the optic nerves and spinal cord.

KEY POINTS

1. MS variants include Balo's concentric sclerosis, Marburg's disease, and tumefactive MS.
2. Devic's disease is considered a distinct demyelinating autoimmune disease.

■ EPIDEMIOLOGY

MS affects more women than men, with a female to male ratio of 1.5:2.4. The mean age of onset is 30 in RRMS and 37 in PPMS. The prevalence of MS is generally higher in northern latitudes, and there is rare familial clustering. The prevalence of MS per 10,000 is 30 to 70 in southern Europe, 100 to 200 in Scandinavia, 100 in the United States, 16 to 30 in the Middle East, and fewer than 10 per 10,000 in Asia, Central America, and most of Africa.

KEY POINTS

1. The female to male ratio is 2:1.
2. The mean age of onset in relapsing MS is 30 years.

■ ETIOLOGY

Geographic differences in the prevalence of MS appear to be due to an interaction between undetermined environmental and genetic factors. The children of families who migrate from a country with a low prevalence of MS to a country with a high prevalence have an increased risk compared with that of their parents. Moreover, the genetic risk for the children of patients with MS is low, although higher than in the general population. The concordance of MS in dizygotic twins and siblings is 3% to 5% and in monozygotic twins is 20% to 40%. The *HLA-DR2* allele increases the risk of MS, and its frequency varies similarly among populations at risk. Further identification of genes is ongoing and most likely involves complex genetic and environmental interactions. Several genetic associations found have included the HLA variables DRB1*1501, DQA1*0102, and DQB1*0602.

KEY POINTS

1. The exact cause of MS is unknown.
2. The concordance of MS in dizygotic twins and siblings is 3% to 5%, and in monozygotic twins it is 20% to 40%.

■ PATHOLOGY

Plaques of demyelination are found in the CNS, primarily in the perivenular, periventricular, and deep white matter areas, but also in the brainstem and spinal cord. Plaques are infrequently found within the cortex. There is relative preservation of axons, but early axonal transection has been described and may account for progression in the long term. The development of a plaque begins with alteration of the blood–brain barrier. This includes the uptake of water, lymphocytes, antibodies, and cytokines into the brain parenchyma. The active plaque is characterized by abundant proinflammatory cytokines (interleukin-2, interferon-gamma, and tumor necrosis factor–beta), myelin debris, lipid-laden macrophages, and perivascular infiltration of lymphocytes, predominantly T-cells (both CD4+ and CD8+). Reactive astrocytes are also found within the plaque.

Remyelination is thought to occur, as suggested by thinly myelinated axons, but occurs over months. More rapid clinical recovery is due to the reduction in edema, cytokines, and inflammation. In addition, there is proliferation of the sodium channel along demyelinated axons that helps to propagate electrical conduction along the axon. Recent pathological studies suggest that there is heterogeneity among plaques regarding features other than the common T-cell and macrophage infiltration. These differences include the predominance of one of the following: (a) TNF-alpha, (b) IgG and complement, (c) oligodendrocyte dysfunction, or (d) oligodendrocyte apoptosis. The chronic plaque is well demarcated and lacks signs of inflammation, which, if present, are limited to the plaque's edges. The center of the plaque is characterized by proliferation of astrocytes and absent oligodendrocytes.

KEY POINTS

1. Demyelination is found in the CNS, primarily in the perivenular, periventricular, and deep white matter areas, but also in the brainstem, spinal cord, and occasionally in the cortex.
2. Remyelination occurs over months.

■ DIAGNOSTIC APPROACH

Key Features

MS is primarily a clinical diagnosis based on a consistent clinical presentation with evidence of CNS demyelination *disseminated in time and space not better explained by another disease*. The essentials of diagnosing MS remain the same as the Schumacher criteria developed in 1965. These key features include the following:

- Age 10 to 50 years at onset
- Involvement of the CNS white matter
- At least two sites of CNS involvement
- Lesions are separated by time and space
- Objective abnormalities on examination
- Course is relapsing-remitting or chronic progressive
- There is no better explanation of the symptoms

A relapse entails CNS dysfunction for at least 24 hours, and relapses must be separated in time by at least 1 month. The latter helps to distinguish one relapse in MS in which symptoms are often subacute and evolving, and more specifically from acute disseminated encephalomyelitis (ADEM). In the case of both SPMS and PPMS, progression must occur for at least 6 months.

In 1983, the Poser criteria extended the age of onset to 59 and included laboratory studies such as cerebrospinal fluid (CSF), neuroimaging, and evoked potentials such as visual evoked potentials (VEP), somatosensory evoked potentials (SSEP), and brainstem auditory evoked responses (BAER).

McDonald's Criteria

In 2001, the McDonald criteria specified the MRI features that may be used to establish the diagnosis. These were again revised in 2005 and have a sensitivity of 77% and specificity of over 90% (Tables 19.2 to 19.4). It is important to remember that these criteria will most likely be revised in the future; however, the key features described remain the same. Magnetic resonance imaging (MRI) should be used to assist in the diagnosis; however, a second clinical relapse is the most accurate method of diagnosing MS.

TABLE 19.2 SUMMARY OF THE MODIFIED MCDONALD'S CRITERIA

CLINICAL ATTACKS	CLINICAL LESIONS	PARACLINICAL TESTING NEEDED
Two	Two	None
Two	One	MRI dissemination in space *or* 2 lesions on MRI consistent with MS plus positive CSF
One	Two	MRI dissemination in time
One	One	MRI dissemination in space *or* 2 MRI lesions consistent with MS plus positive CSF *and* MRI dissemination in time

Note: Clinical lesions may be determined by physical examination or evoked potentials. Positive CSF = positive oligoclonal bands (OCB) or elevated IgG Index. MRI. Dissemination in time = new enhancing at least 3 months or new nonenhancing lesion at least 1 month after the initial attack.

CSF, cerebrospinal fluid; MRI, magnetic resonance imaging.

TABLE 19.3 MRI DISSEMINATION IN SPACE

AT LEAST THREE OF THE FOLLOWING LESIONS CONSISTENT WITH DEMYELINATION:

1. Brain or spinal cord: one enhancing lesion or nine T2 hyperintense lesions

2. One infratentorial lesion or one spinal cord lesion

3. One juxtacortical lesion

4. Three periventricular lesions

Differential Diagnosis

Table 19.5 summarizes the differential diagnosis. Essentially, the lack of concomitant symptoms and signs referable to another disease and the unique temporal characteristics of the relapsing-remitting course help to make a diagnosis of MS. ADEM is monophasic and often characterized by fever, encephalopathy, and a recent history of a viral illness or vaccine. The MRI in ADEM typically shows multiple bilateral subcortical lesions with widespread enhancement. In PPMS, often a confirmatory CSF finding, negative serum studies, and brain MRI are needed. Moreover, clinical features that suggest a disease other than MS include an age of onset under 20 or over 60; family history; lower motor neuron, extrapyramidal, or Parkinsonian signs; early dementia, or the predominance of cortical signs (such as aphasia, apraxia, agnosia, or neglect). A child or young adult with a slowly progressive course and peripheral neuropathy should raise suspicion for a leukodystrophy such as adrenoleukodystrophy and metachromatic leukodystrophy.

Tests

Blood tests that are reasonable to obtain on all patients include complete blood count, erythrocyte sedimentation rate, chemistries, liver function tests (LFTs), antinuclear antibody, and B_{12} level. Additional testing to consider includes Lyme disease serology, angiotensin-converting enzyme level, other infectious and collagen-vascular serologies, thyroid function tests, and very-long-chain fatty acids and arylsulfatase A levels. For suspected neuromyelitis optica, testing for the NMO-IgG antibody in the CSF is helpful.

A brain MRI with gadolinium is the most sensitive. Typical features of MS plaques include their location (deep white matter, brainstem, corpus callosum, or periventricular area), their shape (ovoid, punctuate, or finger-like lesions radially oriented toward the ventricles), and, often, enhancement (open ring). A cervical spine or thoracic spine MRI can also be helpful in making the diagnosis and should be obtained if symptoms or signs are referable to the spine. A normal MRI result, especially in the first several years of the disease, cannot be solely used to exclude MS (Fig. 19.1).

Spinal tap and CSF analysis is indicated at the first relapse and where the diagnosis of MS is not definite. The spinal tap may not be needed if the MRI and clinical presentation are classic

TABLE 19.4 DIAGNOSIS OF PPMS

INSIDIOUS PROGRESSION OF DISABILITY FOR OVER 1 YEAR WITH AT LEAST TWO OF THE FOLLOWING:

1. Nine T2 lesions on brain MRI *or* ≥4 T2 lesions *and* a positive VEP

2. ≥2 T2 intramedullary lesions on spine MRI

3. Positive CSF

CSF, cerebrospinal fluid; MRI, magnetic resonance imaging; VEP, visual evoked potential.

TABLE 19.5 SUMMARY OF DIFFERENTIAL DIAGNOSIS OF MS

Autoimmune	• Acute disseminated encephalomyelitis • Clinically isolated syndrome • Transverse myelitis • Optic neuritis • Cerebellitis
Degenerative	• Subacute combined degeneration (B_{12} deficiency) • Parkinson's "plus" syndromes • Spinocerebellar ataxia
Infectious	• Progressive multifocal leukoencephalopathy • Lyme, HTLV-1, HHV-6, mycoplasma, Epstein-Barr • Syphilis, human immunodeficiency virus, cytomegalovirus • Whipple's
Inflammatory	• Systemic lupus erythematosus; Sjögren's, Behçet's syndrome • Sarcoidosis, celiac disease • Vasculitides
Inherited	• Inherited spastic paraparesis • Metachromatic leukodystrophy, adrenoleukodystrophy • Leber's hereditary optic neuropathy; mitochondrial encephalopathy lactic acidosis and stroke-like episodes (MELAS)
Neoplasm	• Central nervous system (CNS) lymphoma • CNS metastases
Vascular	• Subcortical infarcts • Binswanger's disease

for MS. The CSF often has a mild elevation in the protein and lymphocytes. The IgG index and oligoclonal bands (both need to be tested with serum concomitantly) are present in 70% and 90%, respectively, of clinically definite MS. False positive results occur with the IgG index in CNS infections and inflammation, but rarely with oligoclonal bands (a positive result demonstrates at least two oligoclonal bands that are not present in the serum).

Evoked potential studies (VEP, SSEP, BAER) in an attempt to demonstrate a second lesion in a clinically monophasic patient can help when the diagnosis of MS is in question. A result consistent with demyelination will show delayed conduction velocities.

KEY POINTS

1. The key to diagnosing MS is CNS demyelination disseminated in time and space and not better explained by another disease.
2. The differential diagnosis includes primarily infectious and inflammatory disorders.
3. Routine tests include screening serum tests and a brain MRI with and without gadolinium.
4. Spinal tap testing is needed when the diagnosis is not yet definitive. CSF IgG index and oligoclonal bands (paired with serum samples) are examined.

■ MANAGEMENT

Treatment of Relapses

High-dose corticosteroids shorten the clinical recovery from acute relapses within weeks. There appears to be no long-term effect of such treatment. However, one study of serial pulses of high-dose methylprednisolone over 12 months demonstrated reduced atrophy on MRI at 2 years.

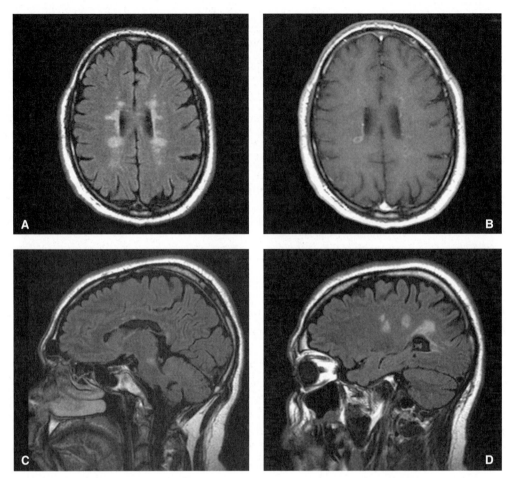

■ **FIGURE 19.1** MRI characteristics in MS. **A.** Axial FLAIR images of the brain demonstrate the classic distribution of lesions radially orientated to the ventricles (Dawson's fingers). **B.** Axial T1-weighted postcontrast images reveal annular enhancement of one such periventricular lesion. **C.** Sagittal FLAIR images are the most useful for evaluation of the corpus callosum, whose involvement is considered highly suggestive of MS. Also seen is a dorsal pontine lesion (infratentorial). **D.** An additional sagittal FLAIR image. (Courtesy of Dr. Gautam Mirchandani.)

Intravenous methylprednisolone is most often given for 4 or 5 days at 1 g per day (or 15 mg per kg per day), often followed by a 7- to 21-day prednisone taper. Some patients do not tolerate oral prednisone well and benefit from a shorter taper.

Immunomodulatory Treatment

First-line disease-modifying therapy for RRMS includes interferon beta-1a (Avonex and Rebif), interferon beta-1b (Betaseron), and glatiramer acetate (Copaxone). Clinical studies have shown that Avonex and Betaseron reduce the probability of conversion to definite multiple sclerosis (44% and 50%, respectively) over 2 years if started at the onset of a clinically isolated syndrome (CIS) or first relapse. It is important to remember that these patients initially also had at least two T2 hyperintense lesions in the white matter on brain MRI.

All four drugs have demonstrated efficacy in reducing relapses by approximately 30%. A direct comparison between Avonex and Rebif demonstrated a 10% greater reduction in relapse rate in the latter over 48 weeks. Unfortunately, there have been no double-blinded, controlled long-term studies that demonstrate a reduction in disability. Despite this, several studies have shown a reduction in disability over a couple years. Avonex has shown a 40% reduction in progression of disability over 2 years, Betaseron by almost 30% over almost 3 years, and Rebif by 30% over 2 years. The progression of disability is defined by the worsening of at least 1 EDSS point over 3 months, yet it is unclear whether this correlates with long-term disability.

Second-line treatments include pulsed intravenous steroids, intravenous immunoglobulin (IVIg), methotrexate, azathioprine, and natalizumab. All of these except natalizumab lack strong evidence-based medicine for their use. Third-line treatments include natalizumab (a monoclonal antibody against alpha-4 integrin present on lymphocytes and monocytes that binds to VCAM-1), cyclophosphamide, and mitoxantrone. Natalizumab (Tysabri) has shown a 68% reduction in relapses at 1 year and a 42% reduction in progression of disability at 2 years. Mitoxantrone (Novantrone) has demonstrated a 68% reduction in relapses over 2 years (although evaluators were not blinded) and a 64% reduction in the progression of disability. Studies involving cyclophosphamide (Cytoxan) have been conflicting. In general, it is thought that patients who respond better to chemotherapy have more frequent relapses, as opposed to a purely progressive course. It is recommended that all third-line treatments are administered with the supervision of an MS specialist.

The main side-effects of the interferons include flu-like symptoms (fever, headache, chills, and myalgias), elevated LFTs, liver failure (rarely), and hypothyroidism. As a result, LFTs should be checked monthly for several months, followed by trimonthly tests. Glatiramer acetate is associated with an unusual tight sensation in the chest, which is not associated with electrocardiographic changes. Both interferons and glatiramer acetate may produce skin rashes and, rarely, skin necrosis. Natalizumab has few side effects (headache, possibly a small increase in the risk of common infections) apart from the rare risk of hypersensitivity reactions and progressive multifocal leukoencephalopathy (PML). PML is generally a fatal disease thought to occur only in the setting of the combined use of natalizumab with interferons or immunosuppressive treatment.

Unfortunately, there is currently no Food and Drug Administration–approved treatment for PPMS. There have been uncertain minimal benefits with the use of oral azathioprine and methotrexate.

Symptom Management

Pseudo-relapses may occur in the setting of hot weather, exercise, fever, or infections. The associated worsening of symptoms will improve with antipyretic medication and treatment of the infection or cooling devices as appropriate.

There is no evidence to suggest that depression in patients with MS should be treated any differently from depression in other patients. There is one controlled study demonstrating a significant response to desipramine over 6 weeks. One study compared the efficacy of cognitive behavioral psychotherapy, sertraline, and a supportive-expressive psychotherapy group. The first two were found to be equivalent and superior to the third treatment group.

Fatigue is poorly understood, but is considered to be of various types. Fatigue can be associated with depression, somnolence, muscle fatigue, or progressive disability. It is best to characterize the type of fatigue and to choose an appropriate treatment accordingly. Commonly used options include amantadine (thought to be dopaminergic), modafinil (most effective for somnolence), and fluoxetine.

Spasticity can cause both spasms and rigidity. These can result in pain and interfere with walking, sleep, and nursing care. Treatments for spasticity include baclofen, tizanidine, dantrolene, diazepam, lorazepam, and intrathecal baclofen. The most commonly used is baclofen, and its main side effects include sedation, with a rare side effect of seizure after its abrupt discontinuation.

Most patients with MS will suffer from pain during their lifetime. More than 30% of patients will report that pain is their most significant complaint. Pain can be due to dysesthesias, muscle spasm, optic neuritis, and trigeminal neuralgia. Typical treatments include gabapentin, carbamazepine, or amitriptyline.

Oxybutynin, tolterodine, and propantheline are used for a spastic bladder. Prazosin is helpful in cases of a spastic external sphincter. In cases of dyssynergia or urinary retention, in which bladder catheterization may be required, it is best to refer the patient to a urologist.

KEY POINTS

1. First-line treatment includes interferon beta-1a (Avonex and Rebif), interferon beta-1B (Betaseron), and glatiramer acetate (Copaxone).
2. Second-line treatment includes pulsed intravenous steroids, IVIg, methotrexate, azathioprine, and natalizumab.
3. The best clinically based evidence for reducing relapses and disability is with natalizumab.
4. Third-line treatment includes mitoxantrone and cyclophosphamide.
5. Symptomatic treatment involves treating spasticity, pain, dysesthesias, fatigue, and urinary urgency, incontinence, and retention.

■ PROGNOSIS

Most patients experience complete or near-complete recovery weeks to months after a relapse.

In regard to long-term disability, prognosis is tremendously varied, but in general occurs faster in PPMS than in RRMS. As a result of the variability, median times to disability are used in population studies. Median times to DSS 3 in SPMS and PPMS are approximately 8 and 3 years, respectively. Median times to DSS 6 in SPMS and PPMS are estimated at 14 and 8 years, respectively. The known prognostic factors are extremely limited in their utility and at best can accurately predict 30% of outcomes in a computerized model. Negative prognostic factors include progressive disease, possibly being male, a higher relapse rate in the first several years, and a faster rate of disability progression in the first several years.

KEY POINTS

1. Most patients experience complete or near-complete recovery weeks to months after a relapse.
2. Predicting outcome is not reliable as clinical courses are highly variable.

■ SUMMARY

In summary, MS is an autoimmune disease with a highly variable course and few disease mimics. Treatments should be tailored to individual patients, their clinical presentation, and their symptoms. There are few highly effective treatments for MS, and the risks should be carefully balanced with the possible benefits. Many additional immunomodulatory treatments are likely to become available over the next decade, and, hopefully, some will include treatment for progressive disease, which is associated with the bulk of long-term disability.

■ SUGGESTED READINGS

CHAMPS Study Group: MRI predictors of early conversion to clinically definite MS in the CHAMPS placebo group. *Neurology* 2002;59:998–1005.

Davies G, Keir G, Thompson EJ, et al. The clinical significance of an intrathecal monoclonal immunoglobulin band: a follow-up study. *Neurology* 2003;60:1163–1166.

Dyment D, Ebers G, Sadovnick A. Genetics of multiple sclerosis. *Lancet Neurol* 2004;3:104–110.

Filippini G, Brusaferri F, Sibley WA, et al. Corticosteroids or ACTH for acute exacerbations in multiple sclerosis. *Cochrane Database Syst Rev* 2000;4:CD0001333.

Goodin D, Arnason B, Coyle P. The use of mitoxantrone (Novantrone) for the treatment of multiple sclerosis. *Neurology* 2003;61:1332–1338.

Goodin D, Frohman E, Garmany G, et al. Disease modifying therapies in multiple sclerosis: report of the Therapeutics and Technology Assessment Subcommittee of the American Academy of Neurology and the MS Council for Clinical Practice Guidelines. *Neurology* 2002;58:169–178.

Jacobs L, Beck R, Simon J, et al. Intramuscular interferon beta-1a therapy initiated during a first demyelinating event in multiple sclerosis. CHAMPS Study Group. *N Engl J Med* 2000;343:898–904.

Johnson K, Brooks B, Cohen J, et al. Copolymer 1 reduces relapse rate and improves disability in relapsing-remitting multiple sclerosis: results of a phase III multicenter, double-blind, placebo-controlled trial. *Neurology* 2001;57:S16–S24.

Kappos L, Polman CH, Freedman MS, et al. Treatment with interferon beta-1b delays conversion to clinically definite and McDonald MS in patients with clinically isolated syndromes. *Neurology* 2006;7:1242–1249.

Kappos L, Weinshenker B, Pozzilli C, et al. Interferon beta-1b in secondary progressive MS: a combined analysis of the two trials. *Neurology* 2004;63:1768–1769.

Kleinschmidt-DeMasters B, Tyler K. Progressive multifocal leukoencephalopathy complicating treatment with natalizumab and interferon beta-1a for multiple sclerosis. *N Engl J Med* 2005;353:369–374.

Korostil M, Feinstein A. Anxiety disorders and their clinical correlates in multiple sclerosis patients. *Mult Scler* 2007;13:67–72.

Kremenchutzky M, Cottrell D, Rice G, et al. The natural history of multiple sclerosis: a geographically based study. *Brain* 1999;122:1941–1950.

Kurtzke J. Rating neurologic impairment in multiple sclerosis: an expanded disability status scale (EDSS). *Neurology* 1983;33:1444–1452.

Lucchinetti C., Bruck W, Parisi J, et al. A quantitative analysis of oligodendrocytes in multiple sclerosis lesions. *Brain* 1999;122: 2279–2295.

Lucchinetti C, Bruck W, Parisi J, et al. Heterogeneity of multiple sclerosis lesions. *Ann Neurol* 2000;47:707–717.

Lynch S, Kroencke D, Denney D. The relationship between disability and depression in multiple sclerosis. *Mult Scler* 2001;7:411–416.

Munari L, Lovati R, Boiko A, et al. Therapy with glatiramer acetate for multiple sclerosis. *Cochrane Database Syst Rev* 2003;4:CD004678.

Noseworthy J, Luchinetti C, Rodriguez M, et al. Multiple sclerosis. *N Engl J Med* 2000;343:938–962.

Panitch H, Goodin D, Francis G, et al. Randomized, comparative study of interferon β-1a treatment regimens in MS: the EVIDENCE Trial. *Neurology* 2002;59:1496–1506.

Patten S, Gordon F, Luanne M, et al. The relationship between depression and interferon beta-1a therapy in patients with multiple sclerosis. *Mult Scler* 2005;11:175–181.

Polman C, O'Connor P, Havrdova E, et al. A randomized, placebo-controlled trial of natalizumab for relapsing multiple sclerosis. *N Engl J Med* 2006;354:899–910.

Polman C, Reingold S, Edan G, et al. Diagnostic criteria for multiple sclerosis: revisions to the McDonald criteria. *Ann Neurol* 2005;58:840–846.

Poser C, Paty D, Scheinberg L, et al. New diagnostic criteria for multiple sclerosis: guidelines for research protocols. *Ann Neurol* 1983;13:227–231.

Prineas J, Kwon E, Cho E, et al. Immunopathology of secondary progressive MS. *Ann Neurol* 2001;50:646–657.

PRISMS Study Group. Randomised double-blind placebo-controlled study of interferon beta-1a in relapsing/remitting multiple sclerosis. *Lancet* 1998;352:1498–1504.

Romani A, Bergamaschi R, Candelor E, et al. Fatigue in multiple sclerosis: multidimensional assessment and response to symptomatic treatment. *Mult Scler* 2004;10:462–468.

Schiffer R, Wineman N. Antidepressant pharmacotherapy of depression associated with multiple sclerosis. *Am J Psychiatry* 1990;147:1493–1497.

Swanton J, Fernando K, Dalton C, et al. Modification of MRI criteria for multiple sclerosis in patients with clinically isolated syndromes. *J Neurol Neurosurg Psychiatry* 2005;830–833.

Thomas P, Thomas S, Hillier C, et al. Psychological interventions for multiple sclerosis (review). *Cochrane Database Syst Rev* 2006;1:CD004431.

Trapp B, Peterson. J, Ransohoff R, et al. Axonal transection in the lesions of multiple sclerosis. *N Engl J Med* 1998;338:278–285.

Weinshenker B, Bass B, Rice GP, et al. The natural history of multiple sclerosis: a geographically based study. *Brain* 1989;133:1419–1428.

Weinshenker B, Rice G, Noseworthy J, et al. The natural history of multiple sclerosis: a geographically based study. *Brain* 1991;114:1045–1056.

Zivadinov R, Rudick R, De Masi R, et al. Effects of IV methylprednisolone on brain atrophy in relapsing-remitting MS. *Neurology* 2001;57:1239–1247.

CHAPTER 20

Stroke and Cerebrovascular Disorders

Sean I. Savitz

■ INTRODUCTION

Stroke results from occlusion or disruption of a blood vessel feeding the brain and has been popularly and incorrectly referred to as a cerebrovascular accident (CVA). Stroke is no more a CVA than a heart attack is a myocardial accident. Strokes present suddenly, in many cases without warning. The effects of stroke are often devastating, and for many patients stroke irrevocably changes their life. It is the leading cause of adult disability, the second cause of death worldwide, and, for certain types, a treatable condition within 3 hours of symptom onset.

■ EPIDEMIOLOGY

No one is spared from potentially having a stroke, which can occur in any age group. The incidence of stroke is higher in the older population because of accumulating and predisposing vascular risk factors over time, including hypertension, diabetes, and hypercholesterolemia. Young patients are at risk for stroke if they have cardiac abnormalities (e.g., patent foramen ovale), experience arterial dissection from trauma, or are hypercoagulable from genetic or medical disorders.

■ RISK FACTORS

The nonmodifiable risk factor for stroke is age. Modifiable risk factors are hypertension, diabetes, smoking, obesity, and increased cholesterol level.

The brain is supplied by anterior and posterior circulations. The vessels for both circulations join at the circle of Willis at the base of the brain. The anterior circulation is fed by the internal carotid arteries (ICAs), which give rise to the middle cerebral artery (MCA) and the anterior cerebral artery (ACA). The posterior circulation is composed of the vertebral arteries joining to form the basilar artery, which gives rise to the posterior cerebral arteries (PCAs) (Fig. 20.1).

There are two major types of stroke—ischemic stroke and intracerebral hemorrhage. The former accounts for 80% of all strokes and the latter for 20%. Each condition is described in detail in the following sections.

■ CEREBRAL ISCHEMIA

Ischemic stroke is classically defined as damage to the brain because of substrate (glucose) and oxygen deprivation. It is caused by either an occlusion of a large or small vessel feeding the brain or decreased cerebral arterial perfusion. The mechanism or cause of ischemic stroke can be described in four categories—embolic, atherothrombotic, small vessel, and hypoperfusion.

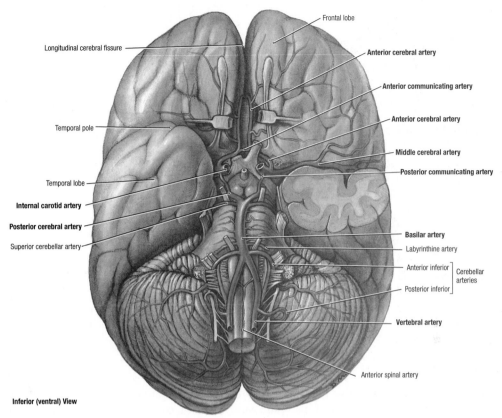

■ FIGURE 20.1 Arteries at the base of the skull (arterial circle of Willis and its branches, basilar artery), inferior (brain) view. (From Agur AMR, Dalley AF. *Grant's Atlas of Anatomy*. 12th ed. Baltimore: Lippincott Williams & Wilkins; 2008, with permission.)

Embolic Stroke

Vessel occlusions are most often due to emboli that have either formed on top of an atherosclerotic plaque or originated and traveled to a cerebral vessel from a proximal site such as the heart. Emboli stick and dock along the endothelial surface and thereby block cerebral blood flow. Figure 20.2 shows the most common origins for emboli in the cerebral circulation.

Atherothrombotic Stroke

Atherosclerosis builds along the vessel wall throughout life in the extracranial and intracranial circulation. In Western society, plaque accumulates in the extracranial carotid and vertebral arteries. Platelet-rich thrombi can form within the plaque and obstruct blood flow.

Small Vessel (Branch Artery or Penetrating Artery Disease) or Lacunar Stroke

The penetrating arteries that branch off the large cerebral vessels (Fig. 20.3) can degenerate over time, leading to distal narrowing. This may be due to chronic hypertension or atherosclerotic plaques in large parent arteries that block the orifices of the small branches. Arterial occlusion leads to small infarcts called lacunae, which is from the French term for "small lakes."

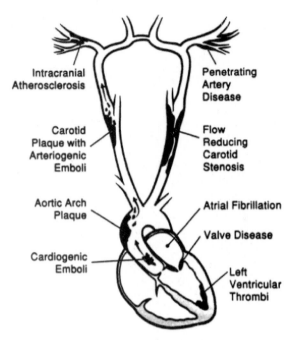

Intracranial
Atherosclerosis

Penetrating
Artery
Disease

Carotid
Plaque with
Arteriogenic
Emboli

Flow
Reducing
Carotid
Stenosis

Aortic Arch
Plaque

Atrial Fibrillation

Valve Disease

Cardiogenic
Emboli

Left
Ventricular
Thrombi

■ **FIGURE 20.2** Most common origins for emboli in the cerebral circulation. (From Albers GW, Amarenco P, Easton JD, et al. Antithrombotic and thrombolytic therapy for ischemic stroke. *Chest* 2001;119:300S–320S, with permission.)

Hypoperfusion

Low cerebral perfusion can cause global ischemia of the entire brain or focal ischemia within a tight artery feeding a specific part of the brain. Most common causes include hypotension and systemic hemorrhage.

Pathophysiology

Under ischemic conditions, neurons can no longer generate adenosine triphosphate (ATP), which leads to cell membrane failure and rises in extracellular glutamate. A complex array of interconnected signaling pathways is unleashed, termed the ischemic cascade, which ultimately leads to degeneration of brain cells. The ischemic cascade includes glutamate excitotoxicity,

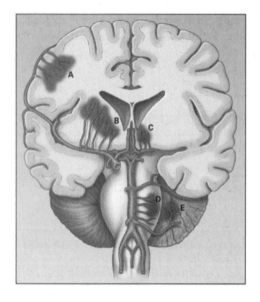

■ **FIGURE 20.3** Small vessel stroke: lacunar infarcts.

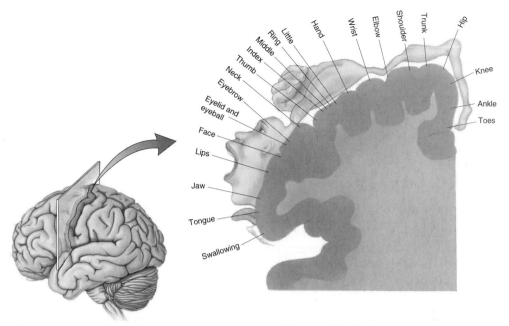

■ **FIGURE 20.4** Diagram illustrating the different kinds of deficits caused by stroke, depending on where in the brain the stroke occurs.

intracellular calcium overload, oxidative stress, apoptosis, and the inflammatory response, all of which in combination result in widespread neuronal, glial, and endothelial cell death. The entire neurovascular unit breaks down, and cerebral edema (both cytotoxic and vasogenic) soon ensues, contributing to the damage.

Clinical Stroke Syndromes

Strokes cause various deficits depending on where they occur in the brain (Fig. 20.4). Classic stroke syndromes resulting from occlusion of specific blood vessels are described in the following section.

Internal Carotid Artery

One of the most localizing signs for internal carotid artery (ICA) occlusions is transient monocular visual loss (amaurosis fugax) caused by ischemia of the retinal artery, which derives from the ophthalmic artery, a major branch of the ICA. ICA occlusions also can cause ischemia in the ipsilateral cerebral hemisphere that often mimic ischemia within the MCA territory but can also cause complete infarction of the anterior circulation, a devastating stroke that leaves the patient paralyzed on the contralateral side with hemianopsia and aphasia (if left hemisphere) or neglect (if right hemisphere).

Middle Cerebral Artery

Occlusion in the MCA typically can cause a mix of signs depending on whether the superior or inferior division of MCA or both is affected.

Signs that occur in the superior division are weakness of the face and arm and sparing of the leg, along with hemisensory loss, Broca's aphasia (if left hemisphere), and neglect (if right hemisphere).

Signs in the inferior division are contralateral visual field deficit, Wernicke's aphasia (if left hemisphere), and visuospatial impairments (if right hemisphere).

Anterior Cerebral Artery

The anterior cerebral artery is a much less common location for vascular occlusion, which causes paresis and sensory loss of the leg.

Posterior Cerebral Artery

The most common finding in the posterior cerebral artery (PCA) is hemianopsia and contralateral hemisensory loss if the thalamus is affected. Alexia without agraphia can occur in left PCA strokes.

Posterior Circulation

Lateral Medullary

Classic clinical features result from damage to the lateral medullary tegmentum and consist of vertigo, ipsilateral facial sensory changes, contralateral loss of pain and temperature sense in the body, ipsilateral Horner syndrome, and oropharyngeal paresis.

Pontine

Bilateral symptoms and signs or crossed findings (involving one side of the face and contralateral side of the body) are the rule in pontine infarcts, which are usually caused by basilar occlusions or its deep perforators feeding the brainstem.

Top of the Basilar Artery

Occlusion of the distal basilar artery causes infarction of the rostral midbrain and bilateral thalami. Clinical features include hypersomnolence, depressed level of consciousness, memory deficits, defective vertical gaze, and small, poorly reactive pupils.

Cerebellum

Ischemia in the cerebellum often causes vertigo, gait instability, headache, and vomiting. The clinical features can resemble those of inner ear disorders.

Small Artery (Lacunar Syndromes)

Lacunar strokes (Fig. 20.3) result from occlusions in the small, deep arteries branching off the large major arteries in the brain. Occlusion causes small infarcts called lacunae in the deep territories of white matter and small gray matter structures of the brain. They do not typically occur in the cortex or cerebellum. Several syndromes are described in the following section.

Pure Motor

Infarcts of the corticospinal and corticobulbar tracts may occur anywhere from the corona radiata to the medulla and occur most commonly the internal capsule and pons.

Pure Sensory

Infarcts of the sensory tracts occur in either the thalamus or the pons.

Sensorimotor

Sensorimotor infarcts produce weakness and sensory changes variably affecting the face, arm, and/or leg. These infarcts most typically occur in the corona radiata.

Ataxic Hemiparesis

Weakness and ataxia of the contralateral body are usually caused by infarcts involving the corticospinal and pontocerebellar tracts, but typically in the pons and internal capsule.

Watershed Infarcts

Watershed infarcts occur at the borderzone between two arterial territories. MCA-ACA watershed strokes cause weakness in the shoulder and hip, along with transcortical motor aphasia. MCA-PCA watershed strokes cause transcortical sensory aphasia and Balint syndrome.

■ HEMORRHAGE

Hemorrhage can occur outside of or inside the brain. Outside of the brain (extra-axial) hemorrhages occur in the epidural, subdural, and subarachnoid spaces. Hemorrhage inside the brain parenchyma is called intracerebral hemorrhage (ICH). This chapter focuses on ICH. The etiology for ICH depends on the location of the hemorrhage in the brain. Deep bleeds such as in the white matter, basal ganglia, thalamus, and pons tend to be caused by hypertension (Fig. 20.5A). Cortical lobar bleeds (Fig. 20.5B) are more likely caused by amyloid angiopathy, vascular malformations, and tumors, but there are many exceptions to this rule.

Pathophysiology

After blood vessel rupture and leakage of blood into the brain parenchyma, the hematoma can expand from continued bleeding within hours of the initial injury. Edema forms from blood-brain barrier breakdown and cytotoxic injury. The blood causes pressure effects on adjacent brain structures and can dissect through the white matter. There is also perihematomal injury caused by the release of inflammatory cytokines and free radicals, and blood products themselves are toxic to the brain.

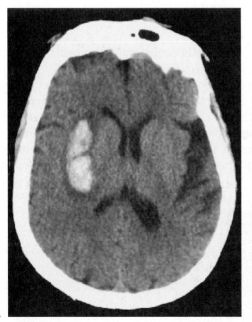
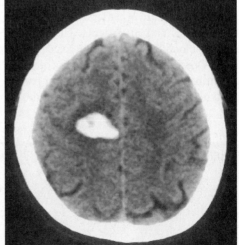

A   B

■ **FIGURE 20.5** Intracerebral hemorrhage. **(A)** Subcortical hypertensive hemorrhage. **(B)** Lobar hemorrhage resulting from cerebral amyloid angiopathy.

Diagnostic Workup

Any patient who presents with sudden focal neurological symptoms should raise concern for an acute cerebrovascular disorder—either ischemia or hemorrhage. Focal in this case implies only that the patient experiences neurological symptoms in the body. Bilateral symptoms are frequently observed in brainstem strokes, for example, as noted previously.

Ischemic Stroke

A clinical diagnosis is made by matching the signs and symptoms to a known pattern that is associated with a particular vessel occlusion (see discussion of clinical stroke syndromes).

Intracerebral Hemorrhage

ICH can mimic an acute vascular occlusion. Few clinical features can reliably distinguish the two, but progression of clinical deficits over minutes to hours might be due to hematoma expansion, whereas vascular occlusions tend to present suddenly, all at once. Specific symptoms depend on the location of the bleed. As the bleed expands, it can lead to raised intracranial pressure, which causes headache, vomiting, and depressed level of consciousness.

Imaging

All patients suspected of stroke or hemorrhage should undergo immediate neuroimaging. Although computed tomography (CT) of the head is the gold standard to visualize an ICH, it may take hours (even 24 hours in some cases) to show signs of an ischemic stroke. Magnetic resonance imaging (MRI) with diffusion weighted sequences (Fig. 20.6) is the most sensitive test available, but even this can be normal in some types of vertebrobasilar infarcts.

If an ischemic stroke is found, it is equally important to obtain vascular imaging to identify vaso-occlusive lesions in the anterior or posterior circulation. CT angiography, magnetic resonance angiography, or transcranial Doppler are the preferred noninvasive methods. Finally, perfusion studies are also available at most comprehensive stroke centers to visualize areas of the brain that are underperfused in ischemic stroke.

Other Studies

Cardiac investigations, including electrocardiography, echocardiography, and rhythm monitoring are important parts of the evaluation to search for cardiac and aortic sources of embolism, especially in patients with no cervicocranial occlusive lesions that explain the signs and symptoms and in patients with multiple brain infarcts in different vascular territories. Screening blood and coagulation tests should include a complete blood count and coagulation studies. Other tests for genetic and acquired coagulopathies and measurement of antiphospholipid antibodies may be appropriate in patients who have a history suggesting prior venous or arterial occlusions or in those in whom no cardiac, aortic, or cervicocranial lesions are found.

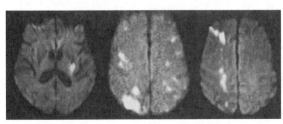

| Lacunar Infarct | Scattered Emboli | Watershed Infarct |

■ FIGURE 20.6 Diffusion imaging: acute stroke.

If hemorrhage is identified, the workup should include a search for the underlying cause. Certain locations will reveal the cause (see previous discussion). In cases in which the cause is unclear, it is important to consider vascular malformations, tumors, and drugs.

Thorough evaluation of a patient's history and findings on physical and neurological examination should always provide guidance regarding appropriate investigations to perform.

■ MANAGEMENT

Ischemic Stroke

Acute Management

Therapies for acute ischemic stroke (AIS) are driven by the concept of the ischemic penumbra—that area of the underperfused brain that is no longer functioning but is still salvageable. The only proven therapy for AIS to salvage the penumbra is reperfusion with the use of tissue plasminogen activator (tPA). A pivotal trial in 1995 showed that 11% more patients treated with intravenous t-PA had achieved full recovery with only mild or no symptoms compared with placebo. Very early therapy is best, and the longer the time from symptom onset to treatment, the less chance there is for a favorable outcome. Currently, the time window for Food and Drug Administration–approved use of t-PA is 3 hours from symptom onset, which severely limits its use. Some studies suggest that imaging can be used to select patients who might benefit from t-PA beyond 3 hours, but this remains experimental. A head CT to rule out an ICH is mandatory before administering t-PA. Various other reperfusion therapies are under investigation, including sonothrombolysis, intra-arterial delivery of lytic agents, and embolectomy. An entirely different therapeutic approach to stroke is neuroprotection, in which drugs or other therapeutic measures are delivered to the ischemic brain and directly target the signaling pathways of the ischemic cascade. This approach has undergone 20 years of testing but has not thus far been proven to enhance recovery from stroke. Hypothermia, however, is one of the most promising strategies currently under investigation.

Prevention

The best therapeutic strategy for ischemic stroke is prevention. Specific secondary prevention strategies rely on the most likely etiology of the initial stroke. Evidence from clinical studies supports the use of warfarin for cardioembolic stroke only. For other causes, such as large artery atherothrombosis, small vessel disease, and embolic stroke from a noncardiac source, antiplatelet therapy is preferable. Emerging evidence also supports using 3-hydroxy-3-methylglutaryl coenzyme A (HMG-CoA) reductase inhibitors, which are marketed to reduce low-density lipoprotein (LDL) levels, but these agents may also help reduce the risk for subsequent cerebral ischemic events and potentially enhance recovery from stroke via mechanisms independent of their effects on cholesterol. Angioplasty and stenting of large artery atherostenosis continue to be tested in clinical trials, but there are no definitive conclusions yet on their indications for stroke prevention.

Hemorrhage

There are no proven therapies for intracerebral hemorrhage. Many agents have been tested in clinical trials and all have fallen by the wayside. Steroids have no proven benefit. Factor VII recently underwent trial for its ability to retard hematoma expansion but was not shown to improve recovery. It is still under investigation as a potential treatment in those patients who show evidence for active bleeding on CT angiography. Surgical evacuation has not been shown to be superior to best medical therapy but is still an option in selected cases. Newer approaches include using lytic agents to soften clots and evacuation of deep bleeds with endovascular approaches. Strict blood pressure control is advised in patients who are recovering from ICH to reduce the probability of subsequent bleeds.

Secondary Measures

Regardless of whether a patient received acute therapy for ischemic stroke or hemorrhagic stroke, hyperglycemia and hyperthermia worsen outcome, and therefore all patients should be aggressively treated for elevated glucose and fever in the acute stages of a cerebrovascular event.

Recovery

Inpatient rehabilitation is recommended for patients who have had an ischemic stroke or hemorrhage who are too disabled to return home but can participate in therapy.

■ PROGNOSIS

Ischemic stroke has a variable prognosis depending on whether the arterial occlusion is recanalized in a timely fashion. Larger strokes with more severe deficits portend a poorer prognosis. Younger patients show remarkable tendencies to improve over older patients. Approximately 80% of patients who participate in acute rehabilitation return home.

■ SUBARACHNOID HEMORRHAGE

Brief mention is given to subarachnoid hemorrhage (Fig. 20.7), which differs in etiology and prognosis. Bleeding occurs in the subarachnoid space. Blood itself can cause vasospasm in arteries, which then lead to ischemic injury. Trauma, aneurysms, and vascular malformations are the most common causes. Patients often present with sudden severe headache (see Chapter 15) and may or may not have neurological deficits. Treatment for those patients with aneurysmal bleeds who survive and have a good prognosis include surgical clipping versus endovascular coiling.

■ CEREBRAL VENOUS THROMBOSIS

Occlusive lesions can also occur in the cerebral veins, causing cerebral venous thrombosis (Fig. 20.8) in both the sinuses and small venous deep channels. Patients with hypercoagulable states, dehydration, and trauma are at risk for venous occlusions. The treatment of choice is anticoagulation.

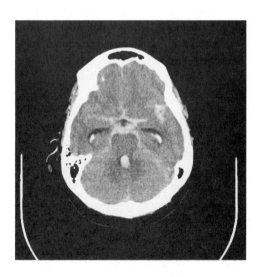

■ FIGURE 20.7 Subarachnoid hemorrhage.

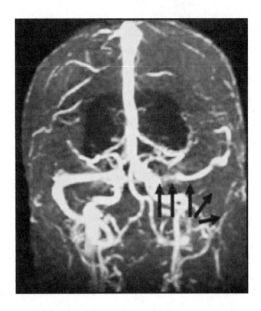

■ **FIGURE 20.8** Cerebral venous occlusion.

KEY POINTS

1. Ischemic stroke is a medical emergency, results from occlusion of a specific cerebral vessel, and causes clinical features depending on the location of the infarct in the brain.

2. The clinical features of intracerebral hemorrhage overlap with those of stroke, can progress because of hematoma expansion, and include vomiting and headache resulting from raised intracranial pressure.

3. Patients suspected of having an acute stroke need immediate evaluation, which includes ascertaining the exact time of onset of symptoms, a head CT to rule out hemorrhage, and assessment whether the patient is a candidate for thrombolytic therapy.

■ **SUGGESTED READINGS**

Caplan LR. *Caplan's Stroke: A Clinical Approach.* Worcester, Mass: Butterworth-Heinemann; 2000.

The National Institute of Neurological Disorders and Stroke rt-PA Stroke Study Group. Tissue plasminogen activator for acute ischemic stroke. *N Engl J Med* 1995;333:1581–1587.

Savitz SI, Caplan LR. Vertebrobasilar disease. *N Engl J Med* 2005;352:2618–2626.

CHAPTER 21

Sleep Disorders

Jean K. Matheson

■ INTRODUCTION

Sleep complaints accompany most psychiatric disorders. Conversely, primary sleep disorders may mimic, exacerbate, or possibly induce psychiatric disease. Sleep disorders may represent a primary disorder of mechanisms regulating sleep or failure of a specific organ system manifesting in a unique way during sleep. Sleep complaints should not be ignored or treated empirically with pharmacological agents without analysis of the etiology.

In practice, some aspects of sleep physiology can be objectively studied with polysomnography (PSG), the simultaneous recording of electroencephalographic, cardiopulmonary, and motor parameters during sleep. The classification of sleep disorders is based on both clinical and physiological criteria; the current classification of sleep disorders is outlined in the *International Classification of Sleep Disorders Diagnostic and Coding Manual* second edition (ISCD-2), a product of a task force of the American Academy of Sleep Medicine. The major diagnostic categories are outlined in Table 21.1.

■ OVERVIEW OF SLEEP

Organization of Sleep Stages

Rapid eye movement (REM) sleep, sometimes called dreaming sleep, and non-REM (NREM) sleep are the two sleep states. REM sleep alternates with NREM in recurring cycles of approximately 90 minutes. Recordings derived from electroencephalography (EEG), eye movements (electro-oculograms [EOGs]), and surface electromyography (EMG) of muscles (typically chin) are necessary to identify sleep states. NREM sleep has classically been divided into four stages (1 to 4), which represent progressive deepening of sleep. A recent revision of staging nomenclature now classifies these stages as N1, N2, and N3 (Fig. 21.1). The waking EEG in quiet wakefulness shows the characteristic alpha rhythm, a posterior predominant 8- to 13-Hz rhythm that attenuates with eye opening. Stage N1 (stage 1) is characterized by the gradual disappearance of alpha rhythms, which are replaced by 4- to 7-Hz theta rhythms and some faster activity. The emergence of sleep spindles (11- to 16-Hz sinusoidal transients lasting at least 0.5 seconds) and K complexes (negative sharp wave followed by positive component lasting ≥0.5 seconds) defines N2 (stage 2). Stages 3 and 4 are now grouped together under the term N3. N3 is characterized by high-voltage slow wave activity with frequencies of 0.5 to 2 Hz. Stage N3 is often referred to as delta sleep, slow wave sleep, or deep sleep. N3 can be characterized as "deep sleep" because subjects are difficult to arouse and typically amnestic for events that occur on arousal from this sleep stage. Although detailed narrative dreaming does not seem to occur, subjects awoken from N3 may report fragmentary dream mentation or that they were "thinking" (see parasomnias below). The normal young adult descends in an orderly progression through the three NREM stages. N3 appears approximately 30 to 40 minutes after sleep onset. The first REM period (stage R) follows this slow wave sleep, approximately 70 to 90 minutes after sleep onset.

TABLE 21.1 INTERNATIONAL CLASSIFICATION OF SLEEP DISORDERS–2 (ICSD-2) DIAGNOSTIC CATEGORIES

I.	Insomnia
II.	Sleep-Related Breathing Disorders
III.	Hypersomnias of Central Origin Not Due to a Circadian Rhythm Sleep Disorder, Sleep Related Breathing Disorder, or Other Cause of Disturbed Nocturnal Sleep
IV.	Circadian Rhythm Sleep Disorders
V.	Parasomnias
VI.	Sleep-Related Movement Disorders
VII.	Isolated Symptoms, Apparently Normal Variants, and Unresolved Issues
VIII.	Other Sleep Disorders

The PSG during REM sleep shows dramatic changes. A sudden loss of EMG activity occurs in the chin muscles, which is indicative of generalized skeletal muscle atonia. Rapid eye movements occur in phasic bursts, and the EEG shows mixed frequencies similar to those in waking and stage 1 sleep, sometimes with a characteristic "saw tooth" pattern.

The first REM period is short, lasting about 10 minutes. The end of the first REM period completes the first sleep cycle. Thereafter, NREM sleep continues to alternate with REM sleep; the healthy adult goes through 4 to 6 cycles (Fig. 21.2).

Sleep architecture is the organization of sleep stages and cycles. The normal young adult spends approximately 5% of the night in stage N1, 50% to 55% in stage N2, 20% in N3, and 20% to 25% in REM. N3 is concentrated in the first third of the night, whereas REM episodes become progressively longer later in the night. N3 decreases as a function of age, whereas REM remains fairly constant after early childhood. Of the newborn's daily 17 to 18 hours of sleep, 50% is REM. Children and early adolescents sleep 10 to 11 hours. Most adults prefer to sleep 7.5 to 8.5 hours. Subjects sleep-restricted to 6 hours show cognitive deficits that are cumulative. Deprivation of REM sleep by medication, sleep disruption, or sleep deprivation results in REM rebound when the cause of the deprivation is removed. Sleep deprivation also induces N3 rebound sleep during recovery sleep.

Sleep Stages

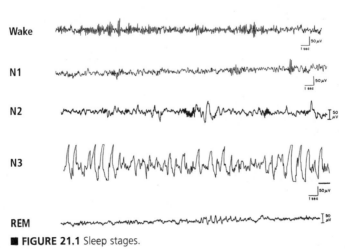

■ **FIGURE 21.1** Sleep stages.

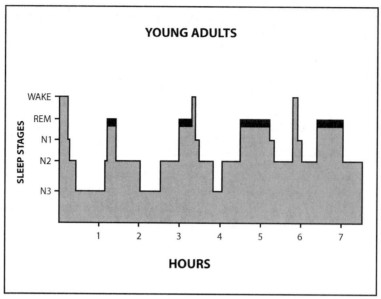

REM and NREM sleep differ physiologically. REM sleep is characterized by both phasic and tonic changes in physiology. The drop in baseline EMG correlates with a tonic change. Rapid eye movements correlate with phasic changes. Tonic physiological changes also include impaired thermoregulation, reduction in ventilatory chemosensitivity, hypotension, bradycardia, increased cerebral blood flow and intracranial pressure, increased respiratory rate, and penile erection. Phasic changes include vasoconstriction, increased blood pressure, tachycardia, and further increases in cerebral blood flow and respiratory rate. During NREM sleep, the physiological state is more stable, with an overall reduction in blood pressure, heart rate, cardiac output, and ventilation. One characteristic feature of N3 is the secretion of growth hormone.

Some disorders are exacerbated by or occur only during certain sleep stages. Sleepwalking, for example, occurs with arousal from NREM, usually N3 sleep. Epileptic seizures tend to be facilitated by NREM sleep but inhibited by REM sleep. Obstructive sleep apnea is typically worse in REM sleep because of REM atonia and decreased respiratory chemosensitivity.

KEY POINTS

1. REM alternates with NREM sleep in cycles of approximately 90 minutes.
2. REM sleep accounts for approximately 20% to 25% of total sleep after infancy.
3. REM sleep is characterized by rapid eye movements, muscle atonia, and detailed narrative dreaming.
4. NREM stage N3 is termed slow wave sleep or deep sleep, decreases with age, and is prominent at the beginning of the night.

■ NEUROBIOLOGY OF SLEEP

There are two sleep drives, one homeostatic (called process S) and the other circadian (process C). A homeostatic drive increases with time spent awake, and the circadian drive is under the influence of the suprachiasmatic nucleus (SCN) of the hypothalamus (see later discussion).

Sleep and wake states represent a complex interaction between wake-promoting arousal and sleep-promoting networks. The ascending arousal system comprises discrete cell groups and their projecting axons originating in brainstem, hypothalamus, and basal forebrain. Neurons of the ventrolateral preoptic nucleus (VLPO) of the hypothalamus are sleep active and sleep promoting and innervate wake-promoting areas, including the neurons of the posterolateral hypothalamus, histaminergic neurons of the tubomammillary nucleus, dopaminergic neurons of the ventral tegmental area, the serotonergic dorsal raphe, norepinephrine-containing neurons of the locus ceruleus, and the cholinergic neurons of the dorsal midbrain and pons. In turn, monoaminergic and cholinergic wake-promoting areas inhibit VLPO, thereby resulting in reciprocal inhibitory relationships that self-reinforce stable periods of sleep and wake. In this model, homeostatic and circadian drives are hypothesized to shift the balance between states by still unknown mechanisms. Adenosine, which accumulates during wakefulness, and whose effect is antagonized by caffeine, may be one of the factors that signals the homeostatic drive to sleep by inhibiting cholinergic arousal systems and activating VLPO. Indirect circadian input into VLPO has been documented.

Brainstem generation of REM sleep is under the influence of the hypothalamus. REM sleep is inhibited by hypocretin-containing cells of the posterior hypothalamus; these cells are lost in narcolepsy.

KEY POINTS

1. The ascending arousal system includes discrete cells groups and their projections originating in brainstem, hypothalamus, and basal forebrain.
2. The most important neurotransmitters within this system include acetylcholine, histamine, hypocretin (orexin) norepinephrine, and dopamine.
3. The VLPO is sleep active and sleep promoting. Activation of VLPO inhibits arousal systems, reducing thalamic transmission of sensory information and allowing sleep to occur.
4. Conversely, wake-promoting areas inhibit VLPO. By virtue of this mutually inhibitory circuit, sleep and wake are self-reinforcing.
5. External circadian and homeostatic influences are thought to shift the balance from stable wake to stable sleep.

■ CIRCADIAN RHYMICITY

Circadian rhythmicity of multiple physiological and behavioral variables, with a period close to 24 hours, is seen in almost all living organisms, even in the absence of environmental cues. Sleep, cortisol secretion, core body temperature, and melatonin secretion by the pineal gland are examples of these rhythms. This internal rhythmicity has long suggested an endogenous clock that can be synchronized by external cues, especially light. The hypothalamic SCN, which receives direct and indirect input from the retinohypothalmic tract, is the major anatomical location of this circadian pacemaker. Intrinsically photosensitive retinal ganglion cells contain the light-sensitive pigment melanopsin, depolarize maximally in response to blue light, and provide the major input into SCN. Rods and cones contribute, but are not required for photic influence of SCN. Melatonin and core body temperature are both good markers of circadian timing (phase) of the SCN. Melatonin levels measured in constant dim light are low during the day; begin to increase in the evening, approximating dusk; are maximal during the night; and abruptly decline in the morning near dawn. Melatonin is secreted by the pineal under the direct influence of the SCN through a circuitous pathway from the hypothalamus to the intermediolateral cell column of the spinal cord, to the superior sympathetic ganglion and finally the pineal. Light serves to activate SCN and immediately turn off melatonin production.

A circadian temperature nadir approximately 2 to 3 hours before a subject's usual awakening is assigned by convention—circadian time zero, which also correlates with peak melatonin levels. Appropriately timed light exposure can shift the phase of the endogenous melatonin and core body temperature rhythm within 2 to 3 days. By way of a feedback loop involving melatonin receptors on the SCN, appropriately timed melatonin can also shift circadian rhythms. Light in the evening delays rhythms, and light in the morning induces phase advances; conversely, melatonin in the afternoon or evening advances rhythms and morning melatonin results in delay. These effects have important clinical implication, as described in the section on circadian disorders. The phase response curve for light, which indicates the degree and direction of phase change at any given time in the circadian day, is well established, but the phase response curve for melatonin is still not completely resolved. The period of the human circadian pacemaker is approximately 24.2 hours.

KEY POINTS

1. The SCN of the hypothalamus is the anatomical location of the circadian pacemaker.
2. The human circadian period is approximately 24.2 hours.
3. Circadian phase is strongly influenced by light via retinohypothalmic tract input into the SCN. Melatonin and body temperature rhythms are markers of underlying circadian phase.
4. Melatonin production is strongly inhibited by light.
5. Light and melatonin are both capable of inducing shifts in circadian phase.

■ SLEEP CLINICAL NEUROPHYSIOLOGY

Polysomnography

PSG is the term applied to the simultaneous and continuous measurement of multiple physiological parameters during sleep. In practice, the term PSG has come to mean a specific type of polysomnographic study in which measurements allow for the identification of sleep stage, monitoring of cardiopulmonary function, and monitoring of body movements during sleep. This study is typically obtained at night in a sleep laboratory for the purpose of identifying, as best as possible given the novel environment, the patient's typical sleep and its associated pathologies. The multiple sleep latency test (MSLT) and the maintenance of wakefulness test (MWT) are more limited daytime sleep studies that are useful in the evaluation of narcolepsy and other causes of daytime sleepiness. The MSLT measures the tendency to fall asleep during the day and screens for the occurrence of inappropriate daytime episodes of REM sleep during multiple daytime naps. The MWT is the inverse of the MSLT and measures the ability to stay awake in multiple daytime naps. Parameters recorded in standard PSG, MSLT, and MWT are indicated in Table 21.2.

The American Academy of Sleep Medicine (AASM) has developed guidelines for the indication for polysomnography. These indications include the following:

1. Suspicion of sleep-related breathing disorders
2. Treatment and follow-up of sleep-related breathing disorders
3. In combination with the MSLT for suspected narcolepsy or idiopathic hypersomnia
4. Evaluation of sleep-related behaviors that are violent, potentially injurious, or do not respond to conventional therapy
5. To assist in the diagnosis of paroxysmal arousals that are suggestive of seizure disorder (with additional video and EEG
6. Evaluation of sleep-related movement disorders.

TABLE 21.2 POLYSOMNOGRAPHY

TEST	PARAMETERS RECORDED
PSG	EEG (F4-M1, C4-M1, O2-M1) Additional EEG if indicated Electro-oculogram (EOG) (eye movement) Electromyography (EMG) (chin) Airflow Respiratory effort Oxygen saturation Electrocardiogram (ECG) EMG limb, anterior tibialis muscles; extensor digitorum muscles when indicated Body position Esophageal pH (rarely)
MSLT and MWT	EEG (F4-M1, C4-M1, O2-M1) EOG (eye movement) EMG (chin) ECG Optional: Respiratory monitoring

F4, C4, O2 refer to frontal, central, and occipital EEG leads, respectively, according to the International 10–20 System; M1 refers to a mastoid reference.

Because sleep-related breathing disorders can have broad clinical presentations and implications, PSG may be indicated in many clinical situations, including congestive heart failure, arrhythmia, coronary artery disease, stroke, hypertension, pulmonary disease, neuromuscular disease, headache, and gastroesophageal reflux. Although PSG is not routinely indicated for the evaluation of chronic insomnias, a history suggestive of a contributing sleep disorder, especially sleep-related breathing or movement disorder, does support the use of PSG. On the other hand, despite research interest in the changes in sleep associated with depression, PSG is not indicated for the primary purpose of establishing a diagnosis of depression because there are no abnormalities of sleep architecture specific to that diagnosis.

Sleep Architecture

A timeline of sleep stages during the night is reported as a hypnogram (Fig. 21.2). Quantitative analysis also includes a number of variables (Table 21.3). Sleep architecture may be distorted by specific disorders and is commonly disturbed by medications (Table 21.4).

Respiratory Measures

The recording of airflow, respiratory effort, and oxygen saturation allows for the determination of abnormal breathing patterns during sleep. These abnormalities underlie the sleep-related breathing disorders. A variety of abnormal breathing events exist, including the following:

Apnea: The absence of airflow for at least 10 seconds. There are three types:
  Obstructive apnea: At least 90% reduction in airflow for at least 10 seconds with evidence of persistent respiratory effort (Fig. 21.3)
  Central apnea: At least 90% reduction in airflow for 10 seconds without evidence of any respiratory effort (Fig. 21.4)
  Mixed apnea: At least 90% reduction in airflow for 10 seconds with initial absence of effort followed by a return of respiratory effort before resumption of airflow.

TABLE 21.3 SLEEP ARCHITECTURE PARAMETERS

VARIABLE	ABBREVIATION	DEFINITION	COMMENTS
Time in bed	TIB	The time from lights out until the subject chooses to end the study.	Excessive time in bed may exacerbate insomnias; common in old age.
Total sleep time	TST	Total time the subject actually slept.	Varies with age: Adult: 7–9 hr Children (5–12): 9–11 hr; (0–2 mo): 10.5–18 hr.
Sleep efficiency index	SE	TST/TIB. Often reported as a percentage. This is an important measure of sleep quality.	Age dependent; average normal adult 85% to 95%; <85% suggests sleep disruption. High efficiency may indicate prior sleep deprivation. Decreases with excessive time in bed, increased wake during sleep or prolonged latency.
Percentage of each stage		This may be reported as a percentage of the TIB or the TST.	Varies with; age approximate; young adult: 5% stage N1, 50% to 55% stage N2, 20%, stage N3, 20% to 25% stage REM.
Sleep onset latency	SL	Time from lights out until the onset of sleep. Sleep onset is usually defined as the onset to the first epoch of any sleep stage. Sometimes reported as latency to 3 epochs of stage one or one epoch of any other sleep stage (unequivocal sleep).	Less than 20 minutes; prolonged in insomnias and delayed sleep phase.
Number of awakenings		Records the number of times the subject returns to stage wake after sleep onset.	Occasional awakenings are common; increased awakenings occur in association with disorders causing arousal.
Number of arousals		Records the number of EEG arousals. Arousal defined as 3 seconds with increased EEG frequency above baseline without awakening.	Increased in disorders such as sleep apnea and periodic limb movements.
REM latency		Reports time from sleep onset to first REM period.	Average 90 minutes in adults. Lower latencies are reported in depression but are nonspecific. Many drugs prolong REM latencies. REM rebound shortens latency.

EEG, electroencephalogram; REM, rapid eye movement.

TABLE 21.4 MEDICATION EFFECTS ON THE POLYSOMNOGRAM

DRUGS	SWS	REM	MISCELLANEOUS
TCAs	⇔	⇓⇓⇓	
SSRIs and SNRIs	⇔?	⇓	SSRIs and SNRIs ⇑ non-REM slow eye movements
Nefazodone	⇔	⇑	
Trazodone	⇑⇔	⇔⇓⇑	
Bupropion	⇔	⇑	NE and DA uptake inhibitor
Mirtazapine	⇔	⇔	
MAOIs	⇔	⇓⇓⇓	
Lithium	⇑⇔	⇓	
BZDs	⇓	⇔⇓	⇑ Spindle activity and stage 2
Zolpidem	⇔	⇔	
Dopaminergic drugs	?	?	Mixed results
Anticonvulsants			Minimal data
Phenytoin	⇑	?	
Carbamazepine	⇑	⇓	
Tiagabine	⇑	⇔	
Gabapentin	⇑	⇑⇔	
Lipophilic beta-blockers	⇓	⇓	
Clonidine	?	⇓	
Opioids	⇓	⇓	Can ⇓ respiratory drive
Amphetamines	⇔⇓	⇓	
Caffeine	⇓	?	Adenosine antagonist Adenosine ⇑ SWS
Alcohol (acute)	⇑	⇓	After the metabolism of alcohol there is a REM rebound, often in second half of night Chronic use ⇓ SWS and REM
Sodium oxybate (GHB)	⇑	⇑⇓	Approved for cataplexy and EDS

BZDs, benzodiazepines; DA, dopamine agonist; EDS, excessive daytime sleepiness; GHB, gamma hydroxybutyrate; NE, norepinephrine; REM, rapid eye movement; SNRIs, selective norepinephrine reuptake inhibitors; SSRIs, selective serotonin reuptake inhibitors; SWS, short wave sleep; TCA, tricyclic antidepressants.

Hypopnea: Abnormal respiratory event lasting at least 10 seconds with at least a 30% reduction in thoracoabdominal movement or airflow compared to baseline and with at least a 4% oxygen desaturation (Fig. 21.5)

Respiratory effort–related arousal (RERA): When airway resistance increases, oxygen saturation and airflow may stay the same as respiratory effort increases to overcome the obstruction. The result of increased respiratory effort may be an arousal that disturbs sleep. These abnormalities are termed RERAs.

Limb Electromyography

Surface recording from the anterior tibialis muscles of the legs identifies body movements and, especially, periodic limb movements, brief bursts of activity 0.5 to 10 seconds in duration that occur in a series of at least four movements. These leg jerks may or may not disrupt sleep.

Obstructive Apnea

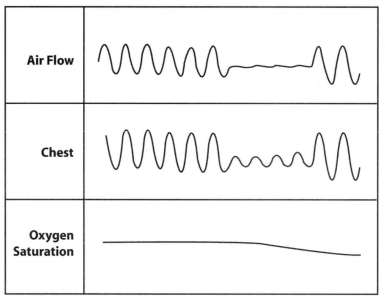

■ **FIGURE 21.3** Obstructive sleep apnea.

Central Apnea

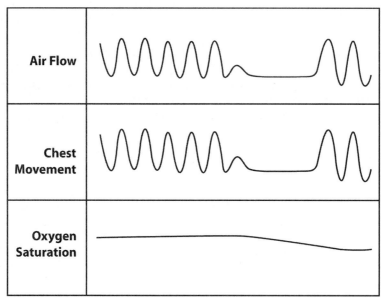

■ **FIGURE 21.4** Central apnea.

Hypopnea

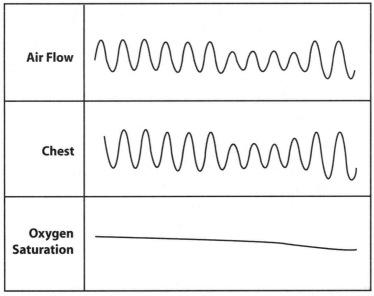

■ **FIGURE 21.5** Hypopnea.

KEY POINTS

1. PSG is the term used for the measurement of multiple physiological measurements during sleep. The usual measurements provide information about sleep stage, respiration, heart rhythm, and leg movements.
2. PSG is the gold standard for the diagnosis of sleep-related breathing disorders, hypersomnias, violent parasomnias, and movement disorders.
3. PSG is not recommended as a diagnostic tool to aid in the diagnosis of depression or other mental illnesses
4. The MSLT and MWT are daytime nap studies used to measure sleepiness and the ability to stay awake during the day, respectively.

■ SLEEP DISORDERS

Insomnias

ISCD-2 specifies general criteria for insomnia with 11 subtypes (Table 21.5). The ISCD general criteria include the following:

A. A complaint of difficulty initiating sleep, maintaining sleep, or waking up too early or sleep that is chronically nonrestorative or poor in quality. In children the sleep difficulty is usually reported by the caretaker and may consist of bedtime resistance or inability to sleep independently.
B. The above difficulty occurs despite adequate opportunity and circumstances of sleep.
C. At least one of the following forms of daytime impairment related to the nighttime sleep difficulty is reported by the patient:
   i. Fatigue or malaise
   ii. Attention, concentration, or memory impairment
   iii. Social or vocational dysfunction or poor school performance

TABLE 21.5 ICSD INSOMNIA CLASSIFICATION
Adjustment insomnia
Psychophysiological insomnia
Paradoxical insomnia
Idiopathic insomnia
Insomnia due to mental disorder
Inadequate sleep hygiene
Behavioral insomnia of childhood
Insomnia due to drug or substance
Insomnia due to medical condition
Insomnia not due to substance or known physiological condition, unspecified (nonorganic insomnia (NOS)
Physiological (organic) insomnia, unspecified

   iv. Mood disturbance or irritability
    v. Daytime sleepiness
   vi. Motivation, energy, or initiative reduction
  vii. Proneness for errors or accidents at work or while driving
 viii. Tension headaches or gastrointestinal symptoms in response to sleep loss
   ix. Concerns or worries about sleep

Adjustment Insomnia

Adjustment insomnia refers to an insomnia that occurs in association with an identifiable stressor lasting less than 3 months.

Psychophysiological Insomnia

In psychophysiological insomnia, patients usually do not have evidence of underlying psychiatric disease, but are highly focused on their insomnia. Overconcern with the process of going to sleep is alerting, induces increased tension, and becomes a sleep-preventing association. The precipitant for this disorder may be an adjustment insomnia. A characteristic pattern emerges: inability to obtain satisfactory sleep for a few nights induces fear that another sleepless night will follow. Patients report that they feel alert as soon as they try to initiate sleep. They toss and turn, watch the clock, and become frustrated that they are unable to sleep. Patients may exhibit anxiety, but the anxiety relates only to sleep and is not generalized. Typically, sleep is better in an environment other than home. The diagnostic criteria require a duration of at least a month.

Paradoxical Insomnia

Paradoxical insomnia was previously termed "sleep state misperception" and sometimes called pseudo-insomnia. In this disorder, patients complain of nearly absent sleep but PSG study does not show objective evidence of the same. This disorder is not a form of malingering. Typically the patient remains convinced that little or no sleep has been obtained, despite the evidence to the contrary on PSG. A clinical clue is the absence of prominent daytime dysfunction, despite the severity of the patient's reported insomnia. Most patients have been treated unsuccessfully and inappropriately with hypnotics for years before the diagnosis is entertained. The underlying mechanism is not understood, but it has been suggested that these patients are hypervigilant, as evidenced by higher frequencies intermixed in the sleep EEG.

Idiopathic Insomnia

Idiopathic insomnia is a chronic insomnia with onset in childhood and of unknown cause, with a persistent course without periods of remission. In contrast to "short sleepers," those who may report a lifelong ability to function well with short sleep durations, those with idiopathic insomnia experience distress and dysfunction consistent with the diagnostic criteria of insomnia.

Insomnia Resulting from a Mental Condition

Insomnia resulting from a mental condition is a category that encompasses the insomnias that occur in association with diagnoses that satisfy mental disorders by DSM criteria. The ISCD-2 diagnostic criteria require that the insomnia is "more prominent than typically associated with the mental disorder as indicated by causing marked distress or an independent focus of treatment." Marked inability to sleep associated with the sense of decreased need to sleep is particularly characteristic of mania and may be prodromic to the full presentation of a manic episode. Schizophrenia also induces prominent insomnia that may precede the onset of psychotic symptoms. Unipolar depression is classically associated with early morning awakening, but that pattern should not be taken as unique to that disorder; sleep disruption is particularly evident at the end of the night in many sleep disorders, especially sleep breathing disorders and advanced sleep phase disorder (see later discussion). Anxiety secondary to inability to sleep should not be confused with the disrupted sleep that may occur in primary anxiety disorders.

Fatal Familial Insomnia

Fatal familial insomnia is a rare disorder caused by a mutation of the prion protein gene *PRNP* located on chromosome 20 in association with a methionine polymorphism at codon 129 of the same gene. The disorder is either familial or sporadic. Patients present with insomnia that is progressive in severity and eventually associated with dream enactment, autonomic hyperactivity, myoclonus, tremor, and cardiac and respiratory dysfunction. The sleep EEG shows loss of sleep spindles, loss of slow wave sleep, and abnormal REM sleep. Pathology shows neuronal loss, with gliosis of the anterior and dorsomedial thalamic nuclei and inferior olives, sometimes with spongiform changes in the cortex. There are deposits of prion proteins in gray matter. Like other prion diseases, the disorder may be transmitted by intracerebral inoculation of brain in experimental animals. The disorder is invariably fatal.

Diagnosis

A careful history is the most important tool. Exploring the patient's day-to-day activities in an orderly fashion is particularly revealing. The schedule of daily activities gives insight into the patient's personality and discloses habits such as alcohol or caffeine use that contribute to poor sleep hygiene. Attention should be directed to the contribution of underlying medical illnesses and medications.

Sleep logs produced by the patient are important in identifying patterns. Occasionally, objective evidence is obtained from actigraphy, in which a device worn by the patient to record body movements over days, enabling by inference the subject's rest-activity cycle. Polysomnograms are obtained when disorders that cause arousals and awakening such as sleep apnea or periodic movements in sleep are suspected.

Treatment

Treatment of the underlying disorder is the first approach. In many cases, history and appropriate studies will identify other treatable sleep disorders, such as circadian rhythm disorders, sleep breathing disorders, and restless legs syndrome; contributing medical illnesses; or exacerbating medications. Even with effective treatment of the underlying etiology, however, insomnia may be self-perpetuating and require directed therapy.

TABLE 21.6 COGNITIVE BEHAVIORAL TECHNIQUES

THERAPY	DESCRIPTION
Stimulus control therapy	A set of instructions designed to reassociate the bed and bedroom with sleep and to reestablish a consistent sleep-wake schedule: (a) Go to bed only when sleepy; (b) get out of bed when unable to sleep; (c) use the bed and bedroom for sleep only (no reading, watching TV, etc.); (d) arise at the same time every morning; (e) no napping.
Sleep restriction therapy	A method designed to curtail time in bed to the actual amount of sleep time. For example, if a patient reports sleeping an average of 6 hours per night, of 8 hours spent in bed, the initial recommended sleep window (from lights out to final arising time) would be restricted to 6 hours. Periodic adjustments in this sleep window are made contingent on sleep efficiency until optimal sleep duration is reached.
Relaxation therapy	Clinical procedures aimed at reducing somatic tension (e.g., progressive muscle relaxation, autogenic training) or intrusive thoughts at bedtime (e.g., imagery training, meditation) interfering with sleep.
Cognitive therapy	Psychological methods aimed at challenging and changing misconceptions about sleep and faulty beliefs about insomnia and its perceived daytime consequences. Other cognitive procedures may include paradoxical intention or methods aimed at reducing or preventing excessive monitoring of and worrying about insomnia and its correlates/consequences.
Sleep hygiene education	General guidelines about health practices (e.g., diet, exercise, substance use) and environmental factors (e.g., light, noise, temperature) that promote or interfere with sleep. This may also include some basic information about normal sleep and changes in sleep patterns with aging.
Cognitive behavior therapy	A combination of any of the above behavioral (e.g., stimulus control, sleep restriction, relaxation) and cognitive procedures.

From Morin CM, Bootzin RR, Buysse DJ, et al. Psychological and behavioral treatment of insomnia: update of the recent evidence (1998–2004). *Sleep* 2006;29:1398–1414, with permission.

The treatment of insomnia includes cognitive-behavioral approaches, hypnotic medications, or a combination of the two approaches. Cognitive-behavioral therapy (CBT) for sleep disorders includes specific techniques (Table 21.6). Randomized controlled studies comparing CBT with hypnotic use (benzodiazepines and nonbenzodiazepine benzodiazepine agonists) have shown that CBT results in better long-term efficacy, even in the elderly.

Hypnotics: Medications approved for treatment of insomnia include benzodiazepines, nonbenzodiazepine receptor agonists, and one melatonin agonist (Table 21.7). Off-label use of sedating antidepressant medications is common, but there are few objective data to support or refute this practice. Whereas benzodiazepine medications bind to widely distributed benzodiazepine receptors (located on the gamma-aminobutyric acid [GABA]-A receptor complex), nonbenzodiazepine benzodiazepine receptor agonists show more selective binding to subsets of benzodiazepine receptors. Zolpidem and zaleplon are known to bind primarily to GABA receptors with an alpha-1 subunit (GABA A1a receptor). The exact binding of eszopiclone is unknown. As a result of this selectivity the nonbenzodiazepine benzodiazepine drugs are less anxiolytic and have fewer myorelaxant and anticonvulsant properties. Important side effects of all benzodiazepine receptor agonists include anterograde amnesia and cerebellar dysfunction that may be manifest as an acute or chronic gait abnormality. It is important to recognize that side effects may strongly correlate with half-life of medications. Drugs with a longer half-life are more likely to induce next-day effects and accumulate, depending on the frequency of dosing. Drugs with a short half-life may wear off too rapidly and result in awakenings during the night. Rebound

TABLE 21.7 HYPNOTICS

MEDICATION	APPROX ONSET OF ACTION	HALF-LIFE
Benzodiazepines, FDA approved as hypnotics		
Flurazepam (Dalmane)	15–45 min	50–120 hr (metabolite)
Quazepam (Doral)	20–45 min	15–120 hr (metabolite)
Estazolam (Prosom)	15–30 min	8–24 hr
Temazepam (Restoril)	45–60 min	4–20 hr
Triazolam (Halcion)	2–30 min	1.5–6 hr
Nonbenzodiazepine benzodiazepine agonists, FDA approved as hypnotics		
Eszopiclone (Lunesta)	≤30 min	5.5–8 hr
Zolpidem (Ambien CR) (bilayer preparation with biphasic release)	≤30 min	Same as zolpidem; but delayed release of second dose
Zolpidem (Ambien)	≤30min	1.5–4.5 hr
Melatonin agonist FDA approved as hypnotic		
Ramelteon (Rozerem)	30 min	1–5 hr (metabolite)

FDA, Food and Drug Administration.

insomnia refers to the phenomenon of insomnia that is worse than baseline, usually lasting 1 to 2 days, following abrupt discontinuation of a hypnotic agent. Withdrawal may also occur, characterized by the appearance of two or more symptoms not present before initiation of the drug, typically including autonomic hyperactivity, restlessness, nervousness, nausea, and muscle tension lasting more than 1 or 2 days. Withdrawal seizures may occur.

Ramelteon is the only Food and Drug Administration (FDA)-approved hypnotic that is not a benzodiazepine receptor agonist. This drug is a melatonin agonist for the human melatonin receptors, MT1 and MT2, which act on the SCN of the hypothalamus. The potency of this drug is much higher than that of over-the-counter melatonin at both receptor types. This drug is not a scheduled drug and has no abuse potential. It has been demonstrated to have a modest effect on sleep initiation but not maintenance. Melatonin receptor agonists have side effects, including elevation of prolactin and depression of testosterone.

All sedative hypnotic drugs now carry an FDA warning concerning the possibility of the development of complex behaviors with amnesia for those behaviors while taking the medication. Sleep driving, that is, driving while apparently still asleep and under the influence of the medication, and sleep eating have been described. These drugs also carry a warning of the possibility of anaphylaxis.

Sedating antidepressant medications have a variety of side effects that should be clearly understood before being prescribed. Anticholinergic symptoms with orthostatic intolerance may be particularly troubling with evening administration in elderly patients.

KEY POINTS

1. A careful history with attention to habits, schedules, and contributing medical and psychiatric disease is the most important diagnostic tool.
2. PSG is primarily employed when there is a suspicion of an underlying sleep disorder, such as sleep apnea or periodic leg movements.
3. The identification of specific insomnia subtypes strongly guides therapy.
4. CBT techniques have been shown to be more effective that hypnotic therapy.

■ SLEEP-RELATED BREATHING DISORDERS

Respiration is abnormal during sleep. PSG is a necessary test in the diagnosis and management of these disorders. Disorders in this classification include central sleep apnea, obstructive sleep apnea, and sleep-related hypoventilation syndromes.

Patients with sleep-related breathing disorders may present with a wide variety of complaints, including daytime sleepiness, insomnia, inattentiveness, cognitive decline, loud snoring, nocturnal gasping, witnessed apneas, nocturnal chest pain, nonrestorative sleep, and morning headaches. Commonly, the behavioral manifestations of sleep-disordered breathing are mistaken for depression.

Obstructive sleep apnea syndromes are characterized by airway obstruction with persistent respiratory effort manifest as obstructive apneas, hypopneas, or RERAs.

Central sleep apnea syndromes are characterized by episodes of decreased respiratory effort that are either cyclic or intermittent, usually with overt central apneas.

Sleep-related hypoventilation syndromes include several disorders that are either primary or secondary to other medical conditions that are associated with sleep-induced or sleep-exacerbated hypoxia and/or hypercarbia, such as chronic obstructive pulmonary disease (COPD) or neuromuscular weakness.

Although PSG in each of these disorders is distinctive, respiratory events of any type tend to fragment sleep. PSG evidence of sleep fragmentation includes increased N1 sleep, delayed REM latency, decreased REM and N3 sleep, increased arousals, increased awakenings, and decreased sleep efficiency. Sleep latency may be prolonged.

Most patients with sleep-disordered breathing have obstructive sleep apnea caused by repetitive collapse at the level of the pharynx, usually at the soft palate or posterior to the base of the tongue. The mechanism of collapse is complex. Sleep relaxes upper airway dilator muscles and impairs reflexes that are critical to maintaining airway patency against the negative pressures induced by the chest wall muscles. Anatomical narrowing because of tonsils, low soft palate, macroglossia, vascular congestion, fat, or structural abnormalities such as micrognathia predisposes to collapse. Dilator muscle activity is inhibited by alcohol and sedating drugs, especially benzodiazepines. Conditions that induce pharyngeal motor or sensory impairment such as myasthenia, muscular dystrophy, stroke, and other brainstem disorders can be predisposing factors. Any cause of increased airway resistance, such as nasal congestion, may induce a compensatory increase in negative pressure in the thorax that promotes further narrowing of the flexible upper airway above. Nocturnal hypoxia exacerbates ischemic heart disease and promotes the development of pulmonary hypertension. Obstructive sleep apnea is known to be associated with excessive daytime sleepiness and the development of hypertension. Increasing evidence shows that sleep apnea has an important influence on insulin resistance, nocturnal arrhythmia, especially atrial fibrillation, stroke, coronary artery disease, and seizure control in patients with epilepsy.

Central sleep apnea syndromes are a manifestation of several forms of respiratory pathophysiology. Episodes may be categorized as those occurring in association with normocapnia or hypocapnia. Normocapnia or hypocapnic central episodes include Cheyne-Stokes breathing, idiopathic central apnea, and high-altitude periodic breathing. These disorders follow from the fact that control of breathing is highly dependent on the chemical responses to PCO_2 and to a lesser extent PO_2. The set point for response to PCO_2 increases variably at the transition to sleep, meaning that a higher PCO_2 is tolerated. If the patient's PCO_2 is below this sleep set point, apnea follows until the PCO_2 rises. Hypoxia or transient wakefulness induced by apnea can transiently increase PCO_2 responsiveness, inducing a brief period of hyperventilation and a PCO_2 that again falls below threshold for values during sleep, continuing the cycle.

Cheyne-Stokes breathing is the most common form of central sleep apnea and is characterized by a waxing and waning respiratory pattern with central apneas and/or hypopneas alternating with periods of hyperpnea. This pattern is particularly characteristic of congestive heart failure, but is also seen in central nervous system (CNS) disease and renal failure. Arousals are prominent during the peak of the hyperpnea, often inducing insomnia. Opioid use is an important cause of central sleep apnea because of centrally mediated respiratory depression. Long-acting opioids such as methadone are particularly implicated. Central apnea associated with hypercarbia is a form of hypoventilation. Bilateral medullary lesions from tumor or infarct, syringobulbia, and surgical cordotomy represent lesions in the pathways involved in automatic breathing that are known to induce this type of central apnea. Central sleep apnea and hypoventilation may also be seen in neuromuscular disease, such as phrenic nerve paralysis, myopathies, and motor neuron disease. The mechanism in these diseases of peripheral neuromuscular disease represents more than end organ failure and is not well understood.

In all of these settings, periods of central apnea also predispose to obstruction. In part, the obstruction occurs because absence of airflow contributes to airway collapse. Combined episodes of central and obstructive apneas are mixed apneas. The coexistence of obstructive, central, and mixed apneas in the same patient is common.

Sleep-related hypoventilation secondary to obesity, with the resultant restriction of chest wall movement, is common and is often seen in association with obstructive sleep apnea. Neuromuscular disorders such as muscular dystrophy and amyotropic lateral sclerosis (ALS) similarly result in hypoventilation because of mechanical dysfunction of breathing. In some neurological disease, such as myotonic dystrophy, there is also abnormality of central chemosensitivity driving respiration. COPD and parenchymal lung disease are also causes of sleep-exacerbated hypoventilation.

Diagnosis

Diagnosis of sleep-disordered breathing begins with an appreciation for the high prevalence of risk factors and wide spectrum of presenting symptoms attributable to these disorders. Excessive daytime sleepiness accompanied by loud snoring are classic symptoms and strong predictors, especially in obese patients. However, there are many risk factors in a general patient population of normal weight, including nasal obstruction secondary to seasonal allergies, septal deviation, retrognathia, high arched palate, macroglossia, long neck, hypothyroidism, pregnancy, menopause, congestive heart failure, pulmonary disease, stroke, and degenerative neurological diseases, among others. Risk increases with age. In a middle-aged population the prevalence of at least mild sleep-disordered breathing, based on a large epidemiological study, is 9% of women and 24% of men. In psychiatric practice, patients may present with insomnia, nonspecific fatigue, lack of initiative, inattention, forgetfulness, and mood disorders.

The gold standard for the diagnosis of sleep-disordered breathing is PSG.

The ISCD-2 provides diagnostic criteria for each of the sleep-related breathing disorders, and the reader is referred to that source for detailed diagnostic criteria.

The diagnosis of obstructive sleep apnea requires either 5 obstructive events per hour, including apneas, hypopneas, or RERAs, with symptoms of one of the following: excessive daytime sleepiness, fatigue, insomnia, unrefreshing sleep, gasping or choking, witnessed apneas or loud snoring; or 15 obstructive events. Primary central sleep apnea requires 5 central apneas per hour of sleep, with one of the following: excessive daytime sleepiness, frequent arousals or awakenings or insomnia, or awakening short of breath. Cheyne-Stokes breathing pattern requires 10 central apneas or hypopneas per hour of sleep with a crescendo-descrescendo pattern accompanied by arousals. Sleep-related hypoventilation syndromes require either evidence of sleep-related elevation of carbon dioxide or oxygen desaturation below 90% for a least 5 minutes, with a nadir of at least 85% and not explained by discrete apneas or hypopneas,

Treatment

Nasal continuous positive airway pressure (CPAP) is the mainstay of treatment for obstructive sleep apnea and for some patients with predominantly central apnea. Airway pressure acts as a pneumatic splint to maintain upper airway patency during sleep. Its effectiveness in central sleep apnea is not well understood, but many of these patients have some component of obstruction that exacerbates the tendency to breathe periodically. Bilevel positive pressure is often better tolerated than CPAP and allows for independent manipulation of inspiratory and expiratory pressures. The prescribed difference between inspiratory and expiratory pressures provides "pressure support" that can be used to increase ventilation in hypoventilation syndromes. Some bilevel devices provide a timed back-up respiratory rate to treat central apneas. New devices based on similar bilevel positive pressure technology automatically detect and respond to changes in airflow or ventilation, thereby functioning as servo-ventilators. These devices are used to treat patients with central or combined central and obstructive sleep-disordered breathing, including Cheyne-Stokes respirations. Oxygen alone is sometimes effective for patients with primarily Cheyne-Stokes respirations. When upper airway anatomical abnormalities are present, surgical correction is considered based on the patient's age, response to positive pressure, and complexity of surgery. Tonsillectomy is an established treatment in children with tonsillar hypertrophy.

KEY POINTS

1. There are three major types of sleep-related breathing disorders: obstructive sleep apnea, central sleep apnea, and sleep-related hypoventilation.
2. All of these disorders induce sleep disruption and important physiological changes that affect multiple organs systems. Patients classically present with excessive daytime sleepiness, but may also display a wide variety of physical and behavioral symptoms, including depression and irritability.
3. Diagnosis is based on PSG.
4. The mainstay of treatment is positive pressure, which can be delivered with a device based on continuous and bilevel technologies.

■ HYPERSOMNIAS OF CENTRAL ORIGIN

Hypersomnias of central origin refer to a group of disorders that result in excessive daytime sleepiness but are not caused by disturbed nocturnal sleep or disorders of circadian rhythms. Excessive daytime sleepiness is defined as the inability to stay awake and alert during the major waking episodes of the day, resulting in unintended lapses into drowsiness or sleep. Patients with these disorders may or may not demonstrate excessive sleep during a 24-hour period.

Narcolepsy

Narcolepsy is the most important and common disorder within the classification of hypersomnias of central origin, with a prevalence of 0.02% to 0.18% in the United States. Onset is usually between the ages of 15 and 25 years and very rarely below the age of 5. Narcolepsy is now classified as narcolepsy with cataplexy, narcolepsy without cataplexy, and narcolepsy secondary to a medical condition. The last is rare. Cataplexy refers to episodes of muscle weakness associated with strong emotion, often laughter. These episodes are typically brief, often involve the knees or face, and are unassociated with a change of consciousness, although sleep sometimes follows immediately. Cataplexy is pathognomonic of narcolepsy, but need not be present. Other common features of narcolepsy include hallucinations at sleep onset (hypnagogic hallucinations), sleep paralysis, inattentive automatic behavior, and poorly maintained nocturnal sleep. Most of the characteristic symptoms of the disorder appear to reflect a disorder of the control mechanisms that regulate REM sleep. Episodes of REM occur at the wrong time, intruding on wakefulness, and the physiological components of REM sleep dissociate and appear independently. Cataplexy and sleep paralysis, for example, are manifestations of the muscle atonia of REM sleep appearing during wakefulness. Recent discoveries strongly suggest that narcolepsy is caused by the loss of hypothalamic neurons containing the neuropeptide hypocretin-1.

Diagnosis

In the past, neurophysiological testing with both the PSG and MSLT provided the only confirmatory evidence for the diagnosis of narcolepsy with and without cataplexy. Using these neurophysiological techniques, the diagnosis of narcolepsy requires a PSG demonstrating 6 hours of sleep, absence of another sleep disorder that could account for symptom and followed the next day by an MSLT that demonstrates REM sleep in at least two naps, and a mean sleep latency across naps of 8 minutes or less. Cataplexy is pathognomonic for narcolepsy with cataplexy; thus unequivocal cataplexy may be used as a sole diagnostic criterion. The MSLT is not valid in the presence of CNS drugs. New diagnostic guidelines include the option of obtaining cerebrospinal hypocretin-1, an assay that can be obtained by sending the sample to specialized centers. Approximately 90% of patients who demonstrate cataplexy have low hypocretin levels; only 10% to 20% of patients classified as having narcolepsy without cataplexy show low hypocretin levels. This study is primarily used in patients with equivocal neurophysiological testing and equivocal cataplexy.

Many patients who carry the diagnosis of narcolepsy without cataplexy are likely to have been misdiagnosed and have another sleep disorder. Narcolepsy resulting from a medical condition, also referred to as symptomatic narcolepsy or secondary narcolepsy, is usually associated with pathology of the hypothalamus and may also result in low hypocretin levels. Although this presentation is rare, a variety of disease processes have been identified in these patients, including tumors, cerebral infarct, sarcoidosis, Neiman-Pick type C, multiple sclerosis, disseminated encephalomyelitis, and paraneoplastic syndromes.

Treatment

The goal of treatment in narcolepsy is to reduce daytime sleepiness to allow a normal level of functioning. Pharmacologic treatment is almost always necessary. Some patients require treatment for both excessive sleepiness and cataplexy; for others, cataplexy is so mild that targeted treatment is unnecessary. The first-line treatment for excessive daytime sleepiness is modafinil, a novel wake-promoting medication with minimal cardiovascular stimulating effects and long half-life, but little disruption of nocturnal sleep. It has no effect on cataplexy. Modafinil renders hormonal birth control unreliable, which can limit its use in young women. Stimulant medications, including methylphenidate and amphetamines, have a long track record in the treatment of narcoleptic excessive daytime sleepiness, are currently less expensive, and can decrease the frequency of cataplexy.

Amphetamines and methylphenidate have side effects consistent with their sympathomimetic properties, including sinus tachycardia and hypertension. Both drugs have abuse potential and can induce toxic psychosis when used in excess. Abuse in the narcoleptic population, however, is rare. Patients generally adopt a fixed dosage schedule in the range of 10 to 60 mg a day using a combination of both long- and short-acting preparations.

Traditionally, cataplexy has been treated with antidepressant medications that demonstrate reuptake inhibition of norepinephrine and serotonin. Tricyclic antidepressants, selective serotonin reuptake inhibitors (SSRIs), and venlafaxine are effective anti-cataplectic medications. Sedating antidepressants such as clomipramine can be given before nocturnal sleep with carryover efficacy during the day.

Sodium oxybate, also known as gamma-hydroxybutyrate (GHB), is approved for both cataplexy and excessive daytime sleepiness; it may have a synergistic effect with modafinil. This drug is a potent CNS depressant whose mechanism of action in narcolepsy and cataplexy is unknown. Sodium oxybate is administered before sleep and again during the night during a planned nocturnal awakening, inducing increased amounts of stage N3 sleep. The drug can be markedly effective in patients with severe cataplexy. Respiratory depression, sodium overload, sleep walking, confusional episodes, and enuresis are important side effects.

Behaviorally, patients can be taught to plan naps during the day—"strategic naps" that decrease episodes of inadvertent sleep and sleepiness, resulting in lower medication requirements. Some patients use only strategic napping, especially during pregnancy, to avoid the use of medications.

Idiopathic Hypersomnia

If no other condition can be identified that explains excessive daytime sleepiness, the diagnosis of idiopathic hypersomnia is applied.

Diagnosis

PSG studies and careful medical, neurological, and psychiatric assessment are particularly important in these disorders to exclude subtle or occult abnormalities. On careful analysis, many of these patients show subtle sleep-disordered breathing that may not be evident with less sensitive recording techniques. Brain magnetic resonance imaging (MRI) is appropriate. The ISCD-2 now classifies these patients as having idiopathic hypersomnia with prolonged sleep time or idiopathic hypersomnia without prolonged sleep times. Prolonged sleep time is defined for this purpose as a usual sleep time of greater than 10 hours.

Treatment

Once underlying contributors are excluded and treated, hypersomnia is treated symptomatically with either the wake-promoting drug modafinil or stimulants, including amphetamines and methylphenidate.

Recurrent Hypersomnia

Recurrent hypersomnia refers to disorders in which episodes of hypersomnia are episodic recurrent and typically eventually resolve over time. There are two syndromes in this category: *Kleine-Levin* and *menstrual-related hypersomnia*. Kleine-Levin, although rare, is well described, but the literature on menstrual-related hypersomnia is limited. Kleine-Levin syndrome is characterized by recurrent episodes of hypersomnia with characteristic behavioral changes, including irritability, inattentiveness, confusion, lack of concern for personal hygiene, hypersexuality, and hyperphagia. Some or all of these behavioral symptoms may be present. Episodes last days or weeks, followed by a return to normal levels of functioning. Diagnostic criteria require that the episodes occur at least once a year. Onset is typically in adolescence, and the male to female ratio is 4:1. The etiology is unknown, but hypothalamic dysfunction of unknown cause and type is theorized. Episodes typically become less frequent and resolve after adolescence.

Menstrual-related hypersomnia is a disorder in which episodes of sleepiness occur approximately a week before the menstrual cycle and resolve with menses. These patients often present soon after menarche. The presumed hormonal mechanisms have not been identified.

Diagnosis

The diagnoses of both Kleine-Levin and menstrual-related sleep disorders are based on the characteristic clinical presentations and the exclusion of other CNS disorders. A careful neurological investigation includes at least MRI and EEG; spinal tap may be indicated. Endocrinological screening is appropriate and is expected to be normal in these syndromes. Recurrent sleepiness may be seen in bipolar disease and seasonal affective disorder. Other primary disorders contributing to sleepiness should be considered and are usually evaluated by polysomnography and MSLT.

Treatment

Multiple medications have been tried for Kleine-Levin for both the behavioral changes and sleepiness. Only amphetamines have proven effective for sleepiness. Lithium has been reported to be effective in reducing relapses in some patients. Antidepressants, anticonvulsants, and antipsychotic medications have not been effective.

Menstrual-related hypersomnia is reported to improve with oral contraceptive use.

KEY POINTS

1. The most important hypersomnia of central origin is narcolepsy. Narcolepsy with cataplexy and narcolepsy without cataplexy are categorized as separate disorders. The narcolepsies are not rare, typically presenting in adolescence and young adulthood.
2. Narcolepsy with cataplexy and some cases of narcolepsy without cataplexy are associated with loss of hypothalmic neurons containing hypocretin (orexin). The etiology of the neuronal loss is unknown.
3. The diagnosis of narcolepsy requires either the presence of unequivocal cataplexy or testing that includes a PSG followed by an MSLT, the latter demonstrating a short mean sleep latency and at least two sleep-onset REM periods.
4. Idiopathic hypersomnia is a diagnosis of exclusion.
5. Kleine-Levin and menstrual-related hypersomnias are rare, clinically unique disorders that are episodic and likely secondary to hypothalamic dysfunction.

■ SLEEP-RELATED MOVEMENT DISORDERS

Sleep-related movement disorders include conditions in which simple stereotyped movements are present during sleep and induce sleep disruption. Difficulty initiating and/or maintaining sleep are the typical complaints. Although these movements could be considered a parasomnia, a separate classification is used for these simple motor behaviors.

Periodic Limb Movement Disorder

Periodic limb movement disorder (PLMD) is the most prevalent of these disorders and is characterized by periods of repetitive stereotyped leg movements that disturb sleep (periodic leg movements [PLMs]). The leg movements are similar to the triple flexion response of the Babinski reflex, but arm movements may also occur. Occasionally, PLMs appear in the presence of evidence of upper motor neuron disease or degenerative neurological disease, consistent with activation of the triple flexion response during sleep. Other types of leg movements may be present without periodicity or without sleep disruption, or they may be secondary to other primary sleep disorders, in which case the term PLMs is not appropriate. Leg movements, for example, frequently accompany arousals from sleep-disordered breathing. Many medications are implicated in the induction of periodic and aperiodic leg movements, most commonly SSRIs and tricyclic antidepressants.

Restless Legs Syndrome

Restless legs syndrome (RLS) is a disorder characterized specifically by an urge to move accompanied by uncomfortable sensations, predominantly in the legs, that is worse when sedentary, relieved by movement, and maximal in the evening. This syndrome is closely associated with PLMD because 80% to 90% of patients with this disorder have PLMs. Some of these patients also demonstrate PLMs while awake (PLMW). RLS, however, is a syndrome based on clinical, not PSG, criteria. The disorder is familial in 50% of cases. Abnormalities of both dopamine and iron metabolism are implicated in the underlying pathophysiology.

Diagnosis

PLMs are often found incidentally on sleep studies and are not generally treated unless accompanied by symptomatic restless legs or clearly contributing to arousals and awakenings. Occasionally, sleep studies are ordered specifically to try to identify the presence of PLMs as a sleep disruptor contributing to insomnia. Diagnosis requires an index of at least 15 events per hour, with evidence of a sleep complaint. RLS, on the other hand, is a purely clinical diagnosis based on the criteria noted above. The workup and treatment of PLMs are essentially the same as for RLS.

Iron studies, including serum ferritin, should be checked in all patients. A screening neurological examination is appropriate. Many clinicians recommend screening for other treatable neuropathies, such as B_{12} deficiency and diabetes.

Treatment

Iron replacement is recommended for patients with ferritin values below 45 to 50 mcg/mL. Response to iron replacement may not occur in all patients and usually takes months to years; some clinicians advocate intravenous replacement if there is severe iron deficiency. Because antidepressants, especially SSRIs and serotonin-norepinephrine reuptake inhibitors (SNRIs), and antihistamines may exacerbate restless legs, these drugs should be avoided if possible. Dopaminergic agonist drugs in low doses, usually only at night, are the mainstay of treatment. Ropinirole and pramipexole are both FDA approved for RLS. Although dosage may be titrated upward every 2 to 3 days, it is best to use as low a dose as possible. Levodopa was initially thought to be a promising drug in the treatment of both RLS and PLMs, but its use is limited by the fact that many patients develop a syndrome of augmentation. After a period of improvement, patients with restless legs who are taking levodopa often develop symptoms earlier in the day, with increasing severity and further exacerbated by dosage increases. Levodopa should be avoided for daily restless legs treatment, but some clinicians advise occasional use when rapid onset is desired. Augmentation may also occur with dopaminergic agonists, but less frequently and usually at the higher end of the dosage spectrum. Gabapentin and low-dose opioids are useful second-line drugs that can be used alone or in combination with dopaminergic agonists for dosage sparing. Benzodiazepine medications, such as clonazepam, once the mainstay of treatment in the 1980s now tend to be third-line drugs because of limited efficacy and the development of tolerance.

KEY POINTS

1. RLS is a distinct clinical disorder that is diagnosed by clinical history alone.
2. Periodic limb movements (PLMs) usually accompany RLS but also occur independently or with other sleep disorders and may not be symptomatic.
3. Iron deficiency, metabolic disorders, and peripheral neuropathy are important causes. RLS and PLMD are exacerbated by antidepressant medications, especially SNRIs and SSRIs.

■ CIRCADIAN RHYTHM SLEEP DISORDERS

Sleep and wake propensity have circadian rhythms controlled by the SCN of the hypothalamus (see earlier discussion). When there is either intrinsic abnormality of these rhythms or misalignment in relationship to sleep and wake behaviors because of external factors, sleep becomes disrupted and the patient is said to have a circadian rhythm disorder. Typically there are consequences during wake attributable to poor sleep quality and disruption of organ system physiology under circadian influence, such as in the gastrointestinal tract. Social and occupational impairment may be prominent. If sleep complaints are not subjected to analysis in a circadian framework, the symptoms are often misinterpreted as insomnia and treated inappropriately. Both light therapy and melatonin together or independently can be used to shift and stabilize rhythms in these disorders as described in the following section.

Advanced Sleep Phase Syndrome

Advanced sleep phase syndrome is a disorder in which the patient habitually falls asleep earlier than the desired clock time, resulting in early evening sleepiness and early awakening. Patients may not recognize the shift because of evening dozing while reading or watching TV and instead complain of early morning awakening. In rodents, insects, and fungi, mutations that alter the length of the circadian period lead to advances or delays in daily rhythms. A recent report of a family with autosomal dominant advanced phase syndrome led to the discovery of a single point mutation in the human homolog (*hPer2*) of the *Drosophila* clock gene *Per2*. Advanced sleep phase disorder is commonly seen in the elderly, and it has been postulated that the circadian period may shorten with age, but shortening of the period with normal aging has not been demonstrated. Patients can be treated with progressive delay of bedtime or with bright-light therapy in the evening. Although melatonin administration in the morning has theoretical appeal, effective treatment paradigms have not yet been established.

Delayed Sleep Phase Syndrome

Delayed sleep phase syndrome is a disorder in which patients habitually adopt a late bedtime and then wake late in the day. The amount of sleep and its quality are normal. The patient is symptomatic when attempts to advance the bedtime to an earlier hour fail. These patients appear to be less able to advance their circadian rhythms to reset the body's natural tendency to delay endogenous rhythms or to compensate for occasional schedule changes. In addition, there is evidence that these patients tend to sleep at a later time in their circadian phase. Adolescents show a propensity to phase delay that appears to be developmentally mediated. Environmental exposure to light can be an important contributor. Light in the evening, including exposure to reading lights and computer screens, causes rhythms to delay. Light in the morning, timed to occur at the end of the patient's habitual sleep period, serves to advance endogenous rhythms and allow for earlier sleep onset. Bright-light therapy with commercially available light boxes is the most effective treatment for delayed sleep phase, but attention to ambient light exposure is appropriate as initial therapy unless rapid treatment is necessary. Timing of light exposure is critical. In a patient with phase delay the body's temperature minimum, a marker of endogenous circadian time, is shifted later in terms of clock time and may, for example, occur in the middle of the morning hours. Inadvertent or inappropriately prescribed exposure to light before this temperature minimum will delay rather than advance rhythms. Thus patients cannot be simply advised to increase light exposure in the morning. Properly timed melatonin administered 1.5 to 6 hours before bedtime has also been shown to be a useful therapy.

A sleep log is a helpful tool to plot the patient's endogenous schedule, to plan appropriate light or melatonin therapy. Time of habitual nonforced awakening is a more reliable measure of phase than bedtime.

Time Zone Change (Jet Lag) Syndrome

Time zone change (jet lag) syndrome is a temporary circadian disorder induced by transmeridian jet travel across two or more time zones.

Shift Work Sleep Disorder

Shift work sleep disorder refers to inability to initiate and maintain sleep or excessive daytime sleepiness in the context of nonstandard work schedules, which include night, early morning, rotating, and intermittent schedules. As in other circadian rhythm disorders, malaise and somatic complaints are common. Inattentiveness while working or driving home adds significant risk. Entrainment to a fixed shift is impaired because most workers do not maintain their work schedule on days off and because ambient light exposure during commuting is usually inappropriate for entrainment to the work schedule. Bright light exposure during night shifts has been shown to be beneficial, combined with light restriction in the morning. Melatonin or a hypnotic drug before daytime sleep is acceptable. Modafinil, a wake-promoting drug, is FDA approved to enhance alertness during night shift work.

Free-Running Type

The free-running type is characterized by what appears to be an erratic sleep-wake cycle. Sleep logs demonstrate, however, that there is a non–24-hour (instead, slightly longer) periodicity in the sleep-wake cycle. This disorder mimics the prolongation of the sleep cycle that can be seen in experimental environments in which subjects are isolated from time cues and are said to be "free-running." Most patients with this disorder are blind and lack the retinohypothalamic input into the SCN. Not all blind patients are impaired, however, because a nonvisual photic pathway to the SCN exists via intrinsically photosensitive retinal ganglion cells in the retina (see earlier discussion). Rarely, sighted patients develop this syndrome, usually associated with psychiatric disorders resulting in social isolation. In blind patients, melatonin at bedtime can entrain rhythms. In sighted patients, enforced sleep scheduling, appropriate light exposure, and melatonin are all appropriate.

Irregular Sleep-Wake Pattern

Irregular sleep-wake pattern is manifest as an irregular sleep-wake cycle that is erratic, without evidence of a well-defined circadian rhythm. Unlike patients with free-running disorder, sleep logs reveal no underlying periodicity. This disorder usually occurs in patients with developmental or degenerative abnormalities of the brain, especially dementias. Patients complain of fatigue, insomnia, and/or excessive daytime sleepiness. Neither sleep nor wakefulness is well maintained. This disorder is treated with external reinforcement of a normal sleep-wake cycle and daytime bright-light exposure. Melatonin has been tried, with variable results showing some efficacy in children with developmental abnormalities but not in elderly demented patients.

Diagnosis

Circadian rhythm disorders are diagnosed on the basis of history, sleep logs, and, if available, actigraphy. The circadian phase is best estimated by the usual wake-up time. Measurements of salivary melatonin are available but are rarely used clinically to help identify circadian rhythms.

Treatment

Treatment guidelines for each of the circadian disorders is discussed in the previous sections. In general, circadian rhythm disorders can be influenced or treated by light.

An underlying phase-response curve to light is known; the effect of light in advancing or delaying rhythms depends on underlying circadian time. A daily temperature minimum 2 to 3 hours before habitual awakening is termed circadian time zero. Light before this minimum will delay rhythms, and light after this minimum will advance rhythms (there is a cross-over point that defines "before" and "after" at 0 plus or minus 12 hours.) In circadian rhythm disorders it is important to try to identify the probable time of the temperature minimum so that light exposure does not inadvertently shift the patient in the wrong direction. The phase-response curve to melatonin is not as well established as that for light. In general, melatonin can be thought of as the inverse of light: melatonin before sleep induces phase advance, and melatonin after the usual wake time induces phase delay.

KEY POINTS

1. The misalignment of circadian rhythms with sleep-wake behaviors result in circadian rhythm disorders.
2. The cause may be intrinsic, as in dementia, or extrinsic, as in jet lag.
3. History, sleep logs, and actigraphy help distinguish these disorders from other sleep disorders.
4. Treatment strategies with scheduling, timed light, and/or melatonin are helpful.

■ PARASOMNIAS

Parasomnias are undesirable physical events that occur as the individual transitions to sleep, during sleep, or on arousal from sleep. These phenomena are usually sleep stage specific.

Disorders of Arousal

Disorders of arousal refers to behaviors characterized by confusion and automatic behavior following sudden arousal from NREM, usually stage N3, sleep. Behaviors are typically goal oriented, but show lack of judgment and occur without awareness of conscious control. The basic instinctual drives of self-protection, aggression, eating, and sex are dominant themes. Arousal from slow wave sleep (stage N3) in both normal individuals and to an exaggerated extent in patients with this disorder are associated with the following:

- Body movements
- Autonomic activation
- Mental confusion and disorientation
- Automatic behavior
- Relative nonreactivity to external stimuli
- Poor response to efforts to provoke behavioral wakefulness
- Amnesia for many intercurrent events
- Fragmentary recall of dream-like mentation

The tendency to arouse spontaneously from NREM sleep tends to be a familial trait, with first presentation in childhood and resolution by adolescence. However, episodes may occur for the first time or recur with greater severity in adolescence or adulthood. Stress, sleep deprivation, and any factors that may contribute to either sleep disruption or excessive slow wave sleep can exacerbate the problem. Sleep apnea and alcohol are frequent causes of adult recurrence. Occasionally, seizure activity may induce the arousal. There is a long-standing debate as to the contribution of emotional factors. Anxiety, depression, and obsessive-compulsive personality may be overrepresented in this patient population.

Sleep Terrors

Sleep terrors are characterized by a sudden arousal from NREM, usually stage N3, sleep with a piercing scream or cry, accompanied by automatic and behavioral manifestations of intense fear. Typically, the individual arouses within the first 2 hours of sleep, sits bolt upright, and screams. Marked tachycardia, mydriasis, and sweating may be evident. The subject is agitated, confused, and difficult to console or arouse fully. Dream recall is not detailed, but a single terrifying image, such as a demon, insect, or intruder, may be reported. Generally, sleep is resumed in a few minutes with amnesia for the entire event.

Sleepwalking

Sleepwalking refers to of a variety of complex behaviors that are initiated during arousals from NREM, usually stage N3, sleep. Sleepwalkers characteristically arouse during the first third of the night from slow wave sleep, leave the bed in a confused state, and perform complex, automatic acts. Some episodes of sleepwalking are initiated by sleep terror, in which case the behaviors exhibited may be violent and directed toward the bed partner as the subject tries to combat a perceived threat. More routine behaviors, such as eating and urinating, may be performed in a remarkably stereotyped fashion idiosyncratic to the subject. The patient may awaken during the behavior embarrassed and bewildered. Most often the patient returns to bed and has no memory of the episode. Patients are at risk of injuring themselves and their bed partners. The typical inability to awaken the patient fully and stop the behaviors is particularly frightening and dangerous to the bed partner. Attacks specifically directed to the bed partner or inappropriate sexual activity ("sexsomnia") raise difficult forensic issues. It is thought that murders have been committed in this context. Care must be taken to secure the sleep environment to prevent falling from heights and leaving the home. Occasionally, dangerous objects, such as knives and guns, need to be made inaccessible.

Confusional Arousal

Confusional arousal consists of confusion during and following arousal from sleep, most typically from slow wave sleep (stage N3) in the first part of the night but also occurring on awakening in the morning. These episodes are most commonly seen in forced arousals from sleep, particularly in individuals with a family or personal history of sleepwalking or sleeptalking and in children under the age of 5. Amnesia for the events during the arousal is typical. This is predominantly a problem for individuals such as physicians, who are called at night and must react appropriately.

Diagnosis

Occasional parasomnic episodes, with typical family and personal histories, need not require further evaluation. The distinction between these disorders and a REM-related nightmare (see later discussion) can usually be made on the basis of history. In the latter the patient can recount detailed dream activity, whereas in the disorders of arousal, only fragmentary images or fears are recalled. Motoric activity associated with detailed dream recall indicates REM behavior disorder (see later discussion) rather than sleepwalking. Atypical features, especially with recurrent stereotypic behaviors suggest nocturnal seizure.

PSG study with additional EEG derivations and video, as well as routine awake and asleep EEGs, are recommended in patients with violent behavior, frequent disruptive episodes, or atypical clinical features. Routine PSG is indicated for patients with coexistent excessive daytime sleepiness. PSG may confirm sudden arousal from delta sleep, even in the absence of an episode; some sleep laboratories induce arousal with a buzzer to precipitate the clinical syndrome. More importantly, PSG may identify another cause of arousal, such as sleep apnea, that precipitates the behavior in the predisposed patient. Seizure activity, although not frequent, may induce arousal, or seizure itself may mimic the clinical syndrome.

Treatment

The first line of treatment is removal of the possible underlying precipitants of arousal or delta sleep (N3) rebound or both. Improved sleep hygiene helps, with avoidance of sleep deprivation, irregular sleep-wake cycles, caffeine, and alcohol. Stress reduction by relaxation techniques appears to be useful. Hypnosis has been tried with success. Coincident sleep apnea should be treated, even if not severe. The mainstay of treatment for recurrent injurious or disruptive episodes is clonazepam, given before sleep. Many patients use the medication intermittently in settings that are dangerous, embarrassing, or known to precipitate their episodes. Clonazepam and other benzodiazepines appear to increase the arousal threshold and decrease stage N3 sleep.

Rapid Eye Movement Behavior Disorder

The low muscle tone characteristic of REM sleep correlates with the normal paralysis that occurs during dreaming. This temporary paralysis, termed REM sleep atonia, prevents the dreaming subject from enacting dreams motorically. In contrast, REM behavior disorder (RBD) is characterized by incomplete REM sleep atonia. As a result, patients are able to enact dreams without awakening from REM and commit stereotyped motor behaviors, such as reaching, running, and attacking. Dream content incorporates these behaviors. Typically the patient, bed partner, or caretaker complains of violent motoric activity during sleep or the recent onset of nightmares. Sometimes the patient is able to incorporate ongoing conversation and activity into the dream, giving rise to the misperception that he is confused or hallucinating, until he suddenly awakens and appears to "clear" his mental status. Hospital caretakers usually dismiss even detailed dreaming reports as confusion, or "sundowning." Patients are frequently incorrectly diagnosed as having posttraumatic stress disorder. RBD occurs most frequently in older men, with a mean age of 60.

RBD often precedes other clinical signs or symptoms of some degenerative diseases, especially Parkinson's disease, Lewy body dementia, and multisystem atrophy (the "synucleinopathies") by years. The combination of degenerative dementia and RBD is highly correlated with the diagnosis of Lewy body disease, based on clinical and pathological criteria. Medications, especially SNRIs, SSRIs, and tricyclic antidepressants are known to precipitate and exacerbate RBD.

Diagnosis

A careful clinical history is often strongly suggestive of RBD, particularly in patients with synucleinopathies. Recent diagnostic guidelines, however, require lack of normal REM atonia documented on PSG or EEG, a characteristic history of dream enactment behavior or witnessed behaviors during REM sleep, and absence of REM-related seizure activity. RBD is frequently misdiagnosed as posttraumatic stress disorder or "sundowning."

Treatment

For unclear reasons, RBD is remarkably responsive to clonazepam. Although the PSG changes persist, phasic increases in EMG tone and behaviors are markedly attenuated with doses of 0.5 to 2 mg; the effect is long-lasting. There are two small studies showing some efficacy of pramipexole, but, surprisingly, dopaminergic agonists and L-dopa are not very effective in this disorder. There are some limited data that suggest that melatonin is effective at doses of 3 to 12 mg.

Antidepressant medications, especially SSRIs and SNRIs, are known to precipitate and exacerbate RBD; these medications should be discontinued if possible.

Treatment of underlying causes of sleep disturbance such as sleep apnea is also helpful, and it is prudent to identify the degree of sleep-disordered breathing present before escalating the clonazepam dosage. Ensuring safety of the sleeping environment is critical.

Nightmare Disorder

In contrast to sleep terrors and other disorders of arousal, nightmares occur almost always in REM sleep. Unlike in sleep terrors, in which amnesia or only fragmentary recall is typical, patients with nightmare disorder usually wake with clear mentation and detailed recall. Nightmares are also distinguished from sleep terrors by timing during the sleep period. Because REM is more prominent in the second half of the night, episodes more commonly occur then. Sleep terrors on the other hand occur when slow wave sleep is more abundant, in the first third of the night.

Nightmare disorder is associated with a wide range of psychiatric disorders, most prominently posttraumatic stress disorder. However, many drugs used for both psychiatric and nonpsychiatric disorders are implicated, including antihypertensives, especially lipophilic beta-blockers, dopaminergic agonists, and antidepressants. When REM sleep is inhibited by drugs, such as antidepressants, REM rebound occurs after the drug is discontinued. The intense dreaming activity associated with REM rebound often has the quality of a nightmare. Alcohol in the evening may result in REM inhibition early in the night, with rebound and nightmare in the second half of the night after the alcohol is metabolized. Occasionally, nightmares are caused by sleep disruption during REM secondary to obstructive sleep apnea. Nightmares are frequent in patients with narcolepsy who have sleep-onset dreaming, especially when associated with sleep paralysis. Nightmares are a component of RBD, but that disorder is distinguished by the presence of dream enactment and REM sleep without atonia.

Diagnosis

Diagnosis of nightmare disorder is generally made by history, as detailed previously. PSG may be indicated to exclude other disorders disrupting REM sleep or RBD. Diagnostic criteria include recurrent episodes with dysphoric emotional content, little or no confusion on awakening, and detailed dream recall.

Treatment

There is no specific treatment of nightmares per se. Attention should primarily be directed to accurate diagnosis and treatment of the underlying disorders or precipitants.

KEY POINTS

1. The term parasomnia refers to undesirable physical events that occur in relationship to sleep.
2. Many parasomnias are associated with abnormal behaviors that may be injurious.
3. Disorders of arousal occur on arousal from NREM sleep and include sleep terrors, sleepwalking, and confusional arousals.
4. RBD is a disorder characterized by loss of the normal REM atonia with resultant dream enactment; it is a disorder highly associated with the synucleinopathies, such as Parkinson's disease, but may be induced by medication, especially antidepressants.
5. Nightmare disorder is typically associated with underlying psychopathology but may also be induced by a variety of medications.

◼ SLEEP IN SELECTED PSYCHIATRIC DISORDERS

Sleep-Related Dissociative Disorders

Sleep-related dissociative disorders are a variant of the DSM-IV–defined dissociative disorder and classified in the ISCD-2 as a parasomnia. In these patients, complex behaviors emerge during wakefulness, either in the transition to sleep or after awakening from REM or NREM. Behaviors often are stereotyped and prolonged and involve enactment of prior abuse.

DSM-IV criteria of a dissociative disorder must be present. The major differential diagnostic concern is between a dissociative episode and an arousal from NREM sleep. PSG study reveals that dissociative episodes are immediately preceded by an awake EEG, whereas disorders of arousal arise from NREM sleep.

Depression

Depression is characterized by several sleep complaints. Most patients report some difficulty with sleep, including all components of insomnia: difficulty initiating sleep, difficulty maintaining sleep, early morning awakening, and nonrestorative sleep. Patients with bipolar disease may be hypersomnolent when depressed and require less sleep when manic. Sleep disturbances may herald exacerbations of depression or mania. Some PSG findings have been reported in depression, but none is considered reliable enough to recommend a PSG as a diagnostic tool. The most characteristic research findings in depression are a shortened REM latency, increased frequency of eye movements during REM (REM density), increased REM percentage, longer first REM period, and early morning awakening. Other common findings include increased sleep latency, increased wake after sleep, decreased total sleep time, and decreased slow wave sleep. Given the nonspecific nature of sleep complaints in depression, it is important to exclude contributing sleep disorders that may mimic or exacerbate depression. Obstructive sleep apnea may produce a clinical syndrome that shares many of the clinical characteristics of depression, including early morning awakening, sleep disruption, nonrestorative sleep, and lack of motivation.

Schizophrenia

Sleep is disturbed in schizophrenia, typically in parallel with the degree of psychosis. Agitation with sleeplessness is typical of acute psychotic episodes. Poor sleep efficiency, prolonged sleep latency, increased wake after sleep, and early awakening are common. Sleep scheduling may be erratic. Most research studies on this disorder have shown decreased slow wave sleep. REM latency has been reported to be reduced. REM density is not increased. REM times are normal in hallucinating and nonhallucinating patients. A decreased number of sleep spindles has been reported.

KEY POINTS

1. A wide variety of sleep complaints and abnormalities commonly accompany psychiatric disorders; these may herald or parallel disease recurrence and exacerbation.
2. None of the PSG abnormalities seen in these disorders provides adequate specificity to aid in psychiatric diagnosis.
3. It is important to exclude treatable sleep disorders such as obstructive sleep apnea and RBD, which may mimic and exacerbate psychiatric disorders.

■ **SUGGESTED READINGS**

American Academy of Sleep Medicine. *The International Classification of Sleep Disorders: Diagnostic & Coding Manual.* 2nd ed. Westchester, Ill: American Academy of Sleep Medicine; 2005.

Barkoukis T, Avidan AY. *Review of Sleep Medicine.* 2nd ed. Philadelphia: Butterworth Heinemann; 2007.

Benca RM, Obermeyer WH, Thisted RA, et al. Sleep and psychiatric disorders: a meta-analysis. *Arch Gen Psychiatry* 1992;49:651–668, discussion 69–70.

Broughton RJ. Sleep disorders: disorders of arousal? Enuresis, somnambulism, and nightmares occur in confusional states of arousal, not in "dreaming sleep." *Science* 1968;159:1070–1078.

España RA, Scammell TE. Sleep neurobiology for the clinician. *Sleep* 2004;27:811–820.

Fuller PM, Gooley JJ, Saper CB. Neurobiology of the sleep-wake cycle: sleep architecture, circadian regulation, and regulatory feedback. *J Biol Rhythms* 2006;21:482–493.

Kryger MH, Roth T, Dement WC. *Principles and Practice of Sleep Medicine.* 4th ed. Philadelphia: Saunders; 2005.

Morin CM, Bootzin RR, Buysse DJ, et al. Psychological and behavioral treatment of insomnia: update of the recent evidence (1998–2004). *Sleep* 2006;29:1398–1414.

Nofzinger E, Keshavan M. Sleep disturbances and neuropsychiatric disease. In: Davis KL, and the American College of Neuropsychopharmacology, eds. *Neuropsychopharmacology: the Fifth Generation of Progress: An Official Publication of the American College of Neuropsychopharmacology.* Philadelphia: Lippincott Williams & Wilkins; 2002.

Peterson MJ, Benca RM. Sleep in mood disorders. *Psych Clin North Am* 2006;29:1009–1032.

CHAPTER 22

Functional Disease: Hysteria

Michael Ronthal

■ INTRODUCTION

The term "hysteria" has largely been dropped from psychiatric parlance in favor of several other *Diagnostic and Statistical Manual of Mental Disorders,* fourth edition categories, but it continues to be used by neurologists as a descriptor for "functional" or "nonorganic" neurological disease. It is estimated that about one third of new neurological symptoms are regarded by neurologists as "not at all" or only "somewhat" explained by organic disease.

How often is there associated organic disease? Following analysis of a series of 112 patients, Slater (1962) concluded that one third had a hysterical conversion syndrome, as well as organic disease; one third were initially thought to have pure hysteria, of whom eight later developed organic disease; and one third had a psychiatric diagnosis such as schizophrenia, depression, or personality disorder. His findings were influential, and his conclusion that the diagnosis of hysteria was a disguise for ignorance and a fertile source of clinical error has influenced modern neurology.

The diagnosis of hysteria is therefore fraught with danger—not only may the diagnosis be plain wrong, but there is frequently a "kernel" (Charcot) of organic pathology that is overwhelmed by the psychiatric signs and symptoms. Approximately 15% of diagnosed conversion reactions subsequently prove to be due to missed neurological conditions.

These patients require extensive study to exclude an organic nidus, but if the same syndrome keeps repeating itself, the return on repeating the investigative studies is low. A good outcome is associated with a short history, but follow-up is necessary—conversion disorders do not protect the patient from developing other diseases.

Conversion reactions may involve any neurological subsystem, including movement, sensation, and cognitive intellectual abilities.

■ HISTORY

The term "hysteria," based on the Egyptian theory of the wandering uterus, is credited to Hippocrates. Pierre Briquet (1776–1881) considered hysteria to be the product of suffering of the part of the brain destined to receive affective impressions and feelings (*personnalite hysterique*) and influenced Jean-Martin Charcot (1825–1893), who delivered his first lecture on hysteria, a lesson on hysterical contractures, at the Salpêtrière, in June of 1870. In the previous year, Charcot had heard a paper by Russell Reynolds at the British Medical Society meeting in Leeds, England, entitled "Paralysis, and Other Disorders of Motion and Sensation, Dependent on Idea." With an influx of female patients to the neurology wards when a psychiatric ward in the condemned Saint Laure building was closed, Charcot devoted himself to the study of hysteria in his later years. His research and case demonstrations attracted many prominent physicians, including Adolf Meyer, James Jackson Putnam, and Sigmund Freud. The French school also included Charles Lasègue, Ernest Mesnet, and Paul Blocq, who wrote the seminal papers on astasia-abasia in 1888. Freud suggested that an unconscious conflict is symbolically converted into a somatic symptom.

The American Civil War prompted an appraisal of functional signs and symptoms in malingering soldiers trying to avoid the battlefield. Weir Mitchell (1829–1914) first encountered hysteria in these soldiers and subsequently developed his "rest cure" for patients with neurosis and hysteria in civilian practice. His therapeutic efforts would be viewed with distain today; he once remarked, "Yes, she will run out of the door in two minutes; I set her sheets on fire. A case of hysteria." He described the rest cure as: "to lie abed half a day and sew a little, and read a little, and be interesting and excite sympathy, is all very well but when they are bidden to stay in bed a month, and neither to read, write nor sew, and to have one nurse—who is not a relative—then rest becomes for some women a rather bitter medicine and they are glad enough to accept the order to rise and go about when the doctor issues a mandate which has become pleasantly welcome and eagerly looked for."

■ "HYSTERICAL" SIGNS AND SYMPTOMS

The crux of a diagnosis of hysteria is that the symptoms and physical signs do not correlate with known neurological damage patterns (Table 22.1).

"La belle indifference," an apparent lack of concern with or about the nature and implications of the symptoms or disability, has no discriminatory value.

TABLE 22.1 FUNCTIONAL SIGNS

Weakness	*Blindness*
Intermittency	Retained blink to threat
Give-way	Mirror test
Hoover's sign for lower limb weakness	Optokinetic nystagmus retained
Cocontraction	Tunnel vision
Sensory loss	*Nonepileptic seizures*
Stocking or glove loss to the groin or shoulder	Closed eyelids during seizure
Splitting the midline, exactly	Gradual onset
Vibration splits midline on skull or sternum	Asynchronous limb movement
"Yes"/"no" answering test	Side-to-side head shaking
Gait disorder	Rapid postictal reorientation
Fluctuations in gait and stance	Bilateral seizure activity with retained consciousness (but beware of frontal seizures)
Excessive slowness	*Dizziness*
Uneconomic postures	Reproduction with hyperventilation
Walking on ice gait	
Sudden knee buckling without falling	
Astasia abasia	
Movement disorders	
Bizarre movements	
Suggestibility	
Improvement with distraction	
Increase of tremor with weighting	

Although laterality has been suggested as an indicator for hysteria, when put to analysis there is only a slight left-sided preponderance of signs and symptoms (55% to 60%). Nonepileptic seizures are preponderantly right-hemisphere related—71% in one study.

Cognitive Complaints

Unconscious processes and psychological disorders may result in a complaint of amnesia. One possible explanation for global amnesia is hysterical dissociation.

The patient who loses his own identity and refers to his driving license for his name is always functional. Suspicion should be roused by slow, haphazard responses to questions.

A host of neuropsychological tests are available to detect hysteria and malingering but are beyond the scope of this chapter.

Weakness

Waxing and waning weakness or intermittency is suggestive of a nonorganic diagnosis. "Give-way" weakness implies that with continued effort there is progressive or abrupt loss of power. This sign is prominent in functional weakness, but can also be triggered by pain. To get a true feel for weakness or lack thereof, strength must be evaluated in the first second of effort; after that the examination has no validity. "Collapsing weakness" is a phenomenon in which the limb collapses from an instructed position with a light touch and is a variant of give-way weakness.

In patients with lower extremity weakness, Hoover's sign has good sensitivity and specificity. It relies on the principle that one normally extends the hip when flexing the contralateral hip against resistance. With the patient supine, test hip flexion in the weak leg while keeping your hand under the good heel, looking for absence of downward pressure on that side, which implies a functional rather than organic weakness.

Cocontraction of agonistic and antagonistic muscles is nonphysiological, and results in a "wooden" limb. When asked to drop the outstretched and "weak" arm, descent may be jerky or the arm may remain elevated as a pseudo-waxy sign.

Sensory Loss

Stocking or glove sensory loss to a joint, usually to the groin or shoulder, is nonorganic. Exact splitting at the midline is functional because there is normally overlap from the contralateral side for 1 to 2 cm.

Loss of tuning fork vibratory sense that splits the midline when the fork is placed on the forehead or sternum must be functional because vibrations are conducted diffusely in bone. One can ask patients to say "yes" when they feel the stimulus and "no" when they do not—if they comply, they must have sensation, despite the claim of anesthesia.

Functional Gait Disorders

Lempert et al., from an analysis of videotapes, suggested six criteria that support the diagnosis of psychogenesis. The following criteria may occur alone or in combination:

1. Momentary fluctuations of stance and gait, often in response to suggestion
2. Excessive slowness or hesitation of locomotion incompatible with neurological disease
3. A "psychogenic" result from a Romberg test, with a build-up of swaying amplitudes after a silent latency or with improvement by distraction
4. Uneconomic postures with wastage of muscular energy
5. "Walking on ice," characterized by small cautious steps with fixed ankle joints
6. Sudden buckling of the knees, usually without falls.

Camptocormia is a functional exaggerated trunk flexion.

Astasia-abasia was defined by Blocq as the inability to maintain an upright posture despite normal function of the legs in the bed. "The motor powerlessness does not hold to a paralysis of general movements because the patient executes with the aid of the lower limbs, with the greatest precision, diverse acts and he can even jump, in some cases, or walk on all fours, but he has lost the memory of specialized movements necessary to remain standing (astasia) and to walk (abasia)."

The quintessential factor of hysterical gait disorder is excessive slowness and stiffness, or maintenance of postural control on a narrow base with flailing arms and excessive trunk sway without falling (tightrope walking).

Fear of falling is present in approximately 50% of patients who have already fallen, has a rational basis, but can become so severe as to become disabling and qualifies as a phobia—the patient may resort to walking only against the walls, or to crawling on hands and knees, culminating in a wheelchair existence.

Severely depressed patients may develop a hypokinetic gait, lifting their legs but with reduced stride length and poor propulsion.

■ MOVEMENT DISORDERS

The diagnosis of a functional movement disorder is particularly challenging because many organic abnormalities look bizarre. Suspicious features include rapid onset, variability, and improvement with distraction, features common to other functional disorders.

Hysterical contracture may be part of "fixed dystonia." A clenched fist attitude in an adult and pain may be suggestive. Remission after general anesthesia, suggestion, or placebo is usually considered diagnostic.

When the limb with a tremor is weighted, the amplitude of the tremor will decrease in organic syndromes, yet increase if the tremor is functional because of coactivation.

Speech Disorders

Hysterical aphonia is the most common functional disorder of speech and may be misdiagnosed as aphasia. The trick is to speak to the patient in a whisper—the patient will often answer in a whisper. A good strong cough implies normal vocal cords.

Nonorganic Visual Loss

Hysterical Blindness

Approximately 1% of visual problems seen by an ophthalmologist are nonorganic. In patients with nonorganic visual loss, clinical observation is useful. A smooth entrance into the room, an intact blink to threat, flinching with increased illumination, or failure to direct the eyes to the patient's own hands during a manual task are clues. A normal papillary response implies normal anterior visual reflex pathways, but is also present in cortical blindness.

In the mirror test, the examiner holds a mirror to the "blind" eye(s) and then moves it. The eyes almost always follow the mirrored object. The mirror can be rotated to induce a pursuit movement. Optokinetic drum–induced nystagmus indicates a visual acuity of at least 6/60.

The malingerer may be unable to sign his name, but the blind person has no difficulty. It was recently shown that wearing sunglasses without any clear ophthalmic reason to wear sunglasses is highly suggestive of functional visual loss.

The ophthalmologist has other test options, such as the following:

- The fogging test: Visual acuity is reduced in the normal eye by progressively stronger spherical lenses. The patient is asked to read the visual acuity chart. Ultimately, acuity is so reduced in the "good" eye that the patient must be reading with the "bad" eye.

- The prism shift test: Normally a prism induces diplopia in the seeing eye, and the fixating eye makes a small compensatory movement so that the image still falls on the fovea. If such movement is detected or diplopia acknowledged, the "bad" eye can see.
- The reading bar test: The patient reads text at a distance of 14 to 16 inches while a vertical bar (e.g., a tongue depressor) is placed 7 inches in front of the patient's face. If both eyes have good acuity, the patient can read, but if one eye is truly blind, part of the page is obscured.
- Polarizing lens test: Polarizing glasses with one lens at 90-degree axis and one at 180-degree axis are used while the patient looks at projected letters that are visible to one eye only (one axis).

Loss of Field

Psychogenic defects remain unchanged in width when tangent screen testing is performed at varying distances. The examiner can do the same with a small red object to demonstrate tubular fields or tunnel vision.

A Goldmann kinetic perimetry examination may show a spiral field, and another useful finding is the demonstration of a star-shaped field. Standardized electroretinographic tests and visual evoked potentials complement the clinical examination.

There is no clear consensus in the literature on whether or not a psychiatric evaluation is indicated in nonorganic visual loss, but between 45% and 78% of patients experience complete resolution of symptoms with reassurance.

Nonepileptic Seizures

Nonepileptic seizures may take the form of hyperkinetic thrashing attacks or motionless/akinetic attacks. No single observed sign can be taken to make the diagnosis, but closed eyelids during an attack are common in nonepileptic seizures and rare in true seizures.

Other common features in functional seizures include gradual onset, undulating motor activity, asynchronous limb movements, side-to-side head shaking, lack of cyanosis, and rapid postictal reorientation. Opisthotonus, although classic, is rare. Bilateral seizure-like activity with tonic/clonic jerking, yet with retained consciousness, is likely functional.

Serum prolactin is elevated within 15 to 20 minutes of a grand mal seizure, but this elevation can be seen in syncope and can be normal after partial seizures. In specialized centers the test can prove useful.

The gold standard for diagnosis is videotelemetry with electroencephalographic (EEG) monitoring, but again caveats exist for frontal lobe seizures that may not have an EEG counterpart.

Functional Dizziness

In panic attacks, dizziness, chest pain, and tachycardia are usually the target symptoms. In Drachman and Hart's (1982) series of dizzy patients, 25% had hyperventilation as the cause.

If the physical examination is negative, ask the patient to hyperventilate—if the maneuver triggers the symptoms exactly, it is the likely cause.

Bear in mind that partial seizures arising in the temporal lobe can present with dizziness, and it is always worth checking an EEG, even if the symptoms are triggered by hyperventilation.

Beta-blockade with propranolol is often effective.

■ TREATMENT

Reassurance, encouragement, and explanation carry the day in patients with mild symptoms. One or more of the following may be helpful:

- Physical therapy and a graded exercise program.
- Cognitive behavioral therapy (CBT), which emphasizes the interaction of cognitive, behavioral, emotional, and physiological factors that perpetuate the symptoms.

- Antidepressant medications may help, even in the absence of a diagnosis of depression.
- Hypnosis may implant suggestions for normative function.
- Examination under intravenous sedation can be used both diagnostically and therapeutically—the patient can be shown a video to prove normal function in a "paralyzed" limb.
- Psychodynamic and other types of psychotherapy can only be supportive.

■ PATHOPHYSIOLOGY

Various neuropsychological theories have held sway over the years, but functional brain imaging is an evolving tool that helps to explain brain function in hysteria and in some cases supports the psychology.

Ludwig (1972) proposed that "selective corticofugal inhibition of afferent stimulation" operates in hysteria to exclude somatic function from consciousness.

Perception is heavily influenced by emotion and motivation, and preconscious processing of emotional stimuli involves connections between amygdala-hippocampus and insula and orbital and cingulate cortices.

The term "binding" suggests abnormal functional connectivity in conversion disorder. Brown and Marsden (1998) proposed that the primary role for the basal ganglia is to facilitate binding of sensorimotor and dorsolateral prefrontal cortices and supplementary and cingulate motor areas in a coherent sequence of motor activity and thought. As in Parkinsonism, bradykinesia and cocontraction seen in conversion disorders may reflect dysfunction of frontal-subcortical circuits.

Functional brain imaging in patients with hysterical deficits shows lack of activation in the appropriate cortical area, but increased activity in the orbitofrontal area, anterior cingulate, and, sometimes, basal ganglia and thalamus. These areas may operate to inhibit the primary cortical sites.

If conversion reactions are the psychobehavioral manifestations of somatic delusions, functional imaging is beginning to show us this process in action.

■ PROGNOSIS

A short duration of symptoms and coexistent anxiety or depression are associated with a good prognosis. Pending litigation is an indicator of poor prognosis. A change in marital status could go either way. In hemisensory loss the prognosis is almost uniformly benign. Conversely, unilateral functional weakness is of poor prognosis—in one study, 83% of patients reported weakness or sensory symptoms at 12 years. This underscores the idea that recovery is not to be expected if improvement has failed to occur during the initial period in hospital.

KEY POINTS

1. Functional signs may coexist with organic pathology.
2. Patients with functional signs are particularly challenging and usually merit extensive investigation to exclude organic pathology.
3. Fluctuating deficits that cannot be localized based on normal neurophysiology are the signpost of "hysteria."
4. Patients who break down with hysterical signs and symptoms require an inordinate degree of support.
5. A short duration of symptomatology makes for a good prognosis.

■ **SUGGESTED READINGS**

Beatty S. Non-organic visual loss. *Postgrad Med J* 1999;75:201–207.

Black DB, Seritan AL, Taber KH, Hurley RA. Conversion hysteria: lessons from functional imaging. *J Neuropsychiatry Clin Neurosci* 2004;16:245–251.

Brown P, Marsden CD. What do the basal ganglia do? *Lancet* 1998;351:1801–1804.

Crimlisk HL, Bhatia K, Cope H, et al. Slater revisited: 6 year follow up study of patients with medically unexplained motor symptoms. *BMJ* 1998;316:582–586.

Devinsky O, Mesad S, Alper K. Non dominant hemisphere lesions and conversion nonepileptic seizures. *Clin Neurosci* 2001;13:367–373.

Drachman DA, Hart CW. An approach to the dizzy patient. *Neurology* 1982;22:323–330.

Goetz CG. J-M Charcot and simulated neurologic disease. *Neurology* 2007;69:103–109.

Hurwitz TA, Prichard JW. Conversion disorder and fMRI. *Neurology* 2006;67:1914–1915.

Katon W. Panic disorder and somatization. *Am J Med* 1984;77:101–106.

Lempert T, Brandt T, Dieterich M, et al. How to identify psychogenic disorders of stance and gait: a video study in 37 patients. *J Neurol* 1991;238:140–146.

Ludwig AM. Hysteria: a neurobiological theory. *Arch Gen Psychiatry* 1972;27:771–777.

Mace CJ, Trimble MR. Ten-year prognosis of conversion disorder. *Br J Psychol* 1996;169:282–228.

Okun MS, Koehler PJ. Paul Blocq and (psychogenic) astasia abasia. *Mov Disord* 2007;22:1373–1378.

Reynolds CR, ed. *Detection of Malingering During Head Injury Litigation.* New York: Plenum Press; 1998.

Stone J, Carson A, Sharpe M. Functional symptoms in neurology: management. *J Neurol Neurosurg Psychiatry* 2005;76S1:i2–i12.

Stone J, Carson A, Sharpe M. Functional symptoms in neurology: assessment and diagnosis. *J Neurol Neurosurg Psychiatry* 2005;76S1:i3–i21.

Stone J, Sharpe M, Rothwell PM, et al. The 12 year prognosis of functional weakness and sensory disturbance. *J Neurol Neurosurg Psychiatry* 2003;74:591–596.

Stone J, Smyth R, Carson A, et al. La belle indifference in conversion symptoms and hysteria. *Br J Psychol* 2006;188:204–209.

Stonnington CM, Barry JJ, Fisher RS. Conversion disorder. *Am J Psychiatry* 2006;163:1510–1517.

CHAPTER 23

Substance Abuse and Neurotoxicology

Stephen J. Traub

$\mathbf{M}$any substances—both legal and illicit—produce alterations in mental status. To the untrained or uncritical eye, these changes may appear to be psychiatric in origin. It is important, therefore, that the practicing psychiatrist have a working knowledge of common neurotoxicological syndromes to correctly differentiate true psychiatric disease from acute medical conditions.

In addition to understanding common neurotoxicological syndromes, the psychiatrist should also develop an approach to assessing the undifferentiated patient who is "not acting right." Such an approach, with an emphasis on physical examination and a de-emphasis on laboratory testing, can yield important diagnostic information and prevent mistriage of a medical patient to the psychiatric service.

This chapter is divided into two sections. The first is a review of seven important neurotoxicological syndromes. For each syndrome, a brief introduction is followed by a description of that syndrome's characteristic mental status changes, a description of other key physical findings that support the diagnosis, the role of laboratory testing, and brief treatment strategies. The second section provides a general method to approach the patient with a possible neurotoxicological syndrome.

There are several key points that should be kept in mind when thinking about a patient with a potential neurotoxicological syndrome. They are introduced here with minimal explanation so that the reader may be familiar with them and are reiterated throughout the chapter.

- Although minor alterations in vital signs may occur in patients with psychiatric disorders, major alterations in vital signs suggest a medical condition.
- A careful, structured history and physical examination will often provide more diagnostic information than laboratory analysis.
- One cannot rely on either dedicated toxicology tests ("tox screens") or serum alcohol levels to definitively determine whether a patient is under the influence of a given drug.
- When drug toxicity is known or strongly suggested, the basic evaluation should include, in addition to a thorough history and physical examination, a fingerstick glucose level (to rule out hypoglycemia as a cause of any mental status changes), an electrocardiogram (to rule out toxin-induced QRS or QTc changes), and acetaminophen and salicylate levels (to rule out these common coingestions).

■ COMMON NEUROTOXICOLOGICAL SYNDROMES

Opioids

Morphine, a naturally occurring substance of the opium poppy, *Papaver somniferum,* has been used for millennia to relieve pain and suffering. Opioids, the class to which morphine belongs, reliably and effectively relieve acute pain and are therefore among the most important medications in the armamentarium of modern medicine.

Unfortunately, opioids also have a high potential for abuse. Heroin is a chemically modified derivative of morphine, which enters the central nervous system (CNS) faster than morphine and provides users with a greater "rush." Oxycodone is a synthetic opioid used in the treatment of pain; OxyContin is a sustained-release version of this medication that has received recent media attention because of concerns regarding its abuse. Hydromorphone (Dilaudid), hydrocodone (found in Lortab and Vicodin), codeine (found in Tylenol No. 3), and propoxyphene (found in Darvocet) are other examples of opioid-containing preparations.

Mental Status Changes

The mental status changes associated with opioid toxicity are those of general CNS depression and "dozing off." The term *narcotic,* often used as a synonym for opioid, derives from the Greek word *narke,* "to make numb." The typical patient with opioid toxicity may drift off and appear to be sleeping during the interview or even fail to complete sentences while talking.

Additional Physical Examination Findings

Opioids frequently produce a characteristic set of physical examination findings, commonly referred to as the "opioid toxidrome." These findings are the constellation of bradypnea (slow breathing), hypopnea (shallow breathing), and/or apnea (not breathing); pinpoint pupils; and decreased or absent bowel sounds.

Laboratory Testing

A positive urine drug screening for opiates in the setting of symptoms of opioid toxicity supports the diagnosis. A negative urine drug screen in a patient who appears to be intoxicated with opioids does not rule out this diagnosis, however, because several commonly abused opiates (including oxycodone and methadone) fail to react with many commercially available opioid drug screens. A positive drug screen in a patient whose symptoms are not consistent with opioid intoxication likely represents recent use and persistent metabolites in the urine, rather than a true intoxication.

Treatment

Opiate toxicity is effectively reversed with the competitive antagonist naloxone (Narcan). In patients who are not known or presumed to be addicted to opiates, a starting dose of 0.4 to 2.0 mg is reasonable. Naloxone has an extraordinary safety profile.

Indiscriminate dosing of naloxone in the known or presumed opiate addict, however, will quickly precipitate withdrawal and should be avoided. In such patients, we recommend an initial dose of 0.01 mg intravenously, repeated every 1 to 2 minutes until the patient is effectively oxygenating (pulse oximetry of 93% or greater) on room air.

In the setting of presumed opiate toxicity, a positive response to naloxone is essentially diagnostic.

Sedative-Hypnotic Agents

Sedative-hypnotic agents are CNS depressants. Alcohol, benzodiazepines, barbiturates, and gamma-hydroxybutyrate (GHB) are among the most commonly used and abused members of this class.

Sedative-hypnotic agents act predominantly at the gamma-aminobutyric acid (GABA) receptor. The GABA receptor is located on the chloride channel. Binding of GABA to the GABA receptor increases chloride channel opening. Some drugs activate GABA receptors directly, whereas others (such as benzodiazepines) increase the effectiveness of GABA at the GABA receptor. In either event, the end result is an increased flux through the chloride channel, which hyperpolarizes neurons, decreases neurotransmission, and results in CNS sedation.

Mental Status Changes

The hallmark of sedative-hypnotic toxicity is a general decrease in mental status. Thought processes are slowed considerably. Speech may be slurred. Patients may be excessively emotional or angry as a result of the disinhibiting effects of these agents. GHB is somewhat unique in that profoundly sedated patients may rouse easily in response to noxious stimulation, only to become profoundly sedated again after the stimulus is removed.

Additional Physical Examination Findings

Vital sign abnormalities depend in large part on the substance ingested. Benzodiazepines rarely produce significant vital sign abnormalities. Most patients with uncomplicated alcohol toxicity have normal vital signs. Barbiturates are not nearly as safe as benzodiazepines (it is for this reason that they have largely been replaced by benzodiazepines for virtually every clinical indication). Barbiturate toxicity may result in bradycardia, hypotension, and respiratory depression or arrest. GHB toxicity may result in bradycardia, coma, respiratory depression, or apnea.

Patients with alcohol toxicity may have the sweet, characteristic odor of this substance on their breath. Alcohol may also produce a significant horizontal nystagmus. Barbiturate intoxication may be associated with cutaneous blisters. With all of these agents, coordination as assessed on the neurological examination is impaired.

Laboratory Testing

Qualitative urine toxicology screening may identify both barbiturates and benzodiazepines. Care should be taken not to overinterpret such results, however. Urine testing usually identifies metabolites of the drug class in question and does not confirm that the observed behavior is due to the drug identified. For example, a patient who has not taken diazepam for several days may still have a positive urine toxicology screen, despite the fact that he or she is no longer under the influence of that drug.

Care should also be taken not to overinterpret serum ethanol levels. Unlike urine toxicology screens, serum ethanol levels reliably quantify the blood concentration of the substance in question. However, *the serum ethanol level is an imperfect gauge of the degree of the patient's intoxication.*

Ethanol is a substance to which patients may develop functional and physiological tolerance, occasionally to a profound extent. A naïve drinker with a blood alcohol level of 100 mg/dL might be profoundly inebriated, whereas a chronic alcoholic may be awake and conversant with an alcohol level of 300 mg/dL. The latter patient may be in acute ethanol withdrawal when his or her blood alcohol level is 150 mg/dL.

The most appropriate measure of sobriety in a patient who has been consuming ethanol, therefore, is the patient's clinical status. Arbitrary numerical cutoffs designed to "determine" a patient's suitability for discharge from the emergency department or for a psychiatric interview are not based on sound physiological principles. Patients who are awake, responding appropriately, and not slurring their speech and are ambulatory with a steady gait are no longer clinically intoxicated. Serum ethanol levels play virtually no role in that determination.

Treatment

Treatment of the patient with sedative hypnotic toxicity is generally supportive and in mild to moderate cases consists of intravenous fluids and supplemental oxygen. Patients who have used long-acting agents (e.g., phenobarbital) should be admitted (usually to the general medical service) when they are symptomatic, because they are unlikely to regain a clear sensorium in a reasonable time period. Patients who are intoxicated with short-acting agents (such as ethanol) can be observed until resolution of their mental status changes.

Flumazenil, a benzodiazepine antagonist, should almost never be used in the setting of known or questioned benzodiazepine intoxication. When given indiscriminately to a patient who is habituated to benzodiazepines, flumazenil may precipitate acute benzodiazepine withdrawal. This syndrome is clinically similar to—and as dangerous as—ethanol withdrawal. Furthermore, patients to whom flumazenil has been administered may prove refractory to further treatment with benzodiazepines because of the antagonist effects of the flumazenil.

Hallucinogens

Although most commonly associated with the Haight-Ashbury district of San Francisco and the "psychedelic" era of the 1960s, hallucinogens have been used by humans for millennia. Aztecs consumed psilocybin-containing mushrooms that they called "teonanácatl" ("flesh of the gods") as part of their religious ceremonies.

In 1943, a young scientist at Sandoz named Albert Hoffman was experimenting on ergot derivatives as part of a series of experiments to discover new vasoactive substances. After he was inadvertently exposed to one of the compounds, lysergic acid diethylamide (LSD), he began hallucinating. His documentation of his experiences and further work in this area opened the door to the modern era of hallucinogen use.

Several substances are used for their hallucinogenic properties. Psilocybin-containing mushrooms, LSD, the plant *Salvia divinorum*, and mescaline are among the most popular. Most hallucinogens are serotonin analogs and exert their hallucinogenic effects via activity at the serotonin-2A receptor.

Mental Status Changes

Patients who are intoxicated with hallucinogens usually complain of vivid visual hallucinations, in contradistinction to the predominantly auditory hallucinations that characterize the primary psychoses or intoxication with sympathomimetic substances. When asked, patients frequently describe the appearance of geometric patterns. Inanimate objects may seem to pulsate or move, and concrete boundaries may be described as "melting." Synesthesias, a melding of sensory perceptions, are also common; patients may "hear" colors or "see" sounds. Time perception may be distorted or completely lost.

Additional Physical Examination Findings

Hallucinogens produce few peripheral physical examination findings; the presence of such findings should prompt a search for other substances or medical conditions. There are exceptions to this general rule, however. Ingestion of nutmeg, for example, typically produces severe nausea and vomiting before the onset of hallucinogenic symptoms.

Laboratory Testing

Laboratory testing is generally unremarkable in patients who have used hallucinogens. These medications produce no pathognomonic metabolic or other laboratory abnormalities. The presence of significant laboratory abnormalities should prompt a search for a concurrent or alternative condition.

■ TREATMENT

Treatment of patients who are using hallucinogens is almost entirely supportive. Agitation is best treated with benzodiazepines. Placing the patient in a calm, quiet room has been advocated for almost 40 years and remains an excellent intervention.

In addition to the supportive measures discussed, care should be taken to prevent the patient from inflicting harm to others or self as a result of impaired judgment. Patients under the influence of hallucinogens have been reported to stare into the sun or attempt to fly, with resultant blindness or death.

Dissociative Agents

Dissociative agents are so named because they produce a state in which the patient seems removed, or dissociated, from himself or herself. Patients who are intoxicated with dissociative agents may have an "otherworldly" or "out of body" experience. These agents have a complex pharmacology, including blockade at the N-Methyl-D-Aspartate (NMDA)-type glutamate receptor. Dissociative agents that are commonly used and abused today include phencyclidine (PCP or "angel dust"), ketamine, and the over-the-counter cough medication dextromethorphan.

Mental Status Changes

Patients who are intoxicated with dissociative agents may present in different ways, depending on the extent of intoxication. Patients who are mildly intoxicated may appear confused and aggressive, whereas severe intoxication may produce complete dissociation and unresponsiveness. Phencylcidine users may alternate between severe agitation and an outwardly calm exterior. Ketamine users try to self-titrate to a level of perceptual distortions without producing complete dissociation. When such users overshoot, they describe the dissociative state as a "K-hole."

Additional Physical Examination Findings

Dissociative agents, particularly phencyclidine and ketamine, frequently produce hypertension and tachycardia. One important corroborative physical examination finding is vertical and/or rotatory nystagmus. Vertical or rotatory nystagmus strongly suggests intoxication with one of a few drugs, including the dissociative agents. Ketamine may also produce excessive salivation.

Laboratory Testing

Urine tests for phencyclidine are commonly available, but the results must be interpreted with caution. Some patients ingest phencyclidine congeners, which possess all of the chemical activity of phencyclidine but do not react with the phencyclidine screening test. Although the results of such a test are truly negative (because the patient did not actually ingest phencyclidine), they may mislead the clinician from the true diagnosis of dissociative agent toxicity. Alternatively, dextromethorphan (in doses used to treat cough, not doses used in abuse) may generate a false positive test because of cross-reactivity with the phencyclidine assay.

There are no other laboratory tests that help confirm dissociative agent toxicity or routinely guide management. Patients who are severely agitated and physically aggressive should be screened for rhabdomyolysis via testing for urine myoglobin (which cross-reacts with the hemoglobin test of the urine dipstick) or serum creatinine kinase.

Treatment

Dissociative agent toxicity rarely requires aggressive treatment. A calm, supporting atmosphere may suffice. Severe agitation may require sedation with benzodiazepines. Aggressive patients may require physical restraint to protect themselves and staff.

Amphetamines, Cocaine, and Other Sympathomimetic Agents

Sympathomimetics are agents that mimic the activity of the sympathetic arm of the autonomic nervous system. Cocaine, amphetamines (such as methamphetamine), and amphetamine analogs (such as methylenedioxymethamphetamine, or "ecstasy") are the most commonly abused members of this class.

Sympathomimetic agents produce much of their effects by increasing brain synaptic levels of dopamine, norepinephrine, and serotonin, neurotransmitters that are implicated in reward and mood centers.

Sympathomimetic use and abuse are not recent phenomena. Indigenous peoples in South and Central America have chewed coca leaves and brewed coca tea for hundreds of years to stave off fatigue and hunger. The original formula for Coca-Cola, which was not modified until the early 20th century, contained cocaine (as suggested by the product's name).

Sympathomimetic use has exploded in recent decades. Cocaine abuse became epidemic in the late 1970s and 1980s, and methylenedioxymethamphetamine ("ecstasy") surged in popularity in the 1990s. Although the use of both drugs is lower today than it was during the height of their popularity, both are still concerns. Methamphetamine abuse has soared in recent years, and "meth" is one of the more important toxicological and social problems of this decade.

Mental Status Changes

Sympathomimetic agents may produce a spectrum a mental status changes.

Recreational users are frequently animated, hyperkinetic, and loquacious; they may seem extremely friendly and hypersexual. Euphoria is common. To the untrained eye, such a patient may simply seem to be in a very good mood.

Heavier use may produce more significant symptoms. Cocaine and amphetamines may produce a psychotic state whose features are virtually indistinguishable from those of the primary psychotic disorders such as schizophrenia. Elevated synaptic dopamine levels may be the principal cause or a contributing factor.

Additional Physical Examination Findings

Sympathomimetic agents frequently produce a characteristic set of physical examination findings, commonly referred to as the "sympathomimetic toxidrome." These findings are the constellation of dilated pupils, tachycardia, hypertension, and diaphoresis, in addition to the mental status changes noted previously. When a patient presents with auditory hallucinations, severe paranoia, and/or religious grandiosity, the presence or absence of these peripheral physical examination findings is a crucial component of the decision to have the patient managed by a medical team or a psychiatric team.

Laboratory Testing

Urine tests for cocaine and amphetamines are commercially available, but the results of these tests must be interpreted with caution.

Urine tests for these drugs typically remain positive long after the drug has been cleared from the patient's system. Cocaine, as one example, remains positive in the urine for several days after recreational use and for up to 10 days in heavy users, despite the fact that the drug produces symptoms for a few hours at most. Therefore a patient with known schizophrenia with psychotic symptoms, who has normal vital signs, dry skin, and midrange pupils, is probably suffering from decompensated mental illness, not cocaine toxicity, even if the urine test is positive for cocaine.

Alternatively, not all sympathomimetics are identified by urine toxicology testing. Some amphetamine analogs will not react with commercially available amphetamine screens. Therefore, patients intoxicated with drugs such as methylenedioxymethamphetamine ("ecstasy") may have normal urine tests.

Treatment

Benzodiazepines are first-line agents in the treatment of sympathomimetic toxicity. They are powerful sedatives and have an outstanding safety profile and a high therapeutic index (meaning they can be given in very high doses without concern for toxicity). Butyrophenones (such as haloperidol and droperidol) interfere with heat dissipation and may prolong the corrected QT (QTc) interval on the electrocardiogram and thus should be avoided.

Sympathomimetic agents such as cocaine and amphetamines are associated with myriad medical complications, including uncontrolled hypertension, hyperthermia, ischemic and hemorrhagic cerebrovascular accidents, myocardial infarction, thoracic aortic dissection, and intestinal ischemia. An important principle in the management of these patients is that somatic complaints require a thorough evaluation before the patient can be "medically cleared" for management by the psychiatric service.

Sedative-Hypnotic Withdrawal

Sedative-hypnotic withdrawal, whether from alcohol, benzodiazepines, barbiturates, or GHB, is a life-threatening illness. Alcohol is, without question, the most commonly used drug in the world and the most commonly implicated drug in sedative-hypnotic withdrawal.

Alcohol is frequently used in the United States and abused by a substantial minority of those who drink. A smaller but still significant number of those who abuse alcohol are physically addicted to alcohol; in these patients, an abrupt decrease or cessation of alcohol intake produces alcohol withdrawal.

There are several alcohol withdrawal syndromes. Not all persons who withdraw from alcohol will experience all of these syndromes, and syndromes may overlap temporally. These syndromes are as follows:

- Alcoholic tremulousness, in which the patient's tremors are accompanied by hypertension and tachycardia. This state generally occurs hours after alcohol abstinence. Patients are usually lucid, unless an intervening medical problem is affecting mental status. In this stage, patients (when asked) will frequently state that they "need a drink." Such patients are frequently (and incorrectly) described as experiencing delirium tremens ("DTs").
- Alcoholic withdrawal seizures, which are almost always generalized tonic-clonic seizures. These are usually single seizures. Any deviation from this pattern should prompt a search for an alternative explanation for the seizures.
- Alcoholic hallucinosis, in which patients complain of hallucinations regardless of whether they have recently been drinking or abstaining. Alcoholic hallucinosis may reflect a "hardwiring" of the brain as much as a state of alcohol abstinence.
- DTs, a state of profound autonomic dysregulation characterized by hypertension, tachycardia, diaphoresis, and profound confusion. DTs usually occurs after days of alcohol abstinence in heavy drinkers. It is a life-threatening problem that must be managed in an intensive care setting.

Mental Status Changes

The mental status changes seen in alcohol withdrawal depend on the syndrome the patient is experiencing at the time. Patients with alcoholic tremulousness typically appear agitated or anxious. Patients with alcoholic withdrawal seizures have a brief postictal state similar to that in patients with seizures of other etiologies. Patients with alcoholic hallucinosis describe vivid hallucinations. Patients with DTs are (as the condition suggests) acutely delirious and may be described by the untrained observer as "crazy" or "out of their mind."

Additional Physical Examination Findings

Like mental status changes, the peripheral physical examination findings in alcohol withdrawal are largely a function of the syndrome the patient is experiencing.

Alcoholic tremulousness is commonly accompanied by hypertension and tachycardia, as well as diaphoresis. Tongue fasciculations, which can be seen when the patient sticks out his or her tongue, strongly suggests alcoholic tremulousness. Diaphoresis may also be seen in this stage.

Patients with alcoholic withdrawal seizures do not have characteristic physical examination findings per se. Such patients may display examination findings consistent with those in other syndromes (such as alcoholic tremulousness) if the seizure occurs concurrently with that syndrome. Tongue lacerations, which may occur with seizures of any etiology, may be seen in patients with alcoholic withdrawal seizures as well.

Laboratory Testing

Laboratory testing plays a limited role in cases of simple alcohol withdrawal. Alcohol levels are usually obtained, but must be interpreted with caution. A level of zero does not confirm that the patients' symptoms are due to alcohol withdrawal, and a positive value does not preclude the diagnosis because alcohol withdrawal may be seen at virtually any level. There is a common misconception that alcohol levels above an arbitrary number (i.e., 100 mg/dL) preclude the diagnosis of alcohol withdrawal. This line of thinking fails to appreciate that many alcoholics typically go through their day with an alcohol level of 200 to 300 mg/dL and that levels in the 100-mg/dL range will produce significant symptoms. The greatest utility of alcohol levels in these patients probably lies in the prediction of the severity of the patient's withdrawal. Patients who manifest moderate to severe withdrawal symptoms with relatively high alcohol levels will probably have a more complicated course than those who manifest minor symptoms with a level of zero.

Laboratory testing may prove helpful in determining why the patient stopped drinking. Alcohol is ubiquitous and inexpensive, and the drive to drink in alcoholics is profound. The abstaining alcoholic should be assumed to have a major medical condition that prevents him or her from drinking until proven otherwise. Occasionally, a history and physical examination are all that are necessary to exclude major medical illnesses. In patients with somatic complaints, however, further testing is usually warranted, such as serum lipase and liver function tests for patients complaining of abdominal pain and a chest radiograph for patients complaining of a cough and fever.

Treatment

Benzodiazepines are the mainstay of treatment for most patients undergoing alcohol withdrawal and are first-line therapy for those with alcoholic tremulousness, alcoholic withdrawal seizures, and DTs. Among the benzodiazepines, diazepam is an excellent choice because it is rapid-acting, has a long serum half-life, and has active metabolites.

Benzodiazepines should be given based on clinical symptoms, not as a standard taper or fixed-dose schedule. Numerous excellent articles have demonstrated that symptom-triggered therapy is equivalent or superior to fixed-dose therapy and usually results in both faster resolution of symptoms and less benzodiazepine administration. The Clinical Institute Withdrawal Assessment (CIWA) scales are frequently (and appropriately) used to help determine the need for benzodiazepine dosing.

Psychiatric patients with minor alcohol withdrawal that responds to low doses of benzodiazepines can safely be managed on the psychiatry service if alcohol withdrawal is a secondary diagnosis. Symptom-triggered therapy based on CIWA scoring is appropriate for such patients.

Patients with moderate to severe alcohol withdrawal, who require high doses of benzodiazepines or frequent dosing of benzodiazepines, or who fail benzodiazepine therapy and require barbiturate or propofol therapy, are more appropriately managed on the medical service.

Alcoholic hallucinosis cannot be treated or cured with benzodiazepine therapy. Such patients are best treated as inpatients on the medical service because they do not have a primary psychiatric condition.

In all patients who present with alcohol withdrawal, parenteral thiamine should be considered. Most if not all alcoholics are thiamine-deficient, and the administration of thiamine is safe. Furthermore, confused alcoholics may be suffering from Wernicke-Korsakoff syndrome, the treatment for which is thiamine repletion.

Anticholinergic Toxicity

Anticholinergic agents may produce an acute, agitated delirium that may be confused for psychiatric illness. Blockade of CNS acetylcholine receptors by the drug in question are responsible for these symptoms.

Many drugs, alone or in combination, can produce anticholinergic toxicity. Diphenhydramine (Benadryl), which is frequently used as a sleep aid and occasionally as a mild sedative, is one of the more common agents to produce anticholinergic toxicity. Although anticholinergic toxicity after isolated therapeutic dosing is uncommon, anticholinergic toxicity can frequently be seen after overdose or when diphenhydramine is given in conjunction with other medications with anticholinergic effects, such as phenothiazines, butyrophenones, and several of the atypical antipsychotic agents.

Jimsonweed is not infrequently smoked for its purported hallucinogenic effects; these effects, however, are the result of anticholinergic toxicity. Such patients frequently present to the emergency department for evaluation.

Mental Status Changes

Patients with anticholinergic toxicity usually present in a state of agitated delirium, which the untrained may confuse with a psychiatric disorder. Visual hallucinations are common, and patients are commonly looking around the room and not focused on the examiner. Picking movements, as if removing small insects from the bed sheets or body, are also common. Patients typically speak as if they have a "mouthful of marbles," which is likely a combination of blockade of central cholinergic transmission and the dry mouth (see below) that frequently accompanies this condition.

Additional Physical Examination Findings

Anticholinergic agents frequently produce a characteristic set of physical examination findings, commonly referred to as the "anticholinergic toxidrome." These findings are the constellation of dilated pupils, tachycardia, normal to mildly elevated blood pressure, dry skin, dry mucous membranes, and decreased or absent bowel sounds in addition to the mental status changes noted above.

Laboratory Testing

There is no laboratory test to determine anticholinergic toxicity; the diagnosis is made on clinical grounds alone. Laboratory evaluation of such patients is driven by coexistent symptoms or conditions.

Treatment

Physostigmine will reverse both the central and peripheral effects of anticholinergic agents. It should be given in a monitored medical setting.

In the event that physostigmine is unavailable or contraindicated, benzodiazepines are an appropriate treatment. Although not as effective as physostigmine, benzodiazepines will help produce sedation in patients with anticholinergic toxicity.

■ ASSESSING THE UNDIFFERENTIATED PATIENT

The previous section was organized to help the clinician understand a known toxin; this section is designed to give the clinician a framework to assess undifferentiated patients for the presence of a neurotoxicological syndrome. Although medical clearance and the exclusion of neurotoxicological conditions is properly the responsibility of the emergency department or general medical service, the practicing psychiatrist is well served to understand the principles of assessment as well, so as to not "miss" a neurotoxicological condition that was not appropriately identified by the initial screening service.

History

When available, the history may provide the diagnosis. Patients who believe that they play a central role in an organized religion and who admit to heavy amphetamine use may have a drug problem, not a psychiatric problem. The known alcoholic who states that he drank too much is likely suffering from alcohol intoxication.

Physical Examination

Frequently, patients refuse to give an active history, give a misleading history, or are unable to give a history as a result of their alteration in mental status. In such patients, the physical examination may prove diagnostic. The "toxidrome-oriented physical examination" consists of a series of items that help identify common neruotoxicological conditions. This examination consists of an assessment of pulse, blood pressure, respiratory rate, mental status, pupils, oral mucous membranes, pulse, blood pressure, respiratory rate, skin findings (dry versus diaphoretic), and bowel sounds.

Resting pulse is usually determined by an interplay of two competing stimuli at the sinoatrial node. Noradrenergic input increases the pulse, and cholinergic input slows it. Sympathomimetic agents, which increase noradrenergic tone, increase the pulse, as do anticholinergic agents. Tachycardia may also be seen with the dissociative agents. Opiates and sedative-hypnotic agents may lower the pulse slightly because of an inhibitory effect of normal sympathetic tone, but this effect is usually minor. Hallucinogens generally do not affect the pulse.

Blood pressure is elevated in sympathomimetic use because sympathomimetics "mimic" the fight-or-flight response of epinephrine and the endogenous sympathetic nervous system. Blood pressure may be elevated in anticholinergic toxicity as a result of agitation; the elevations are usually less than those seen with sympathomimetic toxicity. Sedative-hypnotic withdrawal and dissociative use can also produce elevations in blood pressure. Opiates and sedative-hypnotic agents may lower the blood pressure slightly because of an inhibitory effect on normal sympathetic tone, but, as was the case with the pulse, this effect is usually minor. Hallucinogens generally do not affect the blood pressure.

Respiratory rate may be normal to elevated in sympathomimetic toxicity, anticholinergic toxicity, sedative hypnotic withdrawal, and dissociative use, but variably so. Common sedative-hypnotic agents produce little effect on the respiratory rate unless profound toxicity is present. Opioids consistently and reliably produce a decrease in respiratory rate, ranging from mild hypoventilation to complete apnea. Hallucinogens generally do not affect the blood pressure.

Mental status changes are fully described in the first section of this chapter and will not be repeated here in the interest of brevity.

Pupil size is usually determined by the interplay of two different muscles in the iris. The radial muscle, which acts in response to sympathetic stimulation, makes the pupil wider; the sphincter muscle, which acts in response to cholinergic stimulation, makes the pupil smaller. Both sympathomimetic toxicity (which causes excessive activity of the radial muscle) and anticholinergic toxicity (which stops activity of the sphincter muscle and allows the radial muscle to act unopposed) produce dilated pupils (mydriasis). Opioids act through the third cranial nerve (a cholinergic nerve) to increase tone at the sphincter muscle and thereby produce pin-point pupils. Dissociative agents are the only commonly abused drugs that produce vertical or rotatory nystagmus. Sedative-hypnotic agents and dissociative agents do not have a predictable effect on pupil size.

Oral mucous membranes are usually moist as a result of the baseline activity of salivary glands, which secrete saliva in response to cholinergic stimulation. Anticholinergic agents block these secretions, leading to dry mucous membranes. Ketamine may produce salivation, but other dissociative agents do not commonly do so. Sympathomimetic agents, sedative-hypnotic agents, hallucinogens, and sedative hypnotic withdrawal have little or no effect on mucous membrane turgor.

Human skin typically has a slight amount of perspiration, the result of glands that secrete sweat as a result of cholinergic stimulation. This is particularly notable in certain areas, such as the axilla. Anticholinergic agents block the secretion of sweat, producing skin that is "dry as a bone." Sympathomimetic toxicity reliably produces diaphoresis, as does sedative-hypnotic withdrawal. Dissociative agents, sedative hypnotic agents, and hallucinogens have little to no effect on skin turgor.

Bowel motility (and the bowel sounds that this motility produces) is driven by cholinergic stimulation. Anticholinergic agents reduce bowel motility (and bowel sounds) by blocking cholinergic transmission. Opioids work through a different mechanism to produce reduced or absent bowel sounds. Sympathomimetic agents, sedative-hypnotic agents, dissociative agents, sedative-hypnotic withdrawal, and hallucinogens have virtually no effect on bowel sounds.

The important physical findings of the major toxidromes are listed in Table 23.1. Although not a perfect tool, the toxidrome-oriented physical examination provides important information in the workup of the undifferentiated patient with an alteration in mental status.

Laboratory Evaluation

The critical initial laboratory evaluation of the actually or potentially poisoned patient consists of four important components: fingerstick glucose value, acetaminophen and salicylate levels, and an electrocardiogram. The fingerstick glucose value is useful to exclude hypoglycemia as a cause for any alteration in mental status. Acetaminophen and salicylate levels help to rule out these common coingestants. The electrocardiogram is useful to assess QRS duration (which may be prolonged after ingestion of many drugs, most notably tricyclic antidepressants) and the QT interval (which may be prolonged after ingestion of many substances).

Urine toxicology screens, although usually performed in the workup of most patients with an alteration in mental status, rarely if ever produce a diagnosis that was not already made by history or physical examination. The pitfalls of testing for certain substances are noted earlier in the chapter. Perhaps most importantly, a positive urine drug screen only suggests that the patient was exposed to the substance in question over the last several days or week (depending on the specific drug). It does not confirm that the patient is intoxicated with a certain substance.

That is not to say that toxicology screens are useless, however. The results of these tests can serve as a barometer of the patient's honesty; the patient who denies any history of drug use but is positive for cocaine and marijuana cannot be considered fully reliable. The patient's pattern of recreational drug use is a comorbidity that may affect diagnosis or treatment. What is important to remember is that the toxicology screen is much less accurate than a careful history and physical examination when trying to make a diagnosis in a patient with an acute alteration in mental status.

The remainder of the laboratory workup is driven by the patient's presentation. For instance, a patient with undifferentiated mental status frequently requires an assessment of electrolytes and computed tomography of the head. A febrile patient with altered mental status may require a complete blood count and spinal tap as part of the evaluation.

TABLE 23.1 PHYSICAL EXAM FINDINGS IN COMMON NEUROTOXICOLOGICAL SYNDROMES

FINDING	OPIATES	SEDATIVES	HALLUCINOGENS	DISSOCIATIVE AGENTS	SYMPATHOMIMETIC	SEDATIVE-HYPNOTIC WITHDRAWAL	ANTICHOLINERGICS
	HEROIN	ETHANOL	LSD	PHENCYCLIDINE (PCP)	AMPHETAMINES	ETHANOL WITHDRAWAL	BENADRYL
Pulse	Normal/decreased	Normal/decreased	Normal	Increased	Increased	Increased	Increased
Blood pressure	Normal/decreased	Normal/decreased	Normal	Increased	Increased	Increased	Mildly increased
Respiratory rate	Markedly decreased	Decreased	Normal	Normal	Normal	High normal	Normal
CNS	Sedated	Sedated	Hallucinating	Confusion to unresponsiveness	Agitated	Agitated, tremulous	Agitated delirium
Mucous membranes	Normal	Normal	Normal	Salivation (with ketamine)	Normal	Normal	Dry
Eyes	Constricted pupils	Variable	Normal	Nystagmus (in any direction)	Dilated pupils	Dilated Pupils	Dilated pupils
Skin	Normal	Normal	Normal	Normal	Sweating	Sweating	Dry
Lungs	Normal	Normal	Normal	Normal	Normal	Normal	Normal
Bowel sounds	Decreased	Normal	Normal	Normal	Normal	Normal	Decreased

■ SUMMARY

Patients who use and abuse illicit drugs may present with signs and symptoms that might be confused with psychiatric disease. Although the history in such patients is frequently unobtainable or unreliable, a careful physical examination will often provide useful diagnostic clues. If the diagnosis can be made by history and physical examination, a minimal laboratory workup may be all that is needed. If the diagnosis is unclear, a complete workup for altered mental status may be necessary. Urine toxicology screens, though frequently ordered, rarely make the diagnosis and very infrequently alter management.

KEY POINTS

1. Intoxication with (or withdrawal from) many substances may produce alterations in mental status that can be confused with psychiatric syndromes.
2. History and physical examination are more valuable then alcohol levels or toxicology screens in determining if a patient's condition is drug-related.
3. A structured approach to the patient with an alteration in mental status will help identify neurotoxicological conditions and prevent mistriage of a medical patient to the psychiatric service.

■ SUGGESTED READINGS

Daeppen JB, Gache P, Landry U, et al. Symptom-triggered vs fixed-schedule doses of benzodiazepine for alcohol withdrawal: a randomized treatment trial. *Arch Intern Med* 2002;162:1117–1121.

Flomenbaum NE, Goldfrank LR, Hoffman RS, et al, eds. *Goldfrank's Toxicological Emergencies.* 8th ed. New York: McGraw Hill; 2006.

Nice A, Leikin JB, Maturen A, et al. Toxidrome recognition to improve efficiency of emergency urine drug screens. *Ann Emerg Med* 1988;17:676–680.

CHAPTER 24

Traumatic Brain Injury

Michael P. Alexander

■ INTRODUCTION

Traumatic brain injury (TBI) is one of the more common neurological disorders. The incidence is estimated to be 101 per 100,000 for severe injuries and 540 per 100,000 for mild injuries. Because many patients with TBI are young, and almost all survive, the prevalence is very high—approximately 2% of the U.S. population has some TBI-related disability. The great majority of injuries are mild and recovery is the rule, so the prevalence of symptomatic patients is surely much lower, but not known with certainty. TBI can occur at any age. The common mechanisms of injury differ at different ages: motor vehicle accidents at all ages; accidents and abuse in young children; accidents and sports in school-age children and young adults; and falls in the elderly. Age and mechanism interact to affect outcome. Falls in the elderly have a poorer overall prognosis than other combinations. TBI is often due to alcohol-related accidents.

■ PATHOLOGY

Various mechanisms of injury may produce different profiles of neuropathology, but rapid deceleration is common to most. The skull stops suddenly, but the brain continues to move within the skull. Those parts of the brain tightly tethered to the skull and adjacent to the falx—the venous sinuses and the large basal arteries—probably stop with the skull. Other regions less tightly tethered—particularly the frontal poles, the temporal poles, and the cerebellar hemispheres—may continue to move. The distances are very small but the times are very brief, so deceleration may produce substantial g-forces. Rotational forces produce more injury than purely translational forces.

Deceleration creates gradients of movement or potential movement within the brain, and these gradients generate shearing forces that damage fragile structures—axons and small blood vessels. Rotational gradients are the dominant force. This injury is called diffuse axonal injury (DAI). It is maximal in the frontal and anterior temporal white matter, distributed centripetally from the cortical–white matter boundary into the deeper white matter. Axons are not literally sheared, but the force disrupts function; membrane stability, intracellular transport, and metabolic integrity are all affected. If damaged near the cell body, the nerve may die (apoptosis). Small blood vessels may be damaged enough to leak, contributing to cerebral edema and even small hemorrhages, usually in white matter. The severity of DAI may vary from only transiently interrupted axonal function to severe structural injury, extensive cell death, and multifocal hemorrhages. Concussion is the mildest end of DAI. Based on animal experiments it remains unclear whether a single concussion is often or ever associated with structural brain injury. At a minimum, however, in both concussions and more definitive but mild TBI, there is some injury to axons that can be detected on late diffusion tensor imaging magnetic resonance imaging (DTI MRI) as regional reduction in fractional anisotropy. There is a period of altered cortical function demonstrated on functional MRI (fMRI) by abnormal patterns of activation during working memory tasks.

The same deceleration forces can propel portions of the cortex over rough, bony surfaces. The orbital frontal cortex and temporal poles are particularly susceptible. This injury is focal cortical contusion (FCC). The location of FCC may also be affected by skull deformation at the point of contact (coup) or opposite that point (contrecoup), but brain movement and irregular bony surfaces are the key elements of cortical deformation because anterior contusions are much more common than occipital contusions. In addition, depressed skull fractures can produce FCC underlying a fracture wherever it occurs, although fractures may actually absorb force and reduce brain injury. TBI may result in FCC in patients who otherwise appear to have a mild injury (defined blow), but the presence of FCC customarily excludes a patient from a diagnosis of mild TBI or concussion.

Patients with head injuries may also have subdural hematoma (SDH) or epidural hematoma (EDH). SDHs are commonly associated with subjacent FCC in young people, but in the elderly may occur without direct brain injury. If so, and if properly managed, there need be no brain consequence to the SDH alone. EDHs are usually caused by a fracture across the middle meningeal artery. They are extracerebral and, if recognized and evacuated, do not produce brain injury. Either EDH or SDH may, however, be sufficiently large that it causes underlying compression, vascular compromise (ischemia), and local edema. If very large, particularly if accompanied by FCC and edema, they may lead to increased intracranial pressure (ICP) and even cerebral herniation. These add local and even global hypoperfusion and ischemic injury into the TBI mix. These factors are the main mechanisms of delayed deterioration after TBI.

KEY POINTS

1. The pathology of TBI may be a mixture of different injuries—diffuse axonal injury, focal contusion, secondary hypoxic injury, and various mechanisms of secondary injury from extracerebral hemorrhages.
2. Each pathologic entity has distinct clinical consequences.
3. Concussion is the mildest form of mild injury, but it is unknown whether there is actual DAI.

■ CLINICAL CONSEQUENCES OF THE PATHOLOGY

Diffuse Axonal Injury

The immediate effect of DAI is reduction or loss of consciousness (LOC). The mechanism of LOC is not known with certainty, but it is commonly believed to be due to transient impairment or structural damage to the upper portion of the reticular activating system at the midbrain-thalamic junction. This may be due to transmitted deceleration force or to rotational stress at the junction. At the time of injury there may be brief seizure-like movements or even a brief tonic-clonic seizure. These have no consequence for later development of epilepsy. The depth of initial coma is graded with the Glasgow Coma Scale (GCS) score: mild, 13 to 15; moderate, 9 to 12; severe, 6 to 8; very severe, 3 to 5 (Table 24.1). This acute score carries considerable information for management and prognosis. The customary sense of coma (no purposeful movement, no response to voice, and no eye opening) corresponds to GCS score of 9 or lower. Patients with milder injuries may have had witnessed, unequivocal LOC at the scene but awaken quickly so that the initial GCS score (emergency medical technician or emergency department witness) is greater than 9, any condition from responsive but confused to essentially normal. Concussion blurs into mild TBI at its mildest end. Patients may have no LOC, just a period of dazed confusion for which they subsequently have no memory.

Animal experiments and human clinical studies both demonstrate a strong correlation of duration of coma (DOC), with the quality of eventual recovery. Even the coarsest stratification

TABLE 24.1 INJURY SEVERITY IS DETERMINED BY "INJURY MEASURES" NOT SUBSEQUENT SYMPTOM SEVERITY

INJURY LEVEL/ MEASURE	GLASGOW COMA SCORE (DEPTH OF COMA)	DURATION OF COMA	POSTTRAUMATIC AMNESIA
Very severe	3–5	>1 week	>1 month
Severe	6–8	<1 week	<1 month
Moderate	9–12	<1 day	<1 week
Mild	13–15	<1 hour	<1 day
Concussion	15	0–1 minute	<1 hour

carries management and prognostic information: mild, less than 1 hour; moderate, less than 24 hours; severe, less than 7 days; very severe, more than 7 days.

From coma, patients with DAI progress to a period of wakeful unresponsiveness: eyes open, often brief alerting to voice, and purposeful but random movement. In mild TBI, this phase may be so brief as to be missed by witnesses. In severe injuries with very late emergence from coma, this phase may be very long-lasting or even permanent—the persistent vegetative state. Detection of any responsive behaviors can be very difficult but will distinguish vegetative state from the so-called minimally conscious state. In patients with TBI, as opposed to anoxic injuries, definite evidence of minimally conscious state may emerge very late and first be evident to family or daily caregivers.

Patients next evolve to definitively responsive but confused. In mild TBI, this transition from coma to responsive but confused may take only seconds to minutes, and this confusional state is presumably the initial state in patients with concussion without LOC. During this period, patients may respond coherently, walk, and carry out complex activities or they may be restless and agitated, but they will be amnestic for the period, except for the occasional island of memory. This is posttraumatic amnesia (PTA), although for recording purposes, PTA usually includes the DOC as well. In more severe cases, this period may be quite prolonged and often presents significant management problems.

Confusion clears and the patient enters a stage of awareness and cognitive deficits. When confusion clears, patients become able to form new memories, and the period of PTA ends. In patients with mild injury, this transition may be sharp and the cognitive deficits subtle, escaping notice in the emergency department. In more severely injured patients the transition is blurry—periods of better awareness and attention and slipping back to overt confusion. Specifying the duration of PTA is important because it has strong prognostic value, and, commonly, the end of PTA is declared when the patient is recalling information and events from after the injury. Memory is not normal, but there is coherent recall hour by hour. Determination of PTA may be retrospective, but it is important to establish duration because it is the best indicator of injury severity and prognosis.

Once awareness and orientation improve (PTA ends), patients enter a phase of recovering cognition. The major domains of impairment in all patients—concussion, mild to severe DAI, and typical FCC—are attention and executive function. Attention is a multidimensional domain encompassing speed of processing, preparing to respond, sustaining attention, and shifting attention, which in turn requires switching from or inhibiting prior, competing, or simply salient responses. Keeping information in mind (working memory) might also be considered a dimension of attention. Executive functions are also multidimensional but include all of the controlled cognitive operations: planning, problem solving, and generating and monitoring complex actions. Stages of recovery are summarized in Table 24.2.

TABLE 24.2 STAGES OF RECOVERY

DIFFUSE AXONAL INJURY	FOCAL CORTICAL CONTUSION
Coma	—
Vegetative	—
Minimally conscious	—
Confusion	Confusion
Cognitive impairment	Cognitive impairment
Improvement to executive deficit/recovery	Improvement to focal deficit/recovery

The probability of good recovery is closely correlated with the three severity markers. Patients with the mildest injuries (concussions) usually recover in hours to days. Patients with mild TBI recover in days to weeks, with moderate injuries recovering in weeks to months, and severe and very severe injuries (if they survive) in months to years. More severely injured patients probably never recover completely and always have detectable, often functionally limiting or disabling deficits. These broad claims about recovery times hold for the population of patients with TBI, but a minority of patients diverge from these general conclusions.

Focal Cortical Contusion

FCCs are abrasions of cortical surface. They may occur anywhere as a result of local contact effects, particularly with depressed skull fractures, but they are most commonly orbital frontal and anterior temporal. They are often bilateral. They do not develop as sudden lesions like stroke, but gradually over hours to days from direct mechanical tissue disruption, often with bleeding and associated SAH to more extensive regions of mixed tissue damage, local edema, and hemorrhage. After initial vasospasm, delayed bleeding may occur. There is local loss of cerebrovascular autoregulation, and edema may become malignant, adding to increased ICP. Surgical evacuation of FCC is rarely required and may exacerbate edema. Even evacuation of overlying SDH may exacerbate the local FCC derangements.

Recall that FCCs alone do not cause LOC. The specific effects of FCC are due to their location, but acute determination of those effects may be difficult when there has also been significant DAI. Acute medical and neurosurgical issues are raised by FCC, but relatively less is known about the acute effects and subacute consequences of FCC than is known for DAI.

Evidence about the effects of and recovery from FCC comes from two sources. Patients who have a mild injury by GCS measures (13 to 15), but who have large FCCs on imaging, have occasionally been studied as a group, separate from patients with more severe DAI. This profile has been called "complicated mild TBI." The initial phases of recovery are by definition brief, but the middle phase (confusion/agitation) may be prolonged. The mechanism for this effect is not known but probably reflects the role of the frontal structures in the regulation of attention. The period of cognitive recovery appears to parallel other acute focal lesions, such as infarcts, and reach an asymptote within months, but the outcome may be more limiting than would have been predicted by the initial GCS score.

The second source of evidence comes from cognitive research projects with patients with chronic frontal injuries of various etiologies, often including patients with FCC (but not DAI). The precise impairments of FCC are related to the specific frontal regions involved, but there are common, broad behavioral consequences of these deficits: poor planning of multistep tasks, poor maintenance of task performance (either perseveration or distractibility or both), and poor regulation of interpersonal relationships. Failures are common on standard neuropsychological tests that probe these capacities: Stroop tasks, card sorting, verbal fluency, gambling, and other standard neuropsychological tests.

KEY POINTS

1. There are specific consequences, early and late, of each form of pathology.
2. All clinical measures of severity of DAI—depth of coma, duration of coma, and duration of confusion (PTA)—are correlated with each other and with outcome. The pattern of recovery from DAI is relatively uniform, the length of the separate epochs reflecting severity. Recovery may occur over a long time period.
3. The pattern of deficits after FCC are determined by the lesion site. Because most FCCs are in frontal or anterior temporal structures, the dominant impairments are in attention and executive function. Recovery probably follows the experience with other focal lesions and slows dramatically after 3 months.

■ MANAGEMENT

There are no known interventions that reduce DOC. Neither medications nor sensory stimulation are effective. No interventions are effective for vegetative state, but minimally conscious state (MCS) may respond to stimulants.

If the confusional state is brief, no interventions are warranted. If it is prolonged but the patient is not agitated or a threat to self or staff, no intervention is needed. Agitation is the treatment target, sometimes complicated by other factors. Sleep regulation is frequently disrupted, even after mild injuries, most commonly with sleep phase derangements. Confusion and agitation will rarely clear until sleep phases are approximately restored. When sleep phases are disrupted, agitation will frequently be maximal in the night when staff levels for observation and tolerance of agitation are low. There is no evidence-based support for any specific hypnotic agent. Whatever drug is selected, repeating the dose later in the night may increase morning sedation, further impairing sleep phase restoration. The dose can be increased the next night.

There is also little evidence-based support for specific tranquilizers. Except when TBI confusion is complicated by alcohol withdrawal, benzodiazepines are usually discouraged, causing too much sedation versus tranquilization; the goal is wakeful calm, or the sleep phases will be affected. For episodes of agitated crisis in patients who are intubated, propofol or lorazepam can be effective. Second-generation antipsychotics appear to be effective, although they have not been rigorously studied in the range of clinical situations that arise. Precise dosing schedules will depend on clinical circumstances. If a pattern or precipitants can be detected, behavioral or environmental adjustments should be tried—quiet time before bed, sleep regulation, catheter removal, minimal staff for procedures, etc. Premedication may be useful. If tranquilizers are being used frequently, the daily total can be used to estimate a regular dosing schedule in an attempt to avoid repeatedly dosing for crises. (The principle is exactly the same as for determining effective doses for chronic pain.) For the patient with evening agitation, hypnotics should be given only after tranquilizers so that the patient is calm enough for hypnotics to be effective.

After confusion clears and recovery begins, as many tranquilizers as possible should be withdrawn. Different treatment targets emerge: cognitive—low attention, poor memory, poor executive function; behavioral—fatigue, apathy, irritability, lability; and psychological—depression and anxiety. For patients with severe injury, these will initially be rehabilitation inpatient issues. For patients with mild injury, these may be the issues immediately after injury. They are considered separately.

Severe Injuries

Glasgow Coma Scale Sore Below 12 and Large Focal Cortical Contusion

The phase of recovery in patients with a GCS score below 12 or large FCC usually precipitates discharge planning and transition to inpatient programs. These programs are often labeled cognitive rehabilitation and may take many forms. There is only weak evidence that most are more functionally effective than supervised recuperation with emotional support. Some specific forms of executive rehabilitation based on so-called goal management training are effective and should be incorporated into community- and home-based activities that are meaningful and pertinent to the patient.

Stimulants may improve attention and reduce fatigue; both methylphenidate and amantadine have reported success. They have never been compared to caffeine. Cholinesterase inhibitors are frequently used; they may be effective for memory and general cognitive function, but demonstrated little benefit in a large controlled trial. There are no proven medications to treat apathy, although stimulants are often tried. Dopamine agonists may have a modest benefit for executive functions. Irritability, aggression, and emotional lability may reflect direct neurological damage or frustration, boredom, and depression. Behavioral distractions, such as hobbies, outings, and exercise, should be tried. There is no definitive medication to recommend. Beta-blockers may benefit labile aggression. Anticonvulsants may stabilize lability but are unproven. Depression is common during later recovery stages, with awareness of deficits, persistent disability, loss of work or school contacts, and social isolation. All antidepressants tested have had moderate benefit, albeit with low levels of evidence, but selective serotonin reuptake inhibitors (SSRIs) are usually preferred for side effect profile. In all, there is surprisingly little quality evidence for specific pharmacological interventions. In a recent comprehensive review, only 14 of 101 studies were from 2000 to 2005. There are a lot of "mays" in this discussion.

Pharmacological treatments are summarized in Table 24.3.

TABLE 24.3 TREATMENT ISSUES AND OPTIONS IN NEUROPSYCHIATRY

SLEEP DISTURBANCE	HYPNOTICS ONLY AT BEDTIME
Agitation	Assess sleep, precipitants, diurnal effects
Predictable agitation	Environmental manipulation; premedication
Infrequent, erratic	Antipsychotics when required
Frequent, erratic	Antipsychotics when required; use daily total to estimate a daily regular dosing
Persistent agitation	Daily dose plus as needed for crises; adjust daily dose
Depression	Selective serotonin reuptake inhibitors (SSRIs); bupropion
Anxiety	Regular dosing of benzodiazepines, preferably long half-life, or SSRIs; behavioral therapy
Low arousal	Methylphenidate given morning and early afternoon or in a sustained-release form
Inattention	Methylphenidate or amantadine
Apathy	Unknown, perhaps amantadine
Fatigue	Amantadine; graded exercise program
Executive impairment	Unknown, perhaps cholinesterase inhibitors

Mild Traumatic Brain Injury and Concussion

Patients with mild TBI will usually have been evaluated in an emergency department, perhaps have undergone computed tomography (CT), have other injuries treated, then been discharged home, with various levels of follow-up planned. Patients with concussion without LOC may or may not have an acute evaluation depending on circumstances. The most common setting is probably athletics, particularly football, hockey, and soccer. Most organized athletic programs are quite attentive to the management of concussion. Guidelines for return to play are established. In all circumstances, however, the rapid improvement may defer any immediate attention.

There are additional complications to the recovery and treatment of mild TBI and concussion. First, the patients are much more aware than patients with severe TBI of the accompanying somatic symptoms of injury. This cluster of symptoms plus acute-phase cognitive symptoms is referred to as postconcussive syndrome (PCS). The somatic symptoms (e.g., headache, dizziness, neck pain, tinnitus, nausea) usually are not related to the brain injury. They are usually due to peripheral injuries, that is, cervical strain, vestibular trauma, middle ear trauma, craniofacial injury, and migraine or migraine-like effects (allowing for a central mechanism for true migraine). Treatment is often piecemeal.

The second complication is psychological. Patients may remember most of the circumstances of the injury. Retrograde amnesia is always very brief, so they may recall the circumstances of injury, and PTA is often brief enough to recall frightening circumstances at the scene. Patients with mild TBI have a very high prevalence of depression and anxiety in the months after injury. Both may produce symptoms of distractibility, fatigue, forgetfulness, irritability, and sleep disturbance that are indistinguishable from the TBI symptoms. As the TBI symptoms abate, the psychological symptoms may increase in a manner that makes them seem seamless from the injury. They often believe, and are frequently told, that all symptoms are direct consequences of brain damage, although no vaguely plausible mechanism exists. There is an almost inverse relationship between severity of injury and persistence of PCS symptoms. They are often untreated, perhaps unrecognized by physicians because they are unreported by patients, or they are just swept as a result of brain injury.

The third complication is the absence of support during recovery. Reassurance often alternates with intense attempts to detect brain damage. The patient should be referred for neurological examination, with MRI and electroencephalography (EEG). Coordinated management of anxiety, sleep, pain, and other somatic complaints is not established. On the other hand, there is a burgeoning neuropsychology–industrial complex determined to "medicalize" these patients, often reinforcing the idea that every symptom is due to brain trauma.

Despite the haphazard approach to care, most patients with mild TBI recover. The evidence suggests, in cases uncomplicated by other factors, that the brain injury recovers over days to months. During that time, there are impairments in processing speed and attention. Attention-demanding tasks require more effort, no doubt corresponding to the sense of fatigue patients report, although impairments can be demonstrated on some tasks that do not seem to correlate with the presence of symptoms.

Recalling that the relationship between the PCS and brain injury is tangled, the natural history of PCS has been well described. The prevalence of PCS in patients with mild TBI declines from near 100% acutely (in the first week) to 15% at 1 year, with the steepest decline in the first few weeks. Patients who are still strikingly symptomatic at 3 months have a high probability of being symptomatic at 1 year. Little is known about how much improvement might occur in persistently symptomatic patients.

The PCS is not a diagnostic tool. Unlike standard medical syndromes that have high correlations with a specific disease or lesion location, PCS has no specificity. PCS is an admixture of neurological, somatic, and psychological symptoms, so recovery from PCS may be affected by neurological, somatic, and psychological factors. Distractibility, disturbed sleep, poor memory, and fatigue could characterize depression, anxiety, medication effects, and chronic pain states as readily as TBI sequelae. In fact, population base rates for PCS-like disorders is approximately 15%. PCS may be disabling, but it is not a marker of significant brain injury.

Treatment of the patient with persistent PCS requires parsing of the symptoms. Each of the elements may have treatments. Some are familiar to psychiatrists: antidepressants, preferably SSRIs with monitoring of side effects, anxiolytics, hypnotics, and cognitive-behavioral approaches to "unlearn" disability. Some are familiar to neurologists: headache preventives and symptomatic treatments, judicious use of vestibular suppressants, spine and soft tissue physical therapy, and vestibular rehabilitation. There is absolutely no role for clinic-based memory drills, but a short program of goal management training might help.

There are a few caveats regarding mild TBI and concussion recovery, as follows:

1. Unresolved litigation and compensation are not as pervasively an obstruction to resolution as commonly supposed, although persistent symptoms appear less commonly in insurance systems that do not recognize PCS as a disability. Litigation may motivate patients to prolong, consciously or unconsciously, symptoms of disability.
2. Age is a factor in recovery, although not a well-defined one.
3. Recurrent concussions, which are a problem in contact sports, may also cause prolonged recovery times with each successive concussion (and increased risk of depression and anxiety with each prolonged recovery). Immediately after even a mild TBI, the brain may be quite susceptible to the effects of another metabolically demanding injury. Patients with concussion may recover so quickly that they return to high-risk behaviors before there has been complete recovery. Patients who have had a concussion have an increased rate of further injuries during the days of recovery. Based on extremely rare cases of severe impairment when a second mild injury occurs before complete recovery from the first (second impact syndrome), guidelines for return to play have been developed for athletes. They are generally sensible, but not evidence based, and different guidelines offer different cautions. Recent conferences on sports concussions have suggested evaluating each case individually based on severity, prior concussions, and risk for the sport.

KEY POINTS

1. There are very few evidence-based treatments for mild or severe DAI or for FCC.
2. In the acute phase of severe injuries, the management focus is usually on confusion, agitation, and diurnal rhythm disturbances.
3. In the acute phase of mild injuries, cognitive management is often neglected and somatic symptoms are treated.
4. A minority of patients with apparently mild TBI or concussion have poor functional outcomes. The mechanisms are unknown and probably variable—both psychological and physiological. The management of many of these patients is "overmedicalized."

■ CONCLUSION

TBI can be defined by straightforward clinical measures, but the relative contributions of DAI and FCC, and even hypoperfusion and ischemic injury, are measured independently. The patterns and time course of recovery from each contributing factor are well understood, if not entirely predictable. The appropriate interventions for impairments at each phase of recovery are established, although generally poorly supported by evidence. Recovery from mild TBI (and concussion) is often complicated by nonneurological factors that may become the most functionally limiting.

Given the audience for this text, a number of issues in TBI were not considered. Epilepsy develops in up to 30% of severely injured patients; FCCs are the major risk for epilepsy. Seizures within the first week after injury have a low risk for development of epilepsy. Prolonged prophylactic treatment with anticonvulsants is not indicated. When patients develop late seizures, selection of anticonvulsants follows the same guidelines as for any cause of epilepsy, but sedating side effects may be less well tolerated in these patients. Valproate, leviracetam, and lamotrigine may have the least effect on cognition. Many patients with severe TBI have residual motor impairments, although typical hemiparesis is uncommon. Ataxia, gait problems, tone abnormalities, impaired postural and vestibular reflexes, and dysarthria are all relatively common sequelae of severe TBI.

■ SUGGESTED READINGS

Adams JH, Doyle D, Ford I, et al. Diffuse axonal injury in head injury: definition, diagnosis and grading. *Histopathology* 1989;15:49–59.

Alexander MP. Mild traumatic brain injury: pathophysiology, natural history, and clinical management. *Neurology* 1995;45:1253–1260.

Alexander MP. Minor traumatic brain injury: a review of physiogenesis and psychogenesis. *Semin Clin Neuropsychiatry* 1997;2:177–187.

Alexander MP. In the pursuit of proof of brain damage after whiplash injury. *Neurology* 1998;51:336–340.

American Academy of Neurology. Practice parameter: the management of concussion in sports. Report of the Quality Standards Subcommittee. *Neurology* 1997;48:581–585.

Ayalon L, Borodkin K, Dishon L, et al. Circadian rhythm sleep disorders following mild traumatic brain injury. *Neurology* 2007;68:1136–1140.

Binder LM, Rohling ML. Money matters: a meta-analytic review of the effects of financial incentives on recovery after closed-head injury. *Am J Psychiatry* 1996;153:7–10.

Brooks MM, Patterson DR, Questad KA. The treatment of agitation during initial hospitalization after traumatic brain injury. *Arch Phys Med Rehab* 1997;73:917–921.

Butcher I, McHugh GS, Lu J, et al. Prognostic value of cause of injury in traumatic brain injury: results from The IMPACT Study. *J Neurotrauma* 2007;24:281–286.

Dikmen SS, McLean A, Temkin N. Neuropsychological and psychological consequences of minor head injury. *J Neurol Neurosurg Psychiatry* 1986;49:1227–1232.

Dikmen SS, Temkin NR, Machamer JE, et al. Employment following traumatic head injuries. *Arch Neurol* 1994;51:177–186.

Echemendia RJE. *Sports Neuropsychology.* New York: Guilford Press, 2006.

Fox DD, Lees-Haley PR, Earnest K, et al. Base rates of postconcussive symptoms in health maintenance organization patients and controls. *Neuropsychology* 1995;9:606–611.

Gennarelli TA, Thibault LE, Adams JH, et al. Diffuse axonal injury and traumatic coma in the primate. *Ann Neurol* 1982;12:564–574.

Giacino JT, Ashwal S, Childs N, et al. The minimally conscious state: definition and diagnostic criteria. *Neurology* 2002;58:349–353.

Greiffenstein MF, Baker WJ. Miller was (almost) right: head injury severity related to simulation. *Legal Criminal Psychol* 2006;11:131–145.

Hirtz D, Thurman DJ, Gwinn-Hardy K, et al. How common are the "common" neurologic disorders? *Neurology* 2007;68:326–337.

Inglese M, Makani S, Johnson G, et al. Diffuse axonal injury in mild traumatic brain injury: a diffusion tensor imaging study. *J Neurosurg* 2005;103:298–303.

Katz DI, Alexander MP. Traumatic brain injury: predicting course of recovery and outcome for patients admitted to rehabilitation. *Arch Neurol* 1994;51:661–670.

King NS, Crawford S, Wenden FJ, et al. Early prediction of persisting post-concussion symptoms following mild and moderate head injuries. *Br J Clin Psychol* 1999;38(Pt 1):15–25.

Levin HS, O'Donnell VM, Grossman RG. The Galveston Orientation and Amnesia Test: a practical scale to assess cognition after head injury. *J Nerv Ment Dis* 1979;167:675–684.

Levin HS, Gary HE, Jr, Eisenberg HM, et al. Neurobehavioral outcome 1 year after severe head injury: experience of the Traumatic Coma Data Bank. *J Neurosurg* 1990;73:699–709.

Levine B, Robertson I, Clare L, et al. Rehabilitation of executive functioning: an experimental clinical validation of Goal Management Training. *J Int Neuropsychol Soc* 2000;6:299–312.

Macciocchi SN, Barth JT, Alves W, et al. Neuropsychological functioning and recovery after mild head injury in collegiate athletes. *Neurosurgery* 1996;39:510–514.

McAllister TW, Saykin AJ, Flashman LA, et al. Brain activation during working memory 1 month after mild traumatic brain injury. *Neurology* 1999;53:1300–1307.

McCrory P, Berkovic SF. Concussive convulsions: incidence in sport and treatment recommendations. *Sports Med* 1998;25:131–136.

McCrory PR, Berkovic SF. Second impact syndrome. *Neurology* 1998;50:677–683.

McCrory P, Johnston K, Meeuwisse W, et al. Summary and agreement statement of the 2nd International Conference on Concussion in Sport, Prague 2004. *Br J Sports Med* 2005;39:196–204.

McDowell S, Whyte J, D'Esposito M. Differential effect of a dopaminergic agonist on prefrontal function in traumatic brain injury. *Brain* 1998;1211155–1164.

Meythaler JM, Brunner RC, Johnson A, et al. Amantadine to improve neurorecovery in traumatic brain injury-associated diffuse axonal injury: a pilot double-blind randomized trial. *J Head Trauma Rehab* 2002;17:300–313.

Povlishock JT, Katz DI. Update of neuropathology and neurological recovery after traumatic brain injury. *J Head Trauma Rehabil* 2005;20:76–94.

Ropper AH, Gorson KC. Concussion. *New Engl J Med* 2007;356:166–172.

Ruff RM, Marshall LF, Crouch J, et al. Predictors of outcome following severe head trauma: follow-up data from the Traumatic Coma Data Bank. *Brain Inj* 1993;7:101–111.

Schoenhuber R, Gentilini M. Anxiety and depression after mild head injury: a case control study. *J Neurol Neurosurg Psychiatry* 1988;51:722–724.

Shreiber DI, Bain AC, Ross DT, et al. Experimental investigation of cerebral contusion: histopathological and immuno-histochemical evaluation of dynamic cortical deformation. *J Neuropathol Exp Neurol* 1999;58:153–164.

Silver JM, Koumaras B, Chen M, et al. Effects of rivastigmine on cognitive function in patients with traumatic brain injury. *Neurology* 2006;67:748–755.

Stuss DT, Alexander MP, Shallice T, et al. Multiple frontal systems controlling response speed. *Neuropsychologia* 2005;43:396–417.

Stuss DT, Binns MA, Carruth FG, et al. The acute period of recovery from traumatic brain injury: posttraumatic amnesia or posttraumatic confusional state? *J Neurosurg* 1999;90:635–643.

Stuss DT, Floden D, Alexander MP, et al. Stroop performance in focal lesion patients: dissociation of processes and frontal lobe lesion location. *Neuropsychologia* 2001;39:771–786.

Thurman DJ, Alverson C, Dunn KA, et al. Traumatic brain injury in the United States: a public health perspective. *J Head Trauma Rehabil* 1999;14:602–615.

von Cramon DY, Matthias-von Cramon G, Mai N. Problem-solving deficits in brain-injured patients: a therapeutic approach. *Neuropsychol Rehab* 1991;1:45–64.

Warden DL, Gordon B, McAllister TW, et al. Guidelines for the pharmacologic treatment of neurobehavioral sequelae of traumatic brain injury. *J Neurotrauma* 2006;23:1468–1501.

Warden DL, Salazar AM, Martin EM, Schwab KA, Coyle M, Walter J. A home program of rehabilitation for moderately severe traumatic brain injury patients. The DVHIP Study Group. *J Head Trauma Rehabil* 2000;15:1092–1102.

Whyte J, Hart T, Vaccaro M, et al. Effects of methylphenidate on attention deficits after traumatic brain injury: a multidimensional, randomized, controlled trial. *Am J Phys Med Rehabil* 2004;83:401–420.

Whyte J, Katz D, Long D, et al. Predictors of outcome in prolonged posttraumatic disorders of consciousness and assessment of medication effects: A multicenter study. *Arch Phys Med Rehabil* 2005;86:453–462.

Williams DH, Levin HS, Eisenberg HM. Mild head injury classification. *Neurosurgery* 1990;27:422–428.

Wroblewski BA, Joseph AB, Kupfer J. Effectiveness of valproic acid on destructive and aggresive behaviours in patients with acquired brain injury. *Brain Injury* 1997;11.

Zhang J, Yoganandan N, Pintar FA, Gennarelli TA. Role of translational and rotational accelerations on brain strain in lateral head impact. *Biomed Sci Instrum* 2006;42:501–506.

Zhang L, Plotkin RC, Wang G, Sandel ME, Lee S. Cholinergic augmentation with donepezil enhances recovery in short-term memory and sustained attention after traumatic brain injury. *Arch Phys Med Rehabil* 2004;85:1050–1055.

CHAPTER 25

Pain Syndromes

Bushra Malik • Mark Stillman

■ INTRODUCTION

The International Association for the Study of Pain (IASP) defines pain as "an unpleasant sensory and emotional experience associated with actual or potential tissue damage, or described in terms of such damage." For the experienced clinician at the bedside, pain is what the patient says it is. It is this subjectivity of the individual's pain experience that makes treatment such an inexact science. Unlike other fields of clinical medicine, in which evidence-based methodology and scientific rigor have helped replace the "art of medicine" with greater objectivity, the reliance on patents' subjective reporting in describing pain is the greatest impediment to the advancement of pain as a clinical science. Until recently, much of what practitioners were taught was based on a few scientifically rigorous studies and, more often, on anecdotal reports and consensus opinions.

■ PATHOPHYSIOLOGY

To better understand the clinical approach to diagnosis and evaluation of pain syndromes, the student must understand the basics of pain physiology. It is only with a solid grasp of this knowledge that a rational approach to pain pharmacology can be made.

In the classic neospinothalamic pathway, the first-order neuron, with its nociceptors, transduces and carries impulses to the dorsal horn of the spinal cord (or its counterpart in the brainstem, the trigeminal nucleus caudalis), where it synapses with the second-order neuron. In turn, this second-order nociceptive neuron travels up the spinal cord on the opposite side to synapse with a third-order neuron in the thalamus. From there the third-order neuron travels through the thalamocortical pathway to bring pain to the primary sensory and association cortices. Superimposed on the synaptic connections at the dorsal horn is a descending antinociceptive or analgesic pathway arising from the brainstem (periaqueductal gray, locus ceruleus, and raphe nuclei) and dependent on the monoamines, norepinephrine, and serotonin.

At each synaptic junction, there are interneurons capable of inhibiting the synaptic connection (via gamma-aminobutyric acid [GABA]) or enhancing it (through inhibition of inhibitory interneurons). Each neuron depends on depolarization at the membrane level and relies on voltage-gated sodium and calcium channels that respond to neuropeptides secreted by communicating neurons. Conduction along each neuron in turn depends on the functional integrity of the axon and the insulation surrounding it (Fig. 25.1).

Damage anywhere along this system induces both positive (e.g., paresthesias, increased appreciation of pain, and spontaneous jolts of pain) and negative sensory symptoms (numbness and sensory loss). However, the nociceptive system, unlike other sensory systems in the body, exhibits positive phenomena with afferent sensory damage, which likely emanate from remaining intact synaptic connections on hyperactive brainstem or spinal neurons (see the upper two neurons in Fig. 25.1). Additionally, interference with or damage to the descending

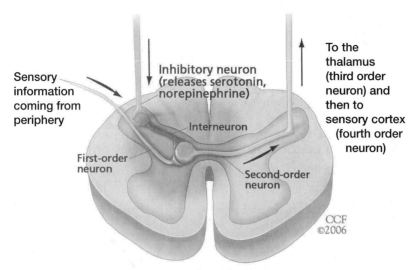

■ FIGURE 25.1 Cross section of the spinal cord showing location of neuronal connections mediating pain.

antinociceptive modulatory pathways can lead to enhancement of pain-conducting traffic along the pathways. This enhancement is dependent on excitatory amino acids, specifically glutamate, secreted by the first-order neuron into the synapse. Glutamate binds to receptors on the second-order nociceptive neuron, opening up the voltage-gated calcium channel and resulting in depolarization (and excitability). Such hyperexcitability is known as sensitization of the second-order neuron and is associated with the phenomena of temporal summation of pain, allodynia, spontaneous pain, and causalgia (burning pain).

Two pain mechanisms are known to be involved in the excitability of neurons, making them more sensitive to stimuli and sensory inputs—peripheral and central sensitization.

Peripheral Sensitization (first order neuronal activation)

Nociception occurs in the context of a number of changes in the chemical environment brought about by local tissue damage and the release of various inflammatory mediators. In the process of *peripheral sensitization,* some of these mediators act to enhance the sensation of pain in response to stimuli in the affected area by decreasing stimulus thresholds and increasing and prolonging nociceptors' firing and intensity of response to suprathreshold stimuli. Prostaglandin E_2, released from arachidonic acid–damaged cells, binds to G protein–coupled prostaglandin receptors to sensitize nociceptors. Interleukin-1b and tumor necrosis factor-α, released by immune system cells involved in the inflammatory response induce the release of cyclooxygenase-2 (COX-2) several hours after the start of inflammation, and COX-2 converts arachidonic acid to prostaglandin H and eventually prostaglandin E_2. Prostaglandin E, bradykinin, nerve growth factor, and leukotrienes also directly sensitize the nociceptors.

Certain peptides released by primary afferent neurons themselves support the process of peripheral sensitization. Substance P, neurokinin A, and calcitonin gene–related peptide (GCRP) released from activated nociceptors act on local mast cells to increase histamine release, further amplifying the process in neurogenic inflammation. Peripheral sensitization is thought to be one of the processes underlying the phenomenon of primary hyperalgesia, whereby injury to peripheral tissues results in an enhanced sensation of pain in response to subsequent suprathreshold painful stimuli. The evolutionary purpose of hyperalgesia is to discourage further contact with damaged tissue, thereby expediting the healing process.

Peripheral sensitization and the consequent hyperalgesia normally resolve as tissue heals. However, chronic pain may occur if the body is unable to restore homeostasis because the initial injury has exceeded the body's capacity for recovery or the injury involves the nervous system itself.

Secondary hyperalgesia—the expansion of hyperalgesia beyond the region of initial tissue damage—is caused by additional nervous system changes secondary to the initial insult and is further described below.

Central Sensitization (second order neuronal activation)

The pathogenesis of central sensitization may be thought of as occurring in two phases. The first stage is triggered by intense nociceptive input to the secondary afferent neurons of the dorsal horn and may thus be considered activity dependent. This excessive input may arise from persistent acute injury, surgical insult, and peripheral sensitization of nociceptors during inflammation, ectopic discharge from nerve injury, a variety of chronic pain syndromes, or other conditions. The activity-dependent stage of central sensitization occurs rapidly; hyperresponsiveness of spinal neurons may be seen within seconds of massive sensory input triggered by an appropriate initial insult in the periphery.

N-Methyl-D-aspartate (NMDA) receptors on secondary afferent neurons of the dorsal horn (or the trigeminal nucleus caudalis in the brainstem) are of critical importance in the pathology of central sensitization. Activation of NMDA receptors by glutamate leads to a number of signaling cascades initiated by increased intracellular calcium influx, activation of G protein–coupled neurokinin receptors, tyrosine kinases, and phosphokinases, leading to phosphorylation of NMDA receptor ion channels and a decrease in the magnesium block of these channels. This release from magnesium blockade acts to functionally open the calcium channel to the influx of extracellular calcium and depolarizes the neuron. As a result, sensitized (depolarized) second-order afferent neurons respond more avidly to continued C fiber afferent input from the periphery; spontaneous or ectopic signal discharge may occur in the context of this loss of gatekeeping function. At some point, the second-order nociceptive neurons in the dorsal horn or trigeminal nucleus caudalis no longer abide by activity-dependent behavior (primary afferent input) and start to exhibit spontaneous activity. To the unfortunate patient, this is interpreted as sudden shooting or tic-like pain, causalgia (unprovoked burning pain), and the appreciation of nonnoxious stimuli as painful (allodynia). In the latter instance, second-order dorsal horn neurons that normally respond to tactile stimuli (wide dynamic neurons) interpret tactile stimuli inside and outside their normal receptive fields as noxious.

Classification of Pain

There are several ways to classify pain. Some specialists arbitrarily separate pain into malignant (cancer-related) and nonmalignant (non–cancer-related) pain. In the daily clinical practice of pain medicine, the experienced practitioner often resorts to a functional classification of pain into two categories: nociceptive (somatic and visceral pain) and nonnociceptive (neuropathic and idiopathic pain).

Somatic pain is caused by the activation of pain receptors in either the cutaneous tissues (body surface) or deep tissues (musculoskeletal tissues). Deep somatic pain is usually described as dull or aching but localized. Surface somatic pain is usually sharper, may have a burning or pricking quality, and is aggravated by movement. Common causes include postsurgical pain and pain related to soft tissue trauma.

The deep somatic nociceptors associated with muscles, tendons, fascia, joints, and periosteum are largely free nerve endings with A delta and C fibers. The afferent fibers carrying pain impulses enter the spinal cord through the ventral and, especially, the dorsal roots. The lightly myelinated A delta fibers terminate primarily in laminae I and V of the dorsal horn of the spinal cord. Unmyelinated, slowly conducting C fibers terminate in laminae II. More rapidly conducting sensory afferents enter the spinal cord by way of the substantia gelatinosa and terminate in lamina I and IV.

Visceral pain results from stimulation of pain receptors in the wall of viscera, and these are sensitive to mechanical distention. Most visceral nociceptors are unmyelinated, slowly conducting polymodal C fibers. In fact, one can burn and cut visceral structures, such as the gut, without inducing pain, but cannot distend it without causing intense discomfort. The pain is described in different terms from somatic pain; it is diffuse, achy, cramping or spasmodic, and generally poorly localized. Visceral pain often is accompanied by the perception of pain arising in somatic structures that share the same spinal level of innervation. This phenomenon, known as referred pain, results from the convergence of nociceptive fibers from different structures onto the same population of cells in the dorsal horn. This explains such recognizable phenomena as pain associated with gastric perforation that causes both upper gastric aching pain and left shoulder pain.

Neuropathic pain is the result of damage or disfunction occurring anywhere along the neuraxis—the peripheral nerve, spinal ganglion, nerve root, spinal cord, brainstem, thalamus, and cortex, but the damage may not be readily detectable at the bedside. The words used by patients to describe the pain help distinguish it from the nociceptive pain types mentioned earlier and incorporate descriptors for both positive and negative sensations—burning, searing or scalding, cold, numb, tingling, shooting, stabbing, crushing, and vice-like. These sensations, which affect not only the sensory system, but also the affective, cognitive, and attention systems, result from the disruption of the body's normal pain-conducting circuitry. A thorough discussion of the theories underlying the generation of neuropathic pain is beyond the scope of this article. Interested readers are referred to recent detailed reviews on the subject.

Neuropathic pain can result from abnormal discharges in injured or regenerating sensory afferents. Injured nerve fibers sometimes develop spontaneous discharges, and afferent impulses may be evoked by electrical activity in surrounding axons in injured nerves. A variety of mechanisms are involved in pain accompanying nerve disease, and multiple mechanisms may be operating simultaneously in any given patient. These mechanisms include the following:

1. Spontaneous discharges in injured nociceptive afferents
2. Induced discharges in injured nociceptors afferents
3. Deafferentation with subsequent changes in dorsal horn or central nociceptive transmission (i.e., loss of inhibitory interneuronal input), leading to central pain generation
4. Activation of sensitized mechanoreceptors by efferent sympathetic activity
5. Specific ion channel changes in primary afferents

Finally, *idiopathic pain* has been used interchangeably with the term psychogenic pain. Idiopathic pain is the more appropriate term because it implies a wider spectrum of poorly understood pain states. The *Diagnostic and Statistical Manual of Mental Disorders,* fourth edition (DSM-IV) refers to "pain disorder associated with psychological factors (acute and chronic)" and "pain disorder associated with both psychological factors and a general medical condition (acute and chronic)." This term has begun to replace the older terminology of psychogenic pain in instances in which no identifiable organic origin could be found. Fibromyalgia, regional myofascial pain, and somatoform pain are examples of idiopathic pain. In addition to the lack of organic origin, the pain and associated symptoms often are thought to be grossly out of proportion to any identifiable disorder.

■ AN APPROACH TO RATIONAL THERAPY

Successful pain management is based on a clear understanding of causation of pain and as complete an understanding of the afferent pathways that serve nociception as possible. This requires a complete history of the nature of the pain, a full accounting of medical history, a directed physical examination, and a personal review of imaging studies.

■ TREATMENT APPROACH TO SOMATIC PAIN

Typical pain is experienced acutely or chronically. Treatment is usually symptomatic and uses a variety of nonspecific, but effective, analgesics. The analgesics interrupt the process of pain impulse formation at any or all of several sites along the process. It should go without saying that effective treatment of the pathological process is a vital component of any treatment regimen.

■ NONOPIOID ANALGESICS

As a group, these agents are indicated for mild-to-moderate nociceptive pain and are particularly useful in the treatment of pain originating in bone and joints. The predominant mechanism of action is probably inhibition of prostaglandin synthesis at the site of tissue injury, thus directly decreasing nociceptor stimulation. Nonsteroidal anti-inflammatory drugs (NSAIDs) may be useful in combination with opiates for more severe pain. Unlike opioid use, NSAID use is not associated with tolerance or physical dependence. Also unlike with opioids, progressive increments of NSAIDs beyond a certain dosage often fail to provide improved pain control (i.e., there is a "ceiling effect" to the analgesia produced by NSAIDs).

Refer to Table 25.1 for information on commonly used nonopioid analgesics.

For minor or self-limited somatic pain, the first choice should be a short-acting agent with a low likelihood of side effects, usually ibuprofen. For persistent or chronic pain, an agent with a longer half-life may be chosen to reduce dosing frequency. For many patients with

TABLE 25.1 NONOPIOID ANALGESICS

CLASS	DRUG	HALF-LIFE (HRS)	DOSE RANGE	MAJOR TOXICITIES
Paraminophenol derivative	Acetaminophen	3	650–1000 mg q4–6h	Hepatotoxicity with high doses
Salicylates (carboxylic acids)	Aspirin	0.5	650–1000 mg q4–6h	GI, including dyspepsia, gastritis, ulceration Increased bleeding time
Propionic acids	Ibuprofen	2	400–1000 mg q6–8h	GI toxicity, may be less common than with acetic acid Renal toxicity, particularly in combination with diuretics
	Naproxen	14	250–500 mg q12h	Similar to ibuprofen
Acetic acids	Indomethacin	45	25–50 mg q8–12h	GI and CNS toxicity, particularly headache Renal toxicity, particularly with triamterene
	Sulindac	14	150–200 mg q12h	GI and CNS effects are less common than with indomethacin; may have less renal toxicity
	Ketorolac	47	15–30 mg IM or 10 mg PO q6h	GI toxicity; for short-term therapy only

CNS, central nervous system; GI, gastrointestinal.

chronic pain, serial trials of different agents are needed to determine the most effective NSAID. A 2-week trial is required to properly assess the response to a given dose. If pain control is inadequate and significant toxicity has not occurred, dose escalation is appropriate. Failure to benefit from one NSAID does not predict the failure to respond to others. Therefore a working knowledge of one or two drugs from each class of NSAIDs is important.

■ CORTICOSTEROIDS

Corticosteroids are used as coanalgesics when inflammation and mass effect of vasogenic edema cause pain. They reduce inflammation by inhibiting phospholipase activity and thus prostaglandin synthesis. In addition, they may reduce axonal sprouting and neurokinin concentration in sensory fibers near injured tissue. Acute neural compression, bony and soft tissue infiltration, and visceral distention cause pain that may respond to steroids.

■ OPIOIDS

The opioids are centrally acting derivatives of opium and are the strongest analgesics in clinical practice. They are initiated when nonopioid analgesics are less effective or the patient presents with more intense or persistent pain. Opioids do not alter the pain threshold of afferent nerve endings to noxious stimuli, nor do they affect the conductance of impulses along peripheral nerves. Analgesia is mediated through changes in the perception of pain at the spinal cord (mu_2, delta, kappa receptors) and at more rostral levels in the CNS (mu_1 and $kappa_3$ receptors). Opioids also modulate the endocrine and immune systems and inhibit the release of vasopressin, somatostatin, insulin, and glucagon.

Commonly Used Opioids

Morphine is the standard opioid against which all others are compared and acts mainly on mu opiate receptors of pain-conducting neurons in the dorsal horn and even the peripheral nociceptors. It decreases the transmission of painful stimuli within the spinal cord and to the spinal cord, causing inhibition of ascending pain pathways and altering the perception of and response to pain. Refer to Table 25.2 for information on commonly used opioids.

Methadone, another classic opioid analgesic, was synthesized in the 1930s. Its affinity for the NMDA receptor is similar to those of dextromethorphan and ketamine. It is also a strong inhibitor of serotonin and norepinephrine reuptake. At high doses, methadone blocks potassium channels required for rapid cardiac muscle repolarization, which may explain the risk for developing torsades de pointes with high doses.

The initial opioid should be a short-acting drug when the patient has severe pain and requires rapid dose titration, when the patient has intermittent pain, or when the patient is opioid naïve and there is concern about delayed toxicity from a long-acting preparation such as methadone, extended-release morphine, or oxycodone and fentanyl. After a basal opioid requirement is determined, a long-acting opioid preparation may be substituted. In the case of cancer-related pain, an additional short-acting opioid is made available for breakthrough pain every 2 to 3 hours as needed. Common adverse side effects from opioids include constipation, nausea, vomiting, mental cloudiness, myoclonus, and respiratory depression.

■ TREATMENT APPROACH TO VISCERAL PAIN

Pain originating from the viscera is familiar to many of us as abdominal cramps or the pain of passing a renal stone. It may be less constant than somatic pain, occurring in sharp waves of pain known as colic. Once the colic dissipates there may be a residual of dull constant pain. Visceral pain is poorly localized and is often referred to a distant cutaneous site, as explained previously.

TABLE 25.2 COMMONLY USED OPIOID ANALGESICS

OPIOID (EQUIANALGESIC DOSES)	RECEPTORS	HALF LIFE (HOURS)	ELIMINATION ROUTE	COMMENT
Morphine 30 mg PO IV or Sub-Q 10 mg	Mu	3–4	Renal	Manipulation of its delivery has enabled longer acting preparations to enter clinical use
*Codeine	Mu	3–4	Renal	Extensively metabolized by liver
Fentanyl TD 25 mcg IV/Sub-Q 25 mcg/hr	Mu	IV: 3–4 Transdermal patch: 12–17 Transmucosal lozenge: 7	Renal, hepatic	Transdermal patch half-life is influenced by absorption rate Increases pain threshold
Hydromorphone: PO 7.5 mg IV or Sub-Q 1.5 mg	Mu	3–4	Renal	Longer acting preparation is in development 5–10 times more potent than morphine Immediate release only
Methadone PO 20 mg IV 10 mg	Mu, delta, NMDA	Varies from few hours to 120 hours	Renal, biliary	Overdose is common given long half-life
Oxycodone PO 30 mg	Mu	3–4	Hepatic, renal	
Buprenorphine SL 0.4 mg IV or Sub-Q 0.4 mcg/hr	Mu	6–8	Renal	Partial agonist antagonist May induce withdrawal

*Acute pain studies performed by Houde et al., in the 1950s did not demonstrate the analgesic potency of codeine or propoxyphene to be any greater than that of aspirin or acetaminophen.

SWITCHING A PATIENT FROM ONE OPIOID TO ANOTHER OPIOID: With the exception of methadone, the clinician should use approximately ½ the equianalgesic dose, provided on a divided, time-contingent basis. With methadone, ¼ or ⅛ the equianalgesic dose should be provided on a q6–q8h prn schedule for the first 48–72 hours. The total daily requirements can then be given on a divided, time-contingent schedule.

NMDA, *N*-Methyl-D-aspartate.

In general, the treatment of visceral pain follows similar guidelines for the treatment of somatic pain, with some exceptions such as the use of antispasmodic drugs. The two anticholinergic drugs most often used are hyoscyamine and glycopyrrolate. The anticholinergic properties of these medications slow peristalsis in the gastrointestinal and genitourinary systems and can help reduce excess secretions. They have found a particularly important role in the palliative management of patients with end-stage cancer-related pain.

■ TREATMENT APPROACH FOR NEUROPATHIC PAIN

Because pain, a decidedly positive phenomenon for the sufferer, is the result of damage or destruction of normal nervous system pathways, it appears to defy management with routine antinociceptive or analgesic maneuvers. In fact, neuropathic pain responds better to medications designed to work in the central nervous system (CNS) for indications such as depression and epilepsy. By limiting excitation and enhancing inhibition, antidepressant, antiarrhythmic, and antiepileptic drugs modulate hypersensitivity-related changes of the nervous system.

Nonopioid Analgesics

There are no randomized, controlled, double-blind studies of nonopioid common analgesics (NSAIDs and non-NSAIDs) in the treatment of neuropathic pain. That should not discount their potential benefit because the NSAIDs have demonstrated not only a peripheral analgesic effect but also a central effect in exerting analgesic efficacy. Using cancer pain treatment as a standard, and keeping in mind that the many presentations of cancer pain represent mixed nociceptive and neuropathic pain states, NSAIDs and non-NSAID analgesics, such as aceta-minophen, have been used as adjuvant agents in patients with neuropathic pain. They exhibit an opioid-sparing effect and work synergistically with the opioids. However, their use comes with risk for complications in a population that is frequently medically fragile.

The role of inflammation and inflammatory cytokines in neuropathic pain is receiving more attention. In patients with exacerbation of pain, a steroid taper can be extremely beneficial. Anti-inflammatory medications such as steroids may induce inhibition of both peripheral prostaglandin pathways and the CNS's glial-based prostaglandin system involved in the response to (neuropathic) pain.

Opioid Analgesics

Classic teaching has traditionally held that neuropathic pain states are opioid resistant and that opioids are best suited for visceral and somatic nociceptive pains. There has been much debate on the topic, and, recently, several carefully conducted trials have demonstrated efficacy of opioid analgesia for neuropathic pain. There are now studies that suggest a benefit from opioid analgesics, presumably related to their ability to inhibit ascending pain impulses centrally. Opioids should be initiated to augment the analgesia of tricyclic antidepressants or anticonvulsants for neuropathic pain. Doses of immediate-release opioids are titrated slowly upward until pain reduction is achieved, and then patients are switched to controlled-release opioids. Most patients with chronic nonmalignant pain can be managed with less than 300 mg daily of oral morphine (or equivalent).

Tramadol, although not a Schedule II opioid analgesic, is a mu opioid agonist, as well as norepinephrine and serotonin reuptake inhibitor. In controlled studies, when doses were carefully titrated to a maximum of 400 mg daily in four divided doses, tramadol fared better than placebo for postherpetic neuropathy and other neuropathic pains, including diabetic neuropathy. Not surprisingly, it has CNS side effects similar to those of opioid analgesics and has been abused by certain populations at risk for addiction and drug abuse.

Antidepressants

Their efficacy is presumed to be due to their potentiation of descending analgesic pathways arising from the periaqueductal gray, the raphe nuclei in the midbrain, the source of serotonin in the brainstem, and the locus ceruleus, the brainstem's locus for norepinephrine. The benefit was initially seen with the tricyclic antidepressants, represented by amitriptyline, imipramine, nortriptyline, and doxepin.

The tricyclic antidepressants continue to fare significantly better than the newer selective serotonin reuptake inhibitors (SSRIs), such as fluoxetine, paroxetine, sertraline, and citalopram. The tricyclic antidepressants are balanced reuptake inhibitors of serotonin and norepinephrine; the SSRI agents inhibit serotonin reuptake at the synapse. Relief can be seen for steady burning or aching pain, as well as tic-like spontaneous pain. The side effect profiles of the tricyclic antidepressants can be problematic, with sedation, confusion, constipation, and more serious cardiovascular adverse effects, such as conduction blocks, tachycardia, and ventricular arrhythmias. These agents also cause weight gain, lowering of the seizure threshold, and orthostatic hypotension. They must be used with special care in the elderly, who are prone to the serious side effects, and obtaining blood levels is recommended to mitigate toxicity in slow drug

TABLE 25.3 CLINICALLY APPROVED ANTIEPILEPTICS FOR NEUROPATHY

ANTIEPILEPTIC	MECHANISMS OF ACTION	ELIMINATION HALF-LIFE	DOSAGES	SIDE EFFECTS	OTHER BENEFITS
Gabapentin	Binds voltage-gated calcium channel's alpha-2 delta subunit, reduces calcium influx and the release of neurotransmitters (glutamate, substance P, and CGRP) at the primary afferent nerve terminals	5–7 hours	1800 mg and 3600 mg/day in divided doses	Fatigue, confusion, and somnolence	Improvements in mood, sleep Lack of interference with other AEDs
Pregabalin	As above	6.3 hours	300 and 600 mg in divided doses	Fatigue, confusion, and somnolence	Lack of interference with other AEDs
Topiramate	Enhances GABA-ergic neurotransmission and blocks glutamate neurotransmission at the AMPA/kainate receptor of the voltage-gated calcium channel	18–24 hours	200 and 400 mg/day	Paresthesias, confusion and forgetfulness, anorexia and weight loss Were responsible for a high drop-out rate.	Weight loss Effective in diabetic and nondiabetic neuropathic pain
Carbamazepine	Blocks voltage-dependent sodium channels	25–65 hours	400 mg/day	Dizziness, nausea, drowsiness, blurred vision, ataxia	Patient-oriented evidence for treatment of trigeminal neuralgia
Lamotrigine	Blocks the activation of voltage-sensitive sodium channels Inhibits the presynaptic release of glutamate	14–30 hours	400 and 600 mg/day	Skin rash (Stevens-Johnson syndrome)	

AEDs, antiepileptic drugs; AMPA, alpha-amino-3-hydroxy-5-methyl-4-isoxazolepropionate; CGRP, calcitonin gene-related peptide; GABA, gamma-aminobutyric acid.

metabolizers. Duloxetine, a newer serotonin and norepinephrine reuptake inhibitor (SNRI), has received Food and Drug Administration (FDA) approval for the treatment of pain associated with diabetic neuropathy on the basis of two large randomized, double-blind, multicenter studies and has also received FDA approval in treating fibromyalgia-related pain.

Local Anesthetics

The local anesthetics are membrane stabilizers that block axonal sodium channels and provide dose-dependent blockade of spontaneous ectopic impulses. This suppression of transduction of nociceptive impulses occurs at concentrations below which normal sensorimotor impulses are suppressed. Local anesthetics are particularly suited to neuropathic conditions emanating from peripheral nervous system injury in which excess voltage-sensitive sodium channels accumulate in the regions of axonal damage or demyelination. Additional mechanisms have been suggested, including postsynaptic modification of NMDA receptor activity and opioid-like effects. Local anesthetics can be administered intravenously, topically, and orally, although the topical preparation of lidocaine remains the best studied agent for neuropathic pain. The lidocaine patch does not appear to function when complete deafferentation has occurred. Aside from local skin reactions, the treatment is well tolerated and systemic blood levels are negligible, obviating concerns of systemic cardiac toxicity.

Antiepileptic Drugs

The most impressive advances in neuropathic pain treatment in the past few years have been seen with the antiepileptic drugs (AEDs). Table 25.3 lists clinically approved antiepileptic agents used for neuropathic pain.

Gabapentin was recognized as an effective drug for neuropathic pain soon after it was introduced as an antiepileptic agent. A similar drug that appears to be equally effective and perhaps even more rapid in onset is pregabalin. By week 1 and in some cases even earlier, it has produced reductions in mean pain scores of more than 50% with dosages of 150 mg daily or higher.

■ IDIOPATHIC (PSYCHOSOMATIC) PAIN

The treatment of idiopathic pain and, for that matter, chronic non–cancer-related pain is beyond the scope of this article. By the very nature of its chronicity, the emotions engendered in suffering, and the complexity and plasticity of the mammalian pain system, such pain defies simplification and categorization. That should not discount the applicability of the principles described above; however, the complexity of the emotive nature of the disorder mandates more than a medicinal approach. These complex pain disorders require a multidisciplinary approach with strong psychological and psychiatric input over extended periods.

■ CONCLUSION

In practice, treatment is based on defining the mechanism(s) by which the pain is generated. A relatively high likelihood of therapeutic success is achieved in the case of nociceptive pain, but only a modest rate of success is obtained in the treatment of neuropathic and idiopathic pain syndromes. The understanding of pain mechanisms, in terms of basic science and as clinical phenomena, remains incomplete. Nonetheless, this mechanistic approach is central to formulating a rational therapeutic strategy. Treatment applied without an understanding of the mechanisms involved has a high likelihood of failure, unnecessary toxicity, and potential for irreversible tissue injury.

KEY POINTS

1. Understanding pathophysiology is important in diagnosis and evaluation of pain.
2. Pain is separated into two categories, nociceptive (somatic and visceral pain) and nonnociceptive (neuropathic and idiopathic pain).
3. Management of pain is based on a clear understanding of causation of pain and requires a complete history of nature of pain.
4. Effective treatment of the pathological process is a vital component of any treatment regimen.

■ SUGGESTED READINGS

Arendt-Nielsen L, Graven-Nielsen T. Central sensitization in fibromyalgia and other musculoskeletal disorders. *Curr Pain Headache Rep* 2003;7:355–361.

Arner S, Meyerson BA. Lack of analgesic effect of opioids on neuropathic and idiopathic forms of pain. *Pain* 1988;33: 11–23.

Backonja M. Anticonvulsants and antiarrhythmics in the treatment of neuropathic pain syndromes. In: Hansson PT, Fields HL, Hill RG, et al, eds. *Progress in Pain Research and Management.* Vol 21. *Neuropathic Pain: Pathophysiology and Treatment.* Seattle: IASP Press; 2001;185–202.

Bonica J. *The Management of Pain.* 2nd ed. Philadelphia: Lea and Febiger; 1990.

Dickenson AH, Matthews EA, Suzuki R. Central nervous system mechanisms of pain in peripheral neuropathy. In: Hansson PT, Fields HL, Hill RG, et al, eds. *Progress in Pain Research and Management.* Vol 21. *Neuropathic Pain: Pathophysiology and Treatment.* Seattle: IASP Press; 2001;85–101.

Dworkin R, Backonja M, Rowbotham M, et al. Advances in neuropathic pain. *Arch Neurol* 2003;60:1524–1534.

Dworkin RH, Corbin AE, Young JP, et al. Pregabalin for the treatment of postherpetic neuralgia: a randomized, placebo-controlled trial. *Neurology* 2003;60:1274–1283.

Eap CB, Buclin T, Baumann P. Interindividual variability of the clinical pharmacokinetics of methadone. *Clin Pharmacol* 2002;41:1153–1193.

Ebert B, Anderson S, Krogsgaard-Larsen P. Ketobemidone, methadone and pethidine are non-competitive NMDA antagonists in the rat cortex and spinal cord. *Neurol Lett* 1995;165–168.

Ebert B, Thorkildsen C, Andersen S, et al. Opioid analgesics as noncompetitive NMDA antagonist. *Biochem Pharmacol* 1998;56:553–559.

England JD, Happel LT, Kline DG, et al. Sodium channel accumulation in humans with painful neuromas. *Neurology* 1996;47:272–276.

Gebhart GF. Visceral pain mechanisms. In: Chapman CR, Foley KM, eds. *Current and Emerging Issues in Cancer Pain: Research and Practice.* Raven Press Ltd, New York; 1993;99–111.

Hansson PT, Lacerenza M, Marchettini P. Aspects of clinical and experimental neuropathic pain: the clinical perspective. In: Hansson PT, Fields HL, Hill RG, et al, eds. *Progress in Pain Research and Management.* Vol 21. *Neuropathic Pain: Pathophysiology and Treatment.* Seattle: IASP Press; 2001;1–18.

Harati Y, Gooch C, Swenson M, et al. Double-blind randomized trial of tramadol for the treatment of the pain of diabetic neuropathy. *Neurology* 1998;50:1842–1846.

Kapur S, Miezkowski T, Mann JJ. Antidepressant medications and the relative risk of suicide attempt and suicide. *J Am Med Assoc* 1992;268:3441–3445.

Mayer EA, Gebhart GF. Basic and clinical aspects of visceral hyperalgesia. *Gastroenterology* 1994;107:271–293.

McMahon SB, Dmitrieva N, Koltzenburg M. Visceral pain. *Br J Anaesth* 1995;75:132–144.

McQuay HJ, Tramer M, Nye BA, et al. A systematic review of antidepressants in neuropathic pain. *Pain* 1996;68: 217–227.

Meeker MH, Rothrock JC. *Alexander's Care of the Patient in Surgery.* St. Louis: Mosby; 1999.

Merskey H, Bogduk N. *Classification of Chronic Pain: Description of Chronic Pain Syndromes and Definitions of Pain Terms.* 2nd ed. Seattle: IASP Press; 1994;222.

Miaskowski C, Cleary J, Burney R, et al. *Guidelines for the Management of Cancer Pain in Adults and Children.* 5th ed. Glenview, Ill: American Pain Society; 2005.

Offenbaecher M, Ackenheil M. Current trends in neuropathic pain treatments. *CNS Spectr* 2005;10:285–297.

Portenoy RK, Lesage P. Management of cancer pain. *Lancet* 1999;353:1695–1700.

Raja SN, Haythornthwaite JA, Pappagallo M, et al. Opioids versus antidepressants in postherpetic neuralgia: a randomized, placebo-controlled trial. *Neurology* 2003;60:927–934.

Samad TA, Moore K, Sapirstein A, et al. Interleuken-1 beta-mediated induction of COX-2 in the CNS contributes to inflammatory pain hypersensitivity. *Nature* 2001;410:471–475.

Sarne Y, Fields A, Keren O, et al. Stimulatory effects of opioids on transmitter release and possible cellular mechanisms: overview and original results. *Neurochem Res* 1996;21:135313–135361.

Schaible HG. Peripheral and central mechanisms of pain generation. *Handb Exp Pharmacol* 2007;177:3–28.

Segal AZ, Rordorf G. Gabapentin as a novel treatment for postherpetic neuralgia. *Neurology* 1996;46:1175–1176.

Sen D, Christie D. Chronic idiopathic pain syndromes. *Best Pract Res Clin Rheumatol* 2006;20:369–386.

Sindrup SH, Jensen TS. Efficacy of pharmacological treatment of neuropathic pain: an update and effect related to mechanism of drug action. *Pain* 1999;83:389–400.

Sindrup SH, Andersen G, Madsen C, et al. Tramadol relieves pain and allodynia in polyneuropathy: a randomized, double-blind, controlled trial. *Pain* 1999;83:85–90.

Watson CPN, Babul N. Efficacy of oxycodone in neuropathic pain: a randomized trial in postherpetic neuralgia. *Neurology* 1998;50:1837–1841.

Watson CPN, Vernich L, Chipman M, et al. Nortriptyline versus amitriptyline in postherpetic neuralgia. *Neurology* 1998;51:1166–1171.

Whitten CE, Donovan M, Cristobal K. Treating chronic pain: new knowledge, more choices. *Permanente J* 2005;9:1.

Yaksh TL. Pharmacology and mechanisms of opioid analgesic activity. *Acta Anaesthesiol Scand* 1997;41(1 Pt 2):94–111.

Yunus MB. Role of central sensitization in symptoms beyond muscle pain, and the evaluation of a patient with widespread pain. *Best Pract Res Clin Rheumatol* 2007;21:481–497.

CHAPTER 26

Central Nervous System Infections

Nicholas J. Silvestri

■ INTRODUCTION

The central nervous system (CNS) is susceptible to a number of infections caused by a broad range of pathogens. The presence of fever in the context of neurological signs or symptoms can be evidence of an underlying CNS infection. In clinical practice, the presentation may also include alteration in mental status, ranging from delirium to dementia, based on underlying etiology. Thus psychiatrists must recognize this possibility and, in the proper clinical setting, keep the diagnosis of a potential CNS infection in their differential diagnosis. In general, once the diagnosis of infection is entertained, appropriate workup includes a spinal tap for analysis of cerebrospinal fluid (CSF). The cellular and biochemical profile of the CSF varies considerably among etiologies (Table 26.1). In addition to laboratory studies, radiological studies are also frequently helpful in the investigation for a suspected infection in the CNS. The findings on computed tomography (CT) and magnetic resonance imaging (MRI) vary widely according to etiology and will be further discussed under each disease entity. With the advent of antibiotics in the middle of the last century, many CNS infections are potentially treatable. Nevertheless, the morbidity and mortality of these conditions remain high. This chapter will focus on the clinical presentation, investigation, and treatment of CNS infections.

■ BACTERIAL MENINGITIS

The annual incidence of bacterial meningitis is approximately 5 per 100,000 adults in the United States. Despite improved diagnostic modalities and treatment, morbidity and mortality remain relatively high. Bacteria reach the CNS by one of two routes. They may travel via hematogenous spread from another area of localized infection within the body, such as pneumonia or osteomyelitis. Alternatively, bacteria may invade the meninges by direct spread from extracranial structures, such as the middle ear or paranasal sinuses. The clinical presentation of bacterial meningitis includes the classic triad of fever, nuchal rigidity (Fig. 26.1), and altered mental status. In a large series of patients with bacterial meningitis, roughly half demonstrated the combination of these three symptoms. If headache is included in the group of presenting complaints, almost all patients with bacterial meningitis will have two of the four symptoms.

As with infections elsewhere in the body, the age of the patient, clinical setting, immune status, and evidence of systemic infection need to be taken into account when determining the organism most likely responsible for the infection (Table 26.2). *Streptococcus pneumoniae* and *Neisseria meningitidis* are the most common causative organisms in infants, children, and adults under 50 years of age. *Haemophilus influenzae* and *Listeria monocytogenes* are less common causes in this age group. In patients over 50 years old, *Streptococcus pneumoniae* remains the most common cause, but *Listeria* species and Gram-negative rods are also often seen. Newborns are susceptible to infection with *Escherichia coli,* group B streptococcus, and *Listeria* species. Nosocomial bacterial meningitis may occur in patients who have undergone a neurosurgical procedure or have sustained severe head trauma within the preceding month, have an

TABLE 26.1 CEREBROSPINAL FLUID FINDINGS IN SELECTED CENTRAL NERVOUS SYSTEM INFECTIONS

DISEASE	OPENING PRESSURE	CELLS/ML	PROTEIN	GLUCOSE	OTHER STUDIES
Normal adult	6–20 cm H$_2$O	0 PMNs <5 lymphocytes 0 RBCs	15–45	At least 50% of serum glucose	
Bacterial meningitis	Normal or elevated	100–10,000 WBCs, mostly PMNs	Elevated	Less than 40% of serum glucose	Positive Gram stain or culture
Viral meningitis	Normal	10–100 WBCs, mostly lymphocytes	Normal to slightly elevated	Normal	PCR available
Viral encephalitis	Normal	10–500 WBCs, mostly lymphocytes Will see RBCs in HSV encephalitis	Normal to slightly elevated	Normal	PCR available
Toxoplasmosis	Normal or elevated	Normal to slightly elevated WBC count	Normal to slightly elevated	Normal to slightly low	PCR available
Cryptococcal meningitis	Normal or elevated	5–20 WBCs, mostly lymphocytes	Elevated	Less than 40% of serum glucose	Positive India ink stain or cryptococcal antigen titers
Tuberculous meningitis	Normal or elevated	10–1000 WBCs, PMNs early and lymphocytes later	Elevated	Less than 40% of serum glucose	Pleocytosis may be mild or absent in immunocompromised patients May see positive AFB stain or culture
Neurosyphilis	Normal	0–300 WBCs	Normal to elevated	Normal	Positive CSF VDRL Positive antitreponemal Ab
Lyme disease	Normal	10–100 WBCs, mostly lymphocytes	Normal to slightly elevated	Normal	IgM or IgG intrathecal antibody production
Neurocysticercosis	Normal	0–100 WBCs, may see eosinophils	Normal	Normal	Positive antibody

AFB, acid-fast bacilli; CSF, cerebrospinal fluid; IgG, immune globulin G; IgM, immune globulin M; PCR, polymerase chain reaction; RBCs, red blood cells; VDRL, Venereal Disease Research Laboratory; WBCs, white blood cells.

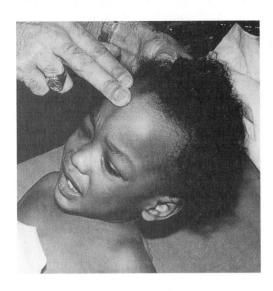

■ **FIGURE 26.1** Nuchal rigidity in a child with bacterial meningitis. (From Fleisher GR, Ludwig W, Baskin MN. *Atlas of Pediatric Emergency Medicine.* Philadelphia: Lippincott Williams & Wilkins; 2004.)

indwelling neurosurgical device, or a CSF leak. Frequently seen organisms under these circumstances include Gram-negative rods, *Staphylococcus aureus,* coagulase-negative staphylococcal species, and streptococcal species.

The workup for bacterial meningitis must be performed promptly because any delay in initiation of therapy may lead to worsened outcome. The moment the diagnosis is entertained based on clinical grounds alone, administration of antibiotics should be done before performing further diagnostic workup. The spinal tap and evaluation of CSF is the single most important diagnostic study in bacterial meningitis, and indeed in most suspected CNS infections. Before performing a spinal tap, elevated intracranial pressure (ICP) must be ruled out with appropriate imaging (usually a CT scan). A funduscopic examination is not adequate because it can take up to 2 weeks for papilledema (Fig. 26.2) to develop in cases of intracranial hypertension. Elevated ICP must be suspected if there are new-onset seizures, if the patient is immunocompromised, if there are signs on neurological examination suspicious for a space-occupying lesion, if papilledema is present, or if there is moderate to severe decrease in consciousness. If elevated ICP is present, treatment of that process as well as empiric treatment for bacterial meningitis should commence. In patients without elevated ICP, a spinal tap should be performed soon after presentation. Opening pressure, as should be measured in every spinal tap, will be high in a majority of cases of bacterial meningitis. Analysis of the CSF demonstrates a predominantly neutrophilic pleocytosis. Typically, there are 100 to 10,000 white cells per milliliter of fluid. The protein will be elevated and glucose will be decreased, less than 40% of the serum glucose when measured concomitantly. Gram stain will often demonstrate the causative organism, as will culture of the CSF. It is also useful to obtain blood cultures at the

TABLE 26.2 CAUSES OF BACTERIAL MENINGITIS

AGE	PATHOGENS
Newborn	*Escherichia coli, group B Streptococcus,* and *Listeria monocytogenes*
Children and adults <50 years	More common: *Streptococcus pneumoniae, Neisseria meningitides* Less common: *Haemophilus influenzae, L monocytogenes*
Adults >50 years	*S pneumoniae, L monocytogenes,* gram-negative rods

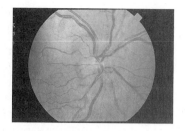

■ **FIGURE 26.2** Acute papilledema. (From Tasman W, Jaeger E, eds. *The Wills Eye Hospital Atlas of Clinical Ophthalmology.* 2nd ed. Philadelphia: Lippincott Williams & Wilkins; 2001.)

time of presentation, because they can also provide insight into the causative organism, especially if the CSF, Gram stain, or culture is negative.

As mentioned previously, early institution of broad-spectrum antibiotics can be life-saving. Studies have demonstrated a clear association between delay in starting antibiotic therapy and a high risk of adverse outcome. It is generally recommended that if imaging is performed before the spinal tap, antibiotic treatment should begin before the scan. Treatment is initially broad spectrum and can be subsequently tailored appropriately once the causative organism is identified. Usually, initial treatment includes a third-generation cephalosporin, vancomycin, and, under appropriate circumstances, ampicillin (if the patient is elderly or immunosuppressed, and therefore susceptible to infection with *L monocytogenes*). Recent studies have also shown that in patients with intermediate disease severity (defined as Glasgow Coma Scale score between 8 and 11) and pneumococcal meningitis, treatment with dexamethasone given shortly before or with the first dose of antibiotics and continued for 4 days reduced the incidence of adverse outcome. Therefore treatment with steroids at the time the diagnosis is entertained as often done in clinical practice.

Untreated, bacterial meningitis is almost universally fatal. Even with prompt treatment, complications of bacterial meningitis are common. In the short term, hyponatremia from the syndrome of inappropriate antidiuretic hormone (SIADH) secretion, cerebral salt-wasting syndrome, or overly aggressive fluid resuscitation may occur. As discussed earlier, increased ICP is another complication of bacterial meningitis, secondary to increased permeability of the blood-brain barrier resulting from release of proinflammatory cytokines. Acute communicating hydrocephalus has also been well-described in patients with bacterial meningitis. Seizures may occur either at presentation or after appropriate therapy and may be due to several etiologies, including increased ICP, the development of encephalitis or cerebritis, or abscess formation. Among seizure types, nonconvulsive status epilepticus has been observed in patients with bacterial meningitis, and the diagnosis must be considered in such patients when encephalopathy develops despite appropriate treatment of underlying infection and other complications. Epilepsia partialis continua (or focal motor status epilepticus) has also been described and may occur secondary to the development of subdural empyema, another potential complication of bacterial meningitis. Stroke can occur, because meningitis may lead to a septic arteritis, venous thrombophlebitis, or general thrombophilia resulting from a proinflammatory state. Nonneurological complications of meningitis occur as a result of the associated bacteremia and include septic shock, disseminated intravascular coagulation, acute respiratory distress syndrome, and septic arthritis.

The outcome of bacterial meningitis has greatly improved over the past 50 years as a result of the development of antibiotics and the improvement in prompt recognition and treatment of this condition. Nevertheless, mortality in pneumococcal meningitis ranges between 20% and 40% and 4% to 13% in meningococcal meningitis. Morbidity, in the form of either focal neurological deficits (such as hearing loss or hemiparesis) or cognitive impairment varies between 10% and 30% of survivors. The presence of coma, seizures, bacteremia, older age, and increasing number of comorbid medical illnesses at presentation are associated with a worse prognosis.

KEY POINTS

1. The clinical presentation of bacterial meningitis includes the classic triad of fever, nuchal rigidity, and altered mental status. Headache is also a very common symptom.
2. *Streptococcus pneumoniae* and *Neisseria meningitidis* are the most common causative organisms in bacterial meningitis in infants, children, and adults under the age of 50.
3. The spinal tap and evaluation of CSF is the single most important diagnostic study in bacterial meningitis, and indeed in most suspected CNS infections. Analysis of the CSF demonstrates predominantly neutrophilic pleocytosis, elevated protein, and decreased glucose level.
4. Despite improved diagnostic modalities and treatment, morbidity and mortality from bacterial meningitis remain relatively high. The workup for bacterial meningitis must be performed promptly because any delay in initiation of therapy may lead to worsened outcome.

■ VIRAL MENINGITIS

The annual incidence of viral meningitis has been reported to be roughly 20 cases per 100,000 adults in the United States. Like in bacterial meningitis, the presentation typically includes a combination of headache, fever, and meningismus. Clinically, meningismus may take the form of nuchal rigidity, pain with eye movement, or the presence of Kernig's or Brudzinski's signs (Fig. 26.3). Patients may also complain of photophobia, lethargy, or irritability. Clinically evident alteration in mental status, seizures, or focal neurological deficits, however, distinguishes viral meningitis from encephalitis (which will be discussed in detail later). The neurological examination is usually normal in cases of viral meningitis, but evidence of a viral infection, such as exanthema, enananthema, or evidence of other systemic involvement (e.g., pneumonia, gastroenteritis) may be present.

Viruses typically invade the CNS via hematogenous spread. Roughly 80% of cases are due to enteroviruses, including echovirus, coxsackievirus, and nonparalytic poliovirus. The peak incidence occurs in the fall months. Other causes of viral meningitis include herpes simplex virus (HSV 2, HSV 1, which more commonly causes encephalitis), varicella-zoster virus (VZV), mumps, adenovirus, human herpesvirus 6, and lymphocytic choriomeningitis virus (Table 26.3). In patients with meningitis due to HSV 2, the characteristic vesicular and ulcerative genital lesions are present approximately 85% of the time and generally precede the onset of neurological symptoms by about 1 week. The initial infection with human immunodeficiency virus (HIV) may present as aseptic meningitis or meningoencephalitis, manifested by headache, altered mental status, seizures, or cranial nerve palsies.

The characteristic findings on analysis of the CSF include a lymphocytic pleocytosis, usually with 10 to 100 cells/mL. Early in the course of the disease, neutrophils may predominate, raising concern for a bacterial process. The Gram stain will be negative in these cases, and CSF chemistry demonstrates normal to slightly elevated protein and normal glucose. There is only modest yield for identification of specific viruses based on viral cultures and specific antibody analysis. Polymerase chain reaction (PCR) for specific viruses, however, has a much better diagnostic yield and is clinically useful. Treatment of viral meningitis is largely supportive. If the underlying etiology is either HSV or VZV, treatment with acyclovir is advocated.

It should be noted that some drugs may lead to the development of aseptic meningitis, which can mimic a viral syndrome. The incidence of drug-induced aseptic meningitis is unknown, but it occurs more frequently in patients with connective tissue or autoimmune disorders. The four major classes of drugs that have been reported to cause this condition include nonsteroidal anti-inflammatory drugs (NSAIDs), antibiotics (including those used to treat various CNS

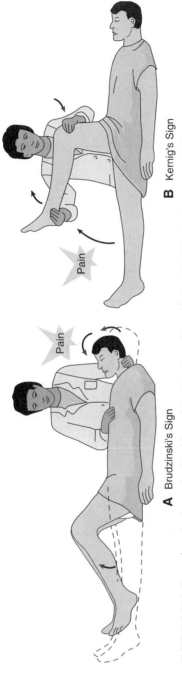

A Brudzinski's Sign

B Kernig's Sign

Pain

Pain

■ **FIGURE 26.3** Signs of meningismus: Brudzinski's and Kernig's signs. (From Nettina SM. *The Lippincott Manual of Nursing Practice.* 7th ed. Philadelphia: Lippincott Williams & Wilkins; 2001.)

TABLE 26.3 CAUSES OF VIRAL MENINGITIS AND ENCEPHALITIS

MENINGITIS	ENCEPHALITIS
- Enteroviruses (including echovirus, coxsackievirus, and nonparalytic poliovirus)	- HSV 1 - Other herpes viruses (including HSV 2, VZV, CMV, CMV, EBV, HHV 6)
- Herpes viruses (including HSV 2 more commonly than HSV 1, VZV, CMV, EBV, HHV 6)	- Arboviruses - Rabies virus
- HIV	
- Mumps virus	
- Adenovirus	
- Lymphocytic choriomeningitis virus	
- Rubella virus	

CMV, cytomegalovirus; EBV, Epstein-Barr virus; HHV 6, human herpes virus 6; HIV, human immunodeficiency virus; HSV, herpes simplex virus; VZV, varicella zoster virus.

infections, such as cephalosporins), muromonab-CD3 (OKT3) (an immunosuppressant agent frequently used in solid organ transplantation), and intravenous immunoglobulin (IVIG). The pathogenesis is poorly understood and is thought to be a hypersensitivity reaction. Clinically, the syndrome is indistinguishable from infectious etiologies and includes fever, meningismus, headache, and alteration in sensorium. The symptoms begin in close temporal relationship to starting the drug. The CSF profile is similar to that seen in infectious etiology, with a neutrophilic pleocytosis (100 to 1000 cells/mL) and elevated protein level. By definition, cultures are negative, and the diagnosis of drug-induced aseptic meningitis is one of exclusion. The outcome is excellent when the offending agent is withdrawn.

KEY POINTS

1. Like in bacterial meningitis, the presentation typically includes a combination of headache, fever, and meningismus. Altered mental status is not a sign of viral meningitis, but rather indicates encephalitis.
2. The vast majority of cases of viral meningitis are due to enteroviruses. Other causes of viral meningitis include HSV 2, HSV 1, VZV, mumps, adenovirus, human herpesvirus 6, and lymphocytic choriomeningitis virus.
3. The characteristic findings on analysis of the CSF in viral meningitis include lymphocytic pleocytosis. The protein and glucose levels are usually normal.
4. Treatment of viral meningitis is largely supportive. If the underlying etiology is either HSV or VZV, treatment with acyclovir is indicated.
5. Four major classes of drugs may cause aseptic meningitis mimicking viral meningitis. These include NSAIDs, antibiotics, OKT3, and IVIg.

■ **VIRAL ENCEPHALITIS**

There are approximately 20,000 cases of viral encephalitis reported annually in the United States. The incidence is increased in immunosuppressed patients, such as those with HIV, who have undergone organ transplantation, or who have an underlying malignancy. The clinical presentation includes headache, fever, seizures, alteration in mental status, and focal neurological deficits (such as hemiparesis). Because of its predilection to involve the temporal lobes, aphasia, anosmia, and behavioral disturbances, including change in personality, may also be present in patients with encephalitis resulting from HSV 1 infection. The diagnostic workup includes excluding other causes of encephalopathy (such as an underlying metabolic derangement), distinguishing an infectious encephalitis from a postinfectious or parainfectious cause (i.e., acute disseminated encephalomyelitis), and, finally, determining the specific viral etiology. All steps are based on history and clinical examination. Analysis of CSF is necessary for the final step. In cases of viral encephalitis, opening pressure will be normal, but lymphocytic pleocytosis will be observed, typically with 10 to 500 cells/mL. As in viral meningitis, protein may be normal to slightly elevated and glucose will be normal. Gram stain is negative, but, again, PCR for specific viruses is usually diagnostic.

Of the various etiologies, HSV 1 is by far the most common, with a reported annual incidence of approximately 1 in 250,000 adults in the United States. Roughly two thirds of cases are thought to result from reactivation of a latent viral infection with intraneuronal spread via either the trigeminal ganglion or the olfactory tract. The onset of HSV encephalitis is characteristically abrupt, with rapid progression. In addition to the other findings on analysis of CSF discussed previously, there is typically a rise in red blood cells in HSV encephalitis because of its necrotizing pathophysiology. PCR of the CSF for HSV is 95% specific if sampled 48 hours to 10 days after symptom onset. There is a high false negative rate if the CSF is sampled before 48 hours. Therapy should start presumptively before the results of the PCR are known, however. Serum HSV antibody analysis is of no clinical utility in this disease. In addition to spinal tap, a number of other ancillary studies are useful in cases of suspected HSV encephalitis. MRI often demonstrates focal T2 hyperintensities and edematous areas in the temporal and orbitofrontal lobes, which enhance with administration of contrast. As mentioned above, this is seen because HSV preferentially causes focal necrosis in these areas. Electroencephalography (EEG) is also useful and characteristically shows periodic lateralized epileptiform discharges originating from the temporal lobe.

The treatment of encephalitis resulting from HSV infection includes prompt initiation of intravenous acyclovir at a dose of 10 mg/kg every 8 hours for at least 14 days. Close monitoring of renal function and administration of intravenous fluids must be undertaken, because treatment with intravenous acyclovir may lead to renal failure. Some authorities advocate repeating the spinal tap after the first 14 days of therapy and continuing for another course if there is evidence of persistent infection. Untreated, the mortality from HSV encephalitis is greater than 70%. With treatment, however, this number falls to 20% to 30%. Factors shown to be predictive of worse outcome include older age, depressed level of consciousness at presentation, long duration of illness, and higher CSF viral load. Morbidity is high in survivors and includes persistent focal neurological deficits, such as hemiparesis, cognitive dysfunction, and epilepsy.

Viral encephalitides caused by infection with arboviruses are also clinically important entities. These infections are mostly mosquito-borne, and specific etiology is geographically dependent. Worldwide, Japanese encephalitis virus is most the common and is typically a disease of children. Among the causes seen in the United States, West Nile virus, St. Louis encephalitis virus, eastern equine encephalitis virus, LaCrosse encephalitis virus, western equine encephalitis virus, and Venezuelan encephalitis virus are commonly seen (Table 26.4). These infections tend to occur in the warm summer months when mosquito breeding is at its highest. In general, infection with these viruses results in a prodromal illness of fever, headache, nausea, and vomiting, typically lasting several days. Only a minority of patients infected with these viruses actually develop encephalitis. Once clinically evident, neurological symptoms begin, however, the disease usually becomes fulminant, with most patients becoming severely encephalopathic to comatose. Focal neurological signs, including cranial nerve palsies and seizures, develop in approximately 50% percent of patients. In patients with West Nile virus encephalitis, symptoms may also include acute flaccid paralysis mimicking poliomyelitis, tremor, myoclonus, or Parkinsonism. In these cases, MRI may demonstrate corresponding abnormalities in the basal ganglia or thalamus.

TABLE 26.4 CHARACTERISTICS OF ARBOVIRUS ENCEPHALITIDES IN THE UNITED STATES

VIRUS	GEOGRAPHIC DISTRIBUTION	AGE MOST OFTEN AFFECTED	MORTALITY
West Nile virus	Nationwide	Adults, most severe in adults >50 years	Low
St. Louis encephalitis virus	Central and Southwest	Adults >50 years	Moderate (~20%)
Eastern equine encephalitis virus	Eastern seaboard and Gulf Coast	All	High (50% to 80%)
LaCrosse encephalitis virus	Eastern and Central	Children	Low
Western equine encephalitis virus	Midwest and West	Infants and adults >50 years	Moderate in infants (10% to 20%), low in adults
Venezuelan encephalitis virus	South	Adults	Low

Laboratory testing often reveals peripheral leukocytosis and hyponatremia, in addition to a lymphocytic pleocytosis in the CSF, except in the case of West Nile virus encephalitis, in which neutrophilic pleocytosis is usually seen. Detection of specific antibodies to the viral pathogen in the CSF is diagnostic. Electroencephalography typically demonstrates anterior-predominant slowing, consistent with an underlying encephalopathic state. Treatment of these infections is largely supportive, and, of the causes mentioned above, infection with eastern equine encephalitis virus has the highest mortality.

Rabies is another cause of viral encephalitis. Infection with rhabdovirus leads to overt CNS findings, which may be predominantly encephalopathic or myelopathic. The virus is transmitted by the bite of an infected animal, usually bats or other wild terrestrial mammals in the United States. Typically, patients develop fever, malaise, and anxiety. Hydrophobia eventually develops and is classic for this disorder. Over a course of days to weeks, encephalopathy progresses to coma, cardiorespiratory failure, and death.

KEY POINTS

1. The clinical presentation of viral encephalitis includes headache, fever, seizures, alteration in mental status, and focal neurological deficits.
2. HSV 1 is by far the most common etiology of viral encephalitis.
3. The treatment of encephalitis resulting from HSV infection includes prompt initiation of intravenous acyclovir, which can be life-saving. Untreated, the mortality from HSV encephalitis is greater than 70% percent.
4. Viral encephalitides caused by infection with arboviruses are also clinically important entities. These infections are mostly mosquito-borne, and specific etiology is geographically dependent. Among the causes seen in the United States, West Nile virus, St. Louis encephalitis virus, eastern equine encephalitis virus, LaCrosse encephalitis virus, western equine encephalitis virus, and Venezuelan encephalitis virus are commonly seen.
5. Treatment of arboviral encephalitides is largely supportive; infection with eastern equine encephalitis virus has the highest mortality.

■ NEUROLOGICAL COMPLICATIONS OF HUMAN IMMUNODEFICIENCY VIRUS INFECTION

It has been estimated by the Joint United Nations Programme on HIV/AIDS that there are over 40 million adults and children living with HIV infection worldwide. Neurological complications are encountered in up to 70% of patients with HIV and acquired immunodeficiency syndrome (AIDS). A clinical distinction must be made between neurological sequelae of the HIV virus itself and those resulting from the opportunistic infections to which AIDS predisposes (Table 26.5).

HIV can lead to neurological symptoms, the most well-described being HIV dementia (also known as HIV encephalopathy or AIDS dementia complex). This syndrome typically occurs in patients with profound immunosuppression and very low CD4 counts. There is also increased risk of developing HIV dementia with advancing age. The incidence, however, has declined since the introduction of highly aggressive antiretroviral treatment (HAART). In 2000 it was estimated that approximately 1% of patients with AIDS suffered from this syndrome. The pathophysiology of the disease is thought to relate to the fact that the presence of HIV within the CNS leads to release of proinflammatory cytokines from microglia, ultimately resulting in neuronal apoptotic death.

The characteristic symptoms develop over the course of months to years. The dementia is subcortical and characterized by behavioral, cognitive, and psychomotor dysfunction that first manifest with psychomotor slowing, reading difficulty, memory loss, and apathy. A prominent gait disorder is also usually present. Eventually, symptoms progress to a state of abulia and global dementia just before death. The differential diagnosis includes opportunistic infections such as progressive multifocal leukoencephalopathy (PML), cytomegalovirus (CMV) encephalitis, primary CNS lymphoma, cryptococcal or tuberculous meningitis (all of which will be described in following sections), or depression. The workup for HIV dementia includes a spinal tap to exclude the aforementioned causes in the differential diagnosis; however, there is no diagnostic CSF profile for this condition alone. MRI of the brain characteristically demonstrates cortical and subcortical atrophy with confluent areas of deep white matter T2 hyperintensity. The treatment of HIV dementia is HAART when CD4 counts are low or the HIV viral load is very high in an attempt to maximally suppress HIV replication within the CNS. This has led to improvement and in some cases reversal of deficits in patients with this symptom complex.

HIV infection can also lead to myelitis or vacuolar myelopathy, primarily involving the thoracic spinal cord. This typically presents as a slowly progressive, painless gait disturbance, with neurogenic bladder dysfunction, evidence of spastic paraparesis, and sensory ataxia on examination. The development of the myelopathy commonly parallels the development of HIV dementia, as discussed earlier. The differential diagnosis for this condition includes infection with syphilis, tuberculosis, human T-lymphotropic virus (HTLV-1), HSV, CMV and vitamin B_{12} deficiency. Unlike HIV dementia, treatment with HAART has not proven to be effective therapy for HIV myelitis or myelopathy.

Neurological disease caused by opportunistic infections is reported to be the first manifestation of AIDS in up to 20% of patients infected with HIV. Previously rare conditions are now

TABLE 26.5 RISK OF OPPORTUNISTIC CENTRAL NERVOUS SYSTEM (CNS) INFECTIONS IN PATIENTS WITH HIV/AIDS BASED ON CD4 COUNT

CD4 COUNT	CNS INFECTION
CD4 count <100	- *Toxoplasma gondii* - *Cryptococcus neoformans* - Progressive multifocal leukoencephalopathy (caused by JC virus)
CD4 count <50	- Primary CNS lymphoma (caused by Epstein-Barr virus) - Cytomegalovirus

commonly seen in this patient population. Toxoplasmosis, cryptococcal meningitis, PML, primary CNS lymphoma, and CMV encephalitis are examples of such opportunistic diseases.

Infection with the parasite *Toxoplasma gondii* is the most common cause of a mass lesion in the brain in patients with AIDS. Toxoplasma causes multifocal necrotizing encephalitis, which predominantly involves the frontal and parietal lobes. It occurs as a result of reactivation of latent infection secondary to loss of cellular immunity, once CD4 counts drop below 100 cells/μL. It is transmitted in undercooked pork products or the handling of cat feces. The clinical presentation varies, and usually includes a combination of headache, focal neurological deficits or signs, encephalopathy, or seizures. Analysis of the CSF may yield normal results or may demonstrate a lymphocytic pleocytosis, elevated protein, and low glucose. PCR for toxoplasma has moderate sensitivity, but high specificity. CT or MRI of the brain characteristically shows multiple lesions (usually more than five), that demonstrate ring contrast enhancement with surrounding edema and mass effect on adjacent structures (Fig. 26.4). If clinical uncertainty exists, the definitive diagnosis is made on brain biopsy. Treatment includes sulfadiazine and pyrimethamine. Most patients with HIV infection and CD4 counts below 100 are treated with trimethoprim-sulfamethoxazole as prophylaxis against toxoplasma.

Cryptococcal meningoencephalitis is the most common fungal infection of the CNS and is the third most common neurological complication in patients with AIDS. It is estimated that up to 10% of patients with HIV will develop cryptococcal meningoencephalitis as their AIDS-defining illness. Like infection with toxoplasma, it occurs in patients with CD4 counts less than 100. It is unclear whether it represents reactivation of a latent infection or is newly acquired via the inhalation of encapsulated fungi. The disease presents with neurological complaints in the absence of any signs or symptoms of systemic disease. The neurological manifestations develop insidiously, are nonspecific, and may include headache, nausea, vomiting, and encephalopathy. Focal neurological signs or seizures are seen in approximately 10% of patients. The diagnosis

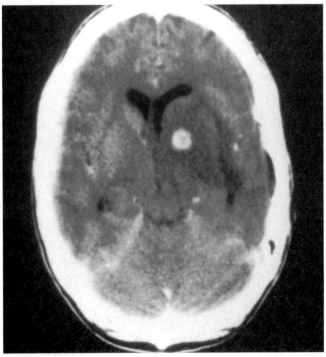

■ **FIGURE 26.4** A CT scan demonstrating a ring-enhancing lesion due to infection with toxoplasmosis. (From Harwood-Nuss A, Linden CH, Sternbach G et al, eds. *The Clinical Practice of Emergency Medicine*. 3rd ed. Philadelphia: Lippincott Williams & Wilkins; 2001.)

rests on demonstration of the organism in the CSF. In approximately 70% of patients, there will be elevated opening pressure and mild mononuclear pleocytosis (usually <20 cells/mL). India ink stain may lead to identification of the organism, but elevated cryptococcal antigen titers or culture of the organism in the CSF clinches the diagnosis. MRI of the brain characteristically shows evidence of a basilar nonexudative meningitis with scattered microadenomas, usually seen in the basal ganglia. Treatment includes intravenous amphotericin B and flucytosine for 2 weeks, followed by a course of oral fluconazole. Unlike in toxoplasmosis, primary prophylaxis against cryptococcus is not recommended in patients with low CD4 counts. With treatment, complete recovery occurs in over 90% of patients. Other fungal infections that may affect the CNS in immunocompromised and immunocompetent patients include coccidiomycosis, aspergillosis, histoplasmosis, and candidiasis.

PML is seen in 1% to 10% of patients with AIDS. First described in patients with chronic leukemia and lymphoma, PML is a fatal demyelinating disease caused by reactivation of a latent polyomavirus known as the JC virus. This virus is ubiquitous and is acquired during childhood. The virus infects oligodendroglial cells and astrocytes, causing cell lysis and multifocal demyelination. PML affects men roughly seven times more frequently than women and is usually seen in patients with CD4 counts less than 100. Because it is multifocal, there are a wide range of neurological signs and symptoms based on the location of the lesions in the CNS. Typically, the disease presents with focal deficits, including hemiparesis, cognitive dysfunction, hemianopia, dysarthria, aphasia, or a gait disorder. Seizures are less common, but can occur. MRI of the brain in PML characteristically demonstrates nonenhancing, primarily white matter disease. Positive status JC virus on PCR in the CSF is highly sensitive and specific for PML. The definitive diagnosis, however, is brain biopsy. HAART has been shown in some studies to prolong duration of survival from time of diagnosis, but without it most patients die within 4 to 6 months from diagnosis. There is no effective treatment against the JC virus itself.

Primary CNS lymphoma is the second most common space-occupying lesion in the CNS, and the incidence is reported to be 2% to 5% of patients with AIDS. It is associated with infection with Epstein-Barr virus and is an extranodal non-Hodgkin's type of lymphoma. It is also an AIDS-defining illness and usually occurs when CD4 counts have dropped below 50 cells/μL. Like in PML, there is a male predominance. The clinical presentation typically includes the insidious development of encephalopathy, focal neurological signs, seizures, and evidence of elevated ICP. The usual delay in diagnosis from initial presentation is usually approximately 2 months. MRI with gadolinium demonstrates single or multifocal enhancing abnormalities, characteristically in a supratentorial distribution. This may appear very similar to toxoplasmosis, and some authorities favor the empiric initiation of therapy against toxoplasmosis if CSF studies are nondiagnostic and reimaging a few weeks after treatment. If there is progression or no change in the lesion, the diagnosis of primary CNS lymphoma should be considered. The CSF may demonstrate elevated protein, beta-2 microglobulin, lactate dehydrogenase, and PCR positive for Epstein-Barr virus DNA. Cytologic examination for malignant cells and flow cytometry should also be performed, but findings are usually positive only later in the course of the illness. Despite treatment with radiation therapy, the mean survival from the time of diagnosis is only 3 to 4 months in the majority of patients.

Infection with CMV in the context of concomitant HIV infection may yield a broad range of neurological syndromes, including encephalitis, polyradiculitis, and peripheral neuropathy. CNS infection with CMV is relatively rare and occurs in patients with CD4 counts less than 50. Unlike in cryptococcus infection, it is a multisystem infection, usually also involving the retina, gastrointestinal tract, and adrenal glands by the time CNS disease is evident. Two distinct neurological syndromes have been described. The first is CMV encephalitis, which presents as a subacute dementia, apathy, and focal neurological deficits, with superimposed periods of encephalopathy. The second is CMV ventriculoencephalitis, which, as the name implies, is an infection of the CSF producing ependymal cells lining the ventricles. In this condition, patients demonstrate rapidly progressive symptoms of encephalopathy and cranial neuropathies. MRI of the brain reveals multifocal areas of T2 hyperintensity in the periventricular white matter with or without ventriculomegaly. These findings are not specific for CMV encephalitis or ventriculoencephalitis, however. Analysis of the CSF leads to variable results, and isolation of CMV in culture is rare, although PCR results positive for CMV DNA may be supportive. Treatment with anti-CMV agents has been disappointing because of poor CNS penetration, and death typically ensues 4 to 6 weeks after initial presentation.

KEY POINTS

1. Neurological complications are encountered in up to 70% of patients with HIV and AIDS. A clinical distinction that must be made is between neurological sequelae of the HIV and those resulting from the opportunistic infections to which AIDS predisposes.
2. HIV can lead to neurological symptoms, the most well described being HIV dementia (also known as HIV encephalopathy and AIDS dementia complex) and vacuolar myelopathy. These syndromes typically occur in patients with profound immunosuppression and very low CD4 counts.
3. Toxoplasmosis, cryptococcal meningitis, PML, primary CNS lymphoma, and CMV encephalitis are examples of opportunistic infections that occur in patients with HIV and AIDS and lead to neurological sequelae.
4. Infection with the parasite *Toxoplasma gondii* is the most common cause of a mass lesion in the brain in patients with AIDS.

■ TUBERCULOUS MENINGITIS

The incidence of tuberculous meningitis has increased over the last 30 years in the United States because of the increased incidence of HIV infection. It is still a common cause of CNS infection in underdeveloped nations. The clinical presentation is relatively nonspecific, and it is difficult to diagnose on clinical history and examination alone. Making the diagnosis requires a high index of suspicion, as in patients with AIDS and low CD4 counts. Symptoms include headache, fever, vomiting, photophobia, and anorexia. These symptoms tend to develop more subacutely than in bacterial or viral meningitis. On examination, patients may have nuchal rigidity, altered mental status (as severe as coma), cranial nerve palsies (especially involving the third, sixth, and seventh cranial nerves), hemiparesis, and, particularly in children, seizures. Examination may also reveal signs of extrameningeal disease, because roughly half of patients with tuberculous meningitis have evidence of active or previous tuberculosis infection elsewhere. The signs and symptoms of tuberculous meningitis relate closely with the underlying pathophysiology of the disease. Infection causes granulomatous inflammation and the development of an inflammatory exudate, primarily in the Sylvian fissures and basal cisterns, as well as around the brainstem, which often leads to cranial nerve palsies and hydrocephalus. In addition, endarteritis may develop and lead to stroke. It should be mentioned that the infection may involve the spinal cord itself and produce a myelopathic picture as well.

Very early in the course of the disease, analysis of the CSF will show polymorphonuclear pleocytosis, but the typical picture once the patient comes to medical attention is a lymphocytic predominance, with cell counts typically varying between 10 and 1000 cells per milliliter. Of note, pleocytosis may be mild or absent in patients with HIV infection or who are otherwise immunocompromised. The opening pressure is characteristically elevated in over half of patients. The protein level is elevated (usually in the range of 100–200), and the glucose level is decreased below 40% of the serum glucose drawn concomitantly in over 95% of patients with tuberculous meningitis. Acid-fast bacilli (AFB) staining of the CSF is seen in close to 60% of patients, and cultures are positive in approximately 70% of patients, although at least 5 mL of

CSF is usually required for these studies. Unfortunately, PCR of the CSF in tuberculosis has low sensitivity and specificity. Findings suggestive of the diagnosis on MRI include basal enhancement, hydrocephalus, presence of tuberculomas, and evidence of infarction. These findings are not necessarily specific for tuberculous meningitis because cryptococcal meningitis, CNS sarcoidosis, viral encephalitis, lymphoma, and carcinomatous meningitis may all have a similar appearance on imaging studies.

There are few clinical data to guide in the choice of drugs or duration of therapy for tuberculous meningitis. Most patients are treated with a combination of four antibiotics, including isoniazid, rifampin, pyrazinamide, and ethambutol, for a duration of 2 months, followed by an additional 8 to 11 months of isoniazid and rifampin. The adjunctive use of corticosteroids is controversial, and strong evidence for their use is lacking. Treatment prevents morbidity and mortality in more than 50% of patients. Coinfection with HIV does not alter the clinical presentation of tuberculous meningitis, but it can lead to greater number and severity of complications and carries a higher mortality.

KEY POINTS

1. The incidence of tuberculous meningitis has increased over the last 30 years in the United States because of increased incidence of HIV infection. It is still a common cause of CNS infection in underdeveloped nations.
2. The clinical presentation is relatively nonspecific; it is difficult to diagnose on clinical history and examination alone. Making the diagnosis requires a high index of suspicion, as in patients with AIDS and low CD4 counts.
3. Infection causes granulomatous inflammation and the development of an inflammatory exudate primarily in the Sylvian fissures and basal cisterns and around the brainstem, often leading to cranial nerve palsies and hydrocephalus.
4. Analysis of the CSF in patients with tuberculous meningitis typically reveals a lymphocytic predominance, elevated protein, and very low glucose levels. The opening pressure is characteristically elevated.

■ INFECTIONS OF THE CENTRAL NERVOUS SYSTEM WITH SPIROCHETES

Neurosyphilis

Syphilis is caused by infection with the spirochete *Treponema pallidum,* and is a sexually transmitted disease. Patients with syphilis may develop neurological symptoms in the secondary or tertiary phases of the disease. Neurosyphilis is rare in the developed world, except in patients with AIDS. In the United States, the rate of syphilis in general was lowest in 2000 since reporting began in 1941. Furthermore, the overall incidence of tertiary syphilis has significantly declined in the latter half of the last century because of adequate antimicrobial treatment. The classic presentations of neurosyphilis include stroke (due to the development of endarteritis), progressive memory loss and dementia, and tabes dorsalis with or without other signs of myelopathy. In modern clinical practice, however, the presenting complaints vary widely. Initial manifestations may include seizures (either generalized or complex partial seizures); neuro-ophthalmologic symptoms, including visual loss and diplopia; hemiparesis or other signs of stroke, personality changes or psychosis; delirium; or the insidious development of symptoms consistent with dementia. The Argyll-Robertson pupil, a small and irregular pupil that will constrict to accommodation but not to light, is also a classic finding in neurosyphilis.

The definitive diagnosis of neurosyphilis depends on the finding of a positive Venereal Disease Research Laboratory (VDRL) assay in the CSF. This, however, is only 50% sensitive. A diagnosis of probable neurosyphilis can be made if a patient has lymphocytic pleocytosis (with

100 to 300 cells/mL) and elevated protein in the CSF, with positive serology for syphilis. Serological tests for syphilis include reactive plasma reagin (RPR), VDRL, and fluorescent treponemal antibody, absorption (FTA-ABS) tests. Of the these tests, it should be noted that VDRL is not specific for syphilis and may be positive in patients with connective tissue disorders, such as systemic lupus erythematosus. In addition, it is relatively insensitive in tertiary disease. The FTA-ABS test is a more sensitive and specific test. High-dose intravenous penicillin G is the treatment of choice.

KEY POINTS

1. Patients with syphilis may develop neurological symptoms in the secondary or tertiary phases of the disease. Neurosyphilis is rare in the developed world, except in patients with AIDS.
2. The classic presentations of neurosyphilis include stroke (as a result of the development of endarteritis or meningovascular disease), progressive memory loss and dementia, and tabes dorsalis.

■ NEUROBORRELIOSIS (LYME DISEASE)

Lyme disease is endemic in Europe and in the Northeast, upper Midwest, and Pacific coast of the United States. The spirochete responsible for the illness, *Borrelia burgdorferi,* is transmitted to humans by the bite of the *Ixodes* tick. The initial manifestation is the development of a characteristic rash, erythema chronicum migrans, and flu-like symptoms. Weeks after the initial symptoms, the spirochete may disseminate into the CNS, where it may remain quiescent for months to years. Once in the CNS, a mild inflammatory response occurs, either directly as a result of the infection or as an overzealous immune response.

Neurological disorders are seen in 15% to 40% of patients with Lyme disease, and the clinical presentation varies broadly. Meningitis, cranial neuropathies (especially facial nerve palsies), and painful radiculitis are the most commonly reported manifestations. In patients with long-standing and untreated disease, a mild chronic encephalopathy has been described. This most often presents with subtle difficulty with concentration and memory. At this point, other symptoms may include generalized fatigue, sleep disturbances, and emotional lability, which may fluctuate in severity over time. Frank psychiatric manifestations of Lyme disease may include anxiety, depression, and psychosis. In addition to neurological symptoms, arthritis and myocarditis are also frequently seen.

The diagnosis of CNS Lyme disease relies heavily on laboratory investigations in patients who are at risk for exposure to the pathogen. Very early or very late in the disease, the CSF may have a normal profile, not suggestive of inflammation or infection. Once the CNS manifestations are apparent, however, there is typically a mononuclear pleocytosis with mildly elevated protein. Up to 90% of patients with CNS Lyme disease will have either immune globulin (Ig)M or IgG intrathecal antibody production. Supportive evidence includes the presence of IgM or IgG antibodies to *B burgdorferi* in the serum. EEG and MRI findings are usually normal. The treatment of choice for CNS Lyme disease is a 4-week course of intravenous ceftriaxone, which leads to improvement in symptoms in the overwhelming majority of patients.

KEY POINT

Neurological disorders are seen in 15% to 40% of patients with Lyme disease, and the clinical presentation varies broadly. Meningitis, cranial neuropathies (especially facial nerve palsies), and painful radiculitis are the most commonly reported manifestations.

■ NEUROCYSTICERCOSIS

Neurocysticercosis is the most common parasitic infection of the nervous system, with an estimated 50 million people suffering from the disease worldwide. The incidence has been on the rise in the United States over the past 20 years because of increased immigration from developing nations where the disease is endemic, as well as improved detection of the disease. Infection with the tapeworm *Taenia solium* is responsible, with pigs acting as the intermediate host. It is transmitted via the fecal-oral route through the ingestion of infective eggs. The larvae may settle anywhere in the body, but they are symptomatic only within the CNS and the eye. The clinical features of the disease are dependent on the number, location, size, and stage of degeneration of the cysts within the CNS. Clinical manifestations frequently develop once an inflammatory response develops around a degenerating cyst. The trigger for this degeneration is unknown, but after an average of 3 to 5 years, the cyst appears to lose its ability to modulate the host immune response, and symptoms may develop. Autopsy studies in endemic areas estimate that up to 80% of lesions are asymptomatic, however. Seizures are the most common manifestation of parenchymal lesions once the host immune response is activated and generates a local inflammatory reaction, including edema. The degenerating and calcified cysts can act as seizure foci. The seizure semiology depends on the location of the lesion and may be simple partial or complex partial, with or without secondary generalization. If cysts are located adjacent to or within the ventricular system, hydrocephalus and its associated signs and symptoms may occur. In addition, if the cysts are located in close proximity to intracranial vessels, local inflammation may lead to vasculitis and stroke.

The diagnosis of neurocysticercosis is made with a high index of clinical suspicion in patients with appropriate epidemiological risk factors. Laboratory studies include positive serology or detection of circulating parasite antigens. Analysis of the CSF usually yields only mildly elevated white cell counts, with normal protein and glucose levels. Eosinophils may be present in the CSF if a cyst is in communication with the subarachnoid space. Findings on CT or MRI of the brain are nonspecific, but can be highly suggestive of the disease. The appearance of the lesions depends on the location, stage of degeneration, and host immune response. On MRI, viable cysts are seen as nonenhancing hypodense lesions, degenerating cysts may enhance with gadolinium and have variable degrees of surrounding edema, and older cysts commonly appear as calcified lesions. The pathognomonic lesion for neurocysticercosis, however, is a scolex that appears as a mural nodule within the cyst. Treatment of neurocysticercosis is individualized and is based on clinical presentation. Symptomatic treatment for seizures and elevated ICP should be undertaken. Treatment against the parasite itself is also performed on a case-by-case basis, with cyst location and degree of inflammatory response taken into account. If the cysts are viable, the treatment of choice is a course of albendazole and dexamethasone.

KEY POINTS

1. Neurocysticercosis is the most common parasitic infection of the nervous system.
2. Seizures are the most common manifestation of parenchymal lesions once the host immune response is activated and generates a local inflammatory reaction.
3. Treatment of neurocysticercosis is individualized and is based on clinical presentation. Symptomatic treatment for seizures and elevated IPC should be undertaken. Treatment against the parasite itself is performed on a case-by-case basis, with cyst location and the degree of the inflammatory response taken into account.

■ BRAIN ABSCESS

Brain abscesses are serious complications of pericranial or distant organ infections. Approximately 40% of abscesses result from extension of sinusitis, otitis media, or mastoiditis. These lesions tend to be unicentric and located in proximity to the site of initial infection.

Abscesses derived from hematogenous spread of distant infections, including bacterial endo-carditis, chronic pulmonary infections, and osteomyelitis, tend to be multifocal and typically occur in the distal territory of the middle cerebral arteries. The latter category accounts for approximately one third of brain abscesses, with the remaining 20% coming from an undetermined source.

Before the development of a capsule around the abscess (at which point the disease is more properly characterized as cerebritis), patients will experience fever and systemic signs of infection. Headache is the most common neurological symptom, with other signs and symptoms including encephalopathy, focal motor or sensory deficits, seizures, aphasia, or ataxia. The clinical presentation depends on abscess location, as well as the presence of potential sequelae of this infection, including hydrocephalus, ventriculitis, or thrombophlebitis, leading to stroke.

The workup for brain abscess involves not only identifying the location of the lesion within the CNS with imaging, but also determining the source of the infection and the responsible pathogens. The latter largely depends on the age and underlying immune status of the patient. The most commonly seen organisms in brain abscesses include streptococcus, coagulase positive staphylococcus, and anaerobic bacteria, such as *Bacteroides* species. The range of organisms, particularly opportunistic pathogens, is considerably broader in immunocompromised patients. Blood cultures should be a part of the workup and are positive in roughly 15% of cases.

In patients with focal signs or symptoms, spinal tap is contraindicated because of concern for the presence of elevated ICP pressure resulting from mass effect and the consequent risk of brainstem herniation. Therefore brain imaging must be undertaken to rule out a focal cerebral lesion if performing a spinal tap is entertained under these circumstances. Typically, MRI is performed to evaluate for location and extent of the lesion, and typically appears as a ring-enhancing mass with surrounding edema. Treatment is against the inciting organisms with appropriate antibiotics and surgical drainage or excision, depending on lesion location. Treatment of complications such as elevated ICP or seizures must also be undertaken. Regardless, approximately 30% of patients are left with some form of neurological sequelae.

KEY POINTS

1. Brain abscesses are serious complications of pericranial or distant organ infections (such as in the heart, lungs, or bone).
2. Headache is the most common neurological symptom, with other signs and symptoms, including encephalopathy, focal motor or sensory deficits, seizures, aphasia, or ataxia. The clinical presentation depends on abscess location, as well as the presence of potential sequelae of this infection, including hydrocephalus, ventriculitis, or thrombophlebitis, leading to stroke.

■ CHRONIC MENINGITIS

Chronic meningitis is defined as predominant leptomeningeal disease with signs of inflammation in the CSF persisting for greater than 4 weeks. Clinically, patients with chronic meningitis usually present with an insidious onset of nonspecific symptoms, including fever, headache, and vomiting, which remain static, fluctuate, or slowly worsen over time. The symptoms and clinical course of this disease are extremely variable between patients. In most patients, many months usually elapse before the diagnosis is made. The incidence of the disease is unknown.

There are various infectious and noninfectious etiologies responsible for the disease. Among infectious etiologies, Lyme disease, coccidioidomycosis, tuberculosis, parasitic infestation, and HIV infection (and associated opportunistic infections) are sometimes responsible. Among non-infectious causes, neoplastic disease, connective tissue disease, sarcoidosis, and drug-induced

TABLE 26.6 CAUSES OF CHRONIC MENINGITIS

INFECTIOUS CAUSES	NONINFECTIOUS CAUSES
- Tuberculosis	- Leptomeningeal metastases
- Lyme disease	- Sarcoidosis
- Syphilis	- Connective tissue diseases (including Sjögren's disease, Behçet's disease, systemic lupus erythematosus)
- Cryptococcus	
- Coccidiomycosis	- Drug-induced meningitis
- Histoplasmosis	
- Candidiasis	
- Cysticercosis	
- Toxoplasmosis	
- HIV	
- Herpes viruses (including HSV, VZV, CMV, EBV)	

CMV, cytomegalovirus; EBV, Epstein-Barr virus; HIV, human immunodeficiency virus; HSV, herpes simplex virus; VZV, varicella zoster virus.

etiologies are also seen (Table 26.6).The CSF profile also depends on etiology, but typical findings include mild lymphocytic pleocytosis and elevated protein. CSF should also be examined on cytology in order to evaluate for underlying malignancy. Other laboratory studies should be based on the clinical features of an individual case and the likelihood that a specific disease entity is the causative factor. Biopsy of the brain or meninges may have a role in patients with a progressive and deteriorating course despite empiric therapy. Treatment is based on underlying cause, and some authorities suggest empiric treatment with antituberculosis agents or steroids is warranted if symptoms are severe or fail to improve after a period of observation. Even despite extensive investigations, the etiology remains unknown in up to one third of patients with chronic meningitis.

KEY POINTS

1. Chronic meningitis is defined as predominant leptomeningeal disease with signs of inflammation in the CSF persisting for more than 4 weeks.
2. Clinically, patients with chronic meningitis usually present with an insidious onset of nonspecific symptoms, including fever, headache, and vomiting, which remain static, fluctuate, or slowly worsen over time.
3. There are various infectious and noninfectious etiologies responsible for chronic meningitis. Among noninfectious causes, neoplastic disease, connective tissue disease, sarcoidosis, and drug-induced etiologies are seen.

■ SUGGESTED READINGS

Davis LE, DeBiasi R, Goade DE, et al. West Nile virus neuroinvasive disease. *Arch Neurol* 2006;60:286–300.

Fallon BA, Nields JA. Lyme disease: a neuropsychiatric illness. *Am J Psychiatry* 1994;151:1571–1581.

Garcia HH, Del Brutto OH, Nash TE, et al. New concepts in the diagnosis and management of neurocysticercosis (*Taenia solium*). *Am J Trop Med Hyg* 2005;72:3–9.

Halperin JJ, Luft BJ, Anand AK, et al. Lyme neuroborreliosis: central nervous system manifestations. *Neurology* 1989; 39:753–759.

Hildebrand J, Aoun M. Chronic meningitis: still a diagnostic challenge. *J Neurol* 2003;250:653–660.

Kennedy PGE. Viral encephalitis. *J Neurol* 2005;252:268–272.

Kupila L, Vuorinen T, Vainionpaa R, et al. Etiology of aseptic meningitis and encephalitis in an adult population. *Neurology* 2006;66:75–80.

Lair L, Naidech AM. Modern neuropsychiatric presentation of neurosyphilis. *Neurology* 2004;63:1331–1333.

MacArthur JC, Brew BJ, Nath A. Neurological complications of HIV infection. *Lancet Neurol* 2005;4:543–555.

Mamidi A, DeSimone JA, Pomerantz RJ. Central nervous system infections in individuals with HIV-1 infection. *J Neurovirol* 2002;8:158–167.

Moris G, Garcia-Monco JC. The challenge of drug-induced aseptic meningitis. *Arch Intern Med* 1999;159:1185–1194.

Tattevin P, Bruneel F, Clair B, et al. Bacterial brain abscesses: a retrospective study of 94 patients admitted to an intensive care unit (1980 to 1999). *Am J Med* 2003; 115:143–146.

Thwaites GE, Hien TT. Tuberculous meningitis: many questions, too few answers. *Lancet Neurol* 2005;4:160–170.

Timmermans M, Carr J. Neurosyphilis in the modern era. *J Neurol Neurosurg Psychiatry* 2004;75:1727–1730.

Tyler KL. Herpes simplex virus infections of the central nervous system: encephalitis and meningitis, including Mollaret's (review). *Herpes* 2004;11(suppl 2):57A–64A.

Van de Beek D, de Gans J, Tunkel AP, et al. Community-acquired bacterial meningitis in adults. *N Engl J Med* 2006;354:44–53.

Van de Beek D, de Gans J, Spanjaard L, et al. Clinical features and prognostic factors in adults with bacterial meningitis. *N Engl J Med* 2004;351:1849–1859.

Whitley RJ, Gnann JW. Viral encephalitis: familiar infections and emerging pathogens. *Lancet* 2002;359:507–514.

CHAPTER 27

Brain Tumors

Jai Grewal • Harpreet K. Grewal • Santosh Kesari

■ INTRODUCTION

On August 1, 1966, Charles Joseph Whitman, a student at the University of Texas in Austin, murdered his wife and mother before ascending to the observation deck of his school's 27-story administration building. Having been trained as a sniper in the Marines, he embarked on a shooting rampage, killing 14 and wounding 31 others before being fatally shot by police. His suicide note requested an autopsy, which revealed glioblastoma in the hypothalamus. Mr. Whitman had seen a psychiatrist several months earlier and he had complained of intense anger and described thoughts about shooting people.

Although this is an exceptionally tragic event involving a brain tumor, it does illustrate the need for psychiatrists to be familiar with neurological conditions that could affect personality and cognition. This chapter provides an overview of those aspects of brain tumors that are frequently tested during in-service and board examinations.

The neurological effects of a brain tumor depend on its location. Brain tumors are divided into those that arise from structures of the central nervous system (CNS) (*primary* brain tumors), and those that are *metastatic* to the brain.

■ CLINICAL FEATURES OF BRAIN TUMORS

The most common presenting symptoms in patients with brain tumors include headaches, seizures, cognitive impairment, personality changes, and focal neurological deficits. The location of the tumor and its histology influence the presentation. Additionally, in neurological diagnosis, the time course is extremely helpful in determining the nature of a lesion. A slow-growing mass lesion is often responsible for subacute cerebral dysfunction, particularly in older individuals.

Headache is a presenting symptom in approximately 35% of newly diagnosed brain tumors. During the course of the disease, headache is reported in up to 70% of patients. It is often dull, nonthrobbing, and intermittent. Supratentorial masses can result in frontal headache. Posterior fossa masses cause headache in occipital and cervical areas. Early morning headache due to increased intracranial pressure (ICP) in the recumbent position, is considered a classic presentation. However, this classic presentation occurs in a minority of patients. When a headache is unilateral or worse on one side, this frequently indicates the side of the lesion. A unilateral or bilateral frontal localization is most common for supratentorial tumors, because most pain-sensitive structures (e.g., large blood vessels and meninges) in the cranium are innervated by the trigeminal nerve. Headache as the sole manifestation of an underlying brain tumor is rare, but certain "red flag" features should raise suspicion for a mass lesion. These are intuitive and include new onset of headache, particularly in older patients; a significant change in character from previous headaches; progressive worsening over days or weeks; pain that is present on awakening or is severe enough to cause awakening; worsening with bending over, coughing, or sneezing; the presence of neurological signs or symptoms; and the presence of nausea, vomiting, or papilledema.

Seizures are the presenting feature of brain tumors in approximately one third of cases. Low-grade tumors, particularly oligodendrogliomas, have a tendency to present with seizures (>70% in some series). Even if seizures do not occur at presentation, they may later occur in 40% to 60% of patients with brain tumors. Seizures tend to be partial, with possible secondary generalization. Seizure semiology may offer clues to the location of the lesion. Seizures involving right gaze deviation and clonic movements of the right arm are likely to originate from the left frontal lobe. Seizures characterized by olfactory hallucinations, déjà vu, impairment of consciousness, and automatisms implicate the temporal lobe. The seizure frequency varies among patients. In patients who have experienced an extensive surgical resection, there may be a marked improvement in seizure frequency (or even complete seizure-freedom) if the active seizure focus has been removed. Conversely, worsening of seizure type or seizure frequency may herald radiological tumor progression.

Altered mental status is a presenting feature in 15% to 20% of cases. Tumors associated with elevated ICP, gliomatosis cerebri, and those located in the frontal lobes are more likely to be associated with altered mental status at presentation. The severity can range from mild inattention to deep coma. Some signs and symptoms also may have localizing value. Frontal lobe tumors can cause progressive change in behavior, mood, and personality, that may be mistakenly attributed to depression; one clue is that these symptoms are relatively resistant to medical therapy.

Focal neurological deficits such as aphasia, hemiparesis, sensory loss, and visual field loss may also occur at presentation and correlate with tumor location. Aphasia is associated with involvement of the dominant hemisphere (usually the left), whereas sensorimotor and visual deficits can occur if the tumor affects the corresponding pathways within the CNS.

Workup of a Patient Suspected of a Brain Tumor

A patient suspected of possibly having a brain tumor should undergo a thorough general and neurological evaluation. Imaging of the brain should be performed in all patients, with magnetic resonance imaging (MRI) preferred over computed tomography (CT) because MRI provides a level of anatomical and pathological detail not possible with CT. Contrast should be given in all patients suspected of having a CNS neoplasm. In certain patients, imaging of the spine may also be considered to exclude drop metastases. The presence of meningeal enhancement on MRI would warrant cerebrospinal fluid (CSF) evaluation to confirm leptomeningeal metastasis. If the patient is suspected of having a metastasis to the brain, a thorough systemic workup for the primary neoplasm should be undertaken. If a diagnosis cannot be established by demonstrating likely metastasis from another primary site of cancer, a brain biopsy or surgical resection may need to be performed.

KEY POINTS

1. Headaches, seizures, altered mental status, and focal neurological deficits are the most common presenting symptoms of a brain tumor.
2. Oligodendrogliomas and dysembryoplastic neuroepithelial tumors (DNETs) commonly present with seizures.
3. MRI of the brain with contrast should be performed in every patient suspected of having a brain tumor.
4. Patients with suspected metastatic disease should have an evaluation for the primary site of cancer. Patients suspected of having a primary brain tumor should have either a brain biopsy or a surgical resection of the tumor, in order to establish a pathological diagnosis.

■ PRIMARY CENTRAL NERVOUS SYSTEM TUMORS

Primary CNS tumors are classified according to the World Health Organization (WHO) 2007 classification. Tumors are graded by the WHO classification from I to IV, with grade IV being the most aggressive. Approximately 70% of pediatric brain tumors are infratentorial, and medulloblastoma is the most commonly diagnosed brain tumor in children under the age of 10. Conversely, 70% of adult brain tumors are supratentorial, and the most common histological categories include meningiomas and high-grade astrocytomas. A summary of the WHO classification is provided in Table 27.1, with notable clinical, radiological, pathological, and molecular features described in Table 27.2.

TABLE 27.1 ABBREVIATED 2007 WORLD HEALTH ORGANIZATION CLASSIFICATION OF BRAIN TUMORS*

TUMORS OF NEUROEPITHELIAL TISSUE	TUMORS OF THE PINEAL REGION
Astrocytic tumors	Pineocytoma
Pilocytic astrocytoma	Pineal parenchymal tumor of intermediate differentiation
Subependymal giant cell astrocytoma	Pineoblastoma
Pleomorphic xanthoastrocytoma	**Embryonal tumors**
Diffuse astrocytoma	Medulloblastoma
Anaplastic astrocytoma	CNS primitive neuroectodermal tumor
Glioblastoma	CNS neuroblastoma
Gliomatosis cerebri	Atypical teratoid/rhabdoid tumor
Oligodendroglial tumors	**Tumors of cranial and paraspinal nerves**
Oligodendroglioma	Schwannoma
Anaplastic oligodendroglioma	Neurofibroma
Oligoastrocytic (mixed) tumors	Malignant peripheral nerve sheath tumor
Oligoastrocytoma	**Tumors of the meninges**
Anaplastic oligoastrocytoma	Meningioma (15 variants)
Ependymal tumors	Hemangioblastoma
Subependymoma	Hemangiopericytoma
Myxopapillary ependymoma	**Primary CNS lymphoma**
Ependymoma	**Germ cell tumors**
Anaplastic ependymoma	Germinoma
Choroid plexus tumors	Embryonal carcinoma
Choroid plexus papilloma	Yolk sac tumor
Choroid plexus carcinoma	Choriocarcinoma
Neuronal and mixed neuronal-glial tumors	Teratoma
Dysplastic gangliocytoma of cerebellum	Mixed germ cell tumor
Dysembryoplastic neuroepithelial tumor	**Tumors of the sellar region**
Gangliocytoma	Craniopharyngioma
Ganglioglioma	Granular cell tumor of the neurohypophysis
Anaplastic ganglioglioma	**Metastatic tumors**
Central neurocytoma	
Paraganglioma	

(Adapted with permission from Louis DN, Ohgaki H, Wiestler OD, et al, eds. *WHO Classification of Tumours of the Central Nervous System*. Lyon, IARC; 2007.)

TABLE 27.2 NOTABLE FEATURES OF SELECTED NERVOUS SYSTEM TUMORS

TUMOR	CLINICAL	RADIOLOGICAL	PATHOLOGICAL
Oligodendroglioma	Often presents with seizures	Calcifications	"Fried egg" appearance 1p and 19q chromosomal deletions
Ependymoma	Peak age 15; may present as obstructive hydrocephalus	Majority are in fourth ventricle or spinal cord; enhancing May spread via CSF pathways	Perivascular pseudorosettes
Meningioma	Most common primary CNS tumor (40%) More common in women Pregnancy may promote growth	Diffuse contrast enhancement, dural tail locations: convexity, parasagittal, sphenoid wing, spinal, cavernous sinus	EMA-positive desmosomes Progesterone receptors Many variants
Primary CNS lymphoma	May shrink or disappear (transiently) with corticosteroids May be associated with HIV	Diffuse contrast enhancement	Most B-cell Perivascular cuffing CD20+
Glioblastoma	Peak age 55 Median survival 14.6 months Chemotherapy shown to prolong survival in RCT	Ring-enhancing necrotic appearing mass	Vascular proliferation Necrosis Pseudopalisading arrangement of tumor cells
Medulloblastoma	Peaks in first and third decades of life May present with obstructive hydrocephalus or cerebellar signs	Posterior fossa enhancing mass May seed via CSF pathways ("drop metastases")	Small, round blue cells (on H-E) Homer-Wright rosettes (characteristic of all PNETs)
Neuroblastoma	First decade of life May present with "dancing eyes" (opsoclonus-myoclonus)	Occurs along the sympathetic chain in chest or abdomen	Similar to medulloblastomas May form "florets"
Ependymoblastoma	First 5 years of life Prognosis poor	Supratentorial enhancing mass with possible CSF seeding	True rosettes
Neurofibromas	Associated with NF1	Dorsal spinal nerve roots	Hyperplasia of Schwann cells
Schwannomas	Tinnitus, hearing loss Bilateral schwannomas may be associated with NF2	Cerebropontine angle mass	Antoni A and B Verocay bodies
Gangliocytoma/ ganglioglioma	First two decades of life Intractable complex-partial seizures	Temporal lobe mass	Gangliocytoma: only neoplastic neuronal cells Ganglioglioma: mixed neoplastic neuronal and glial cells; eosinophilic granular bodies

(continued)

TABLE 27.2   NOTABLE FEATURES OF SELECTED NERVOUS SYSTEM TUMORS (Continued)

TUMOR	CLINICAL	RADIOLOGICAL	PATHOLOGICAL
Dysembryoplastic neuroepithelial tumor	Second and third decades of life; rarely regrows after surgical resection	Medial temporal lobe	Neuronal and glial elements
Choroid plexus papilloma	In adults tumor of choroid plexus more likely to be metastatic	Children: lateral ventricle Adults: fourth ventricle	

CNS, central nervous system; CSF, cerebrospinal fluid; EMA, epithelial membrane antigen; H-E, hematoxylin-eosin; NF, neurofibromatosis; PNET, primitive neuroectodermal tumor; RCT, randomized controlled trial.

Astrocytic Tumors

Astrocytomas are neuroepithelial neoplastic counterparts of the glial cell known as the astrocyte. Their astrocytic lineage is confirmed by positive glial fibrillary acidic protein (GFAP) staining on immunohistochemistry. They can be divided into well-circumscribed and diffuse (infiltrating) categories. Well-circumscribed astrocytomas include pilocytic astrocytoma, pleomorphic xanthoastrocytoma, and subependymal giant cell astrocytoma (all WHO grade I). Infiltrating astrocytomas include diffuse (low-grade) astrocytoma (grade II), anaplastic astrocytoma (grade III), and glioblastoma (grade IV). The latter three neoplasms form an interrelated group, sharing molecular and genetic abnormalities. Over time, diffuse astrocytomas accumulate genetic mutations and can progress to higher grade astrocytomas. The average age at diagnosis increases with increasing grade, with the median age of diagnosis being 34, 41, and 55 years for diffuse astrocytoma, anaplastic astrocytoma, and glioblastoma, respectively.

Pilocytic Astrocytoma

Also known as juvenile pilocytic astrocytoma, pilocytic astrocytomas (PAs) (WHO grade I) tend to occur in the first two decades of life and present as a cyst with an enhancing nodule on MRI. The differential diagnosis for this finding is shown in Table 27.3. Although they can occur throughout the neuraxis, they tend to arise infratentorially in children. They are the most common gliomas in this age group. They are well-circumscribed, slow growing, and characterized by Rosenthal fibers and eosinophilic granular bodies on pathological examination. Surgical resection is usually curative of PA, as well as several other tumors (Table 27.4). Malignant transformation, although possible, is rare.

TABLE 27.3   DIFFERENTIAL DIAGNOSIS OF A CYST WITH ENHANCING MURAL NODULE

Pilocytic astrocytoma
Pleomorphic xanthoastrocytoma
Ganglioglioma
Hemangioblastoma
Glioblastoma (usually cyst wall is enhancing)

TABLE 27.4   TUMORS TREATED BY SURGICAL RESECTION

Pilocytic astrocytoma
Pleomorphic xanthoastrocytoma
Subependymal giant cell astrocytoma
Subependymoma
Myxopapillary ependymoma
Paraganglioma of the filum terminale
Dysplastic gangliocytoma of the cerebellum
Dysembryoplastic neuroepithelial tumor
Ganglioglioma
Central neurocytoma
Meningioma
Hemangioblastoma

Subependymal Giant Cell Astrocytoma

Subependymal giant cell astrocytomas (SEGAs) are associated with tuberous sclerosis (TS), with approximately 10% of patients with TS developing SEGAs at the foramen of Monro by age 20. A typical presentation is hydrocephalus. In about half of all patients with TS, there is no family history, because the TS genes have a high rate of spontaneous mutation.

Pleomorphic Xanthoastrocytoma

Pleomorphic xanthoastrocytomas (PXAs) (WHO grade II) are large cortical tumors with a predilection for the superficial temporal lobes and often present as seizures. The mean age of diagnosis is 14. Brain imaging may reveal a cystic tumor with an enhancing mural nodule. As the name implies, pathology shows pleomorphism, cellular atypia, and lipid-laden multinucleated giant cells. There is GFAP and synaptophysin positivity. Gross total resection may be curative.

Diffuse (Low-Grade) Astrocytoma

As their name implies, diffuse astrocytomas are quite infiltrative and do not have distinct boundaries with normal brain. Based on the prevailing cell type, three major variants can be distinguished. These are fibrillary (most common), gemistocytic, and protoplasmic. The gemistocytic variant carries a worse prognosis and increased tendency for malignant transformation. Unlike circumscribed astrocytomas, diffuse astrocytomas are not curable with surgical resection. However, there are data to suggest that extensive surgical resection may prolong survival.

The average age at diagnosis of diffuse astrocytoma is 34 years. The clinical presentation may include seizures and headaches. The tumor may also be discovered incidentally on brain imaging obtained for other reasons, such as trauma. Brain CT reveals a nonenhancing hypodensity, and MRI typically shows a diffuse, nonenhancing area of T2 hyperintensity (Fig. 27.1A–D). Cyst formation is possible, but calcifications are much less common than oligodendrogliomas. Histologically, the tumor resembles normal brain, but is distinguished by increased cellularity. There is an absence of high-grade features such as high mitotic activity, endovascular proliferation, or necrosis. Mutations of *TP53* (a tumor suppressor gene) can be found.

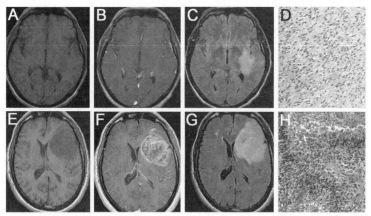

■ **FIGURE 27.1** Magnetic resonance imaging (MRI) and pathological features of an anaplastic glioma **(A–D)** and glioblastoma **(E–H)**: axial T1-weighted images **(A,E)** show no definite abnormality in the case of low-grade glioma and marked hypodensity in the case of glioblastoma; axial T1-weighted post-gadolinium images **(B,F)** show no enhancement in the case of low-grade glioma and marked heterogeneous enhancement in the case of glioblastoma; axial fluid-attenuated inversion recovery MRI images **(C,G)** show T2 hyperintensity within and surrounding tumor, more so in glioblastoma; and pathological specimens from low-grade glioma **(D)** and glioblastoma **(H)** show characteristic features. Low-grade tumors are moderately hypercellular and composed of well-differentiated astrocytes that infiltrate into normal brain. Modest nuclear atypia is present, but mitoses, necrosis, and vascular proliferation are absent. Glioblastoma shows very high cellularity, marked nuclear atypia, vascular proliferation, many mitoses, and geographic necrosis with pseudopalisading. (Reproduced with permission from Norden AD, Kesari S. Cancer neurology: Primary and metastatic brain tumors. In: Atri A, Milligan TA, eds. *Hospital Physician Neurology Board Review Manual.* Wayne, PA: Turner White Communications; 2006.)

A needle or open biopsy may be sufficient to establish a diagnosis; however, extensive surgical resection is preferable when feasible. There are two reasons for this. First, an extensive resection yields more tumor tissue to ensure an accurate pathological diagnosis. An erroneous diagnosis of a grade II astrocytoma (when the tumor is actually higher grade) may result in undertreatment and undersurveillance of the tumor. Second, data suggest that an extensive surgical resection of low-grade astrocytomas may impart a survival advantage.

Additional treatment options for low-grade astrocytomas include radiation therapy and chemotherapy, although there is no class I evidence proving a survival advantage with these modalities for low-grade gliomas. The median survival in patients with diffuse astrocytomas is 6 to 8 years, with marked variations between individuals. Because of this relatively longer survival, there are concerns of long-term cognitive toxicity related to therapy (particularly radiation) in patients with low-grade tumors. After a variable period of slow tumor growth, diffuse astrocytomas may *transform* to a higher grade astrocytoma.

Anaplastic Astrocytoma

Anaplastic astrocytoma (WHO grade III) is a more aggressive malignancy than low-grade diffuse astrocytoma. The median age of diagnosis is older at 41 years. It is histologically characterized by high cellular density and evidence of increased proliferation (mitotic figures). On MRI, the tumor may be associated with more mass effect and may be enhancing. Median survival is 3 to 5 years. After surgery, patients are usually treated with radiation therapy and may receive chemotherapy.

Glioblastoma

Glioblastoma (WHO grade IV) is the most aggressive type of astrocytoma. The median age at diagnosis is 55 years. Neurological symptoms progress rapidly. MRI typically reveals a ring-enhancing, cystic, irregular mass with surrounding vasogenic edema (Fig. 27.1E–H). Histologically, it is characterized by vascular proliferation and necrosis, often exhibiting a "pseudopalisading" pattern. Its astrocytic lineage is confirmed with GFAP positivity. Median survival is 14.6 months with standard therapy. Gliosarcoma, an aggressive variant of glioblastoma, is typically GFAP negative and responds poorly to treatment.

There are two distinct ways in which glioblastomas can arise. Glioblastomas occurring de novo (without any evidence of preexisting lower grade astrocytoma) are considered *primary* glioblastomas and tend to occur in older individuals. Primary glioblastomas are associated with amplification of the epithelial derived growth factor receptor (EGFR). Transformation from a lower grade astrocytoma results in a *secondary* glioblastoma. Compared to primary glioblastoma, secondary glioblastoma is associated with relatively longer survival, younger age at diagnosis, and abnormalities of the platelet derived growth factor receptor (PDGFR) rather than EGFR.

Accepted treatment of glioblastoma consists of maximum feasible surgical resection, followed by the concurrent administration of radiation therapy and chemotherapy with temozolomide. This combined treatment followed by additional temozolomide was shown to prolong survival (compared with radiation alone) in a randomized controlled trial. Additionally, patients who had a methylated O^6-methylguanine-DNA-methyltransferase (MGMT) promoter had a better survival rate than those patients with an unmethylated promoter. The poor prognosis associated with this tumor diagnosis warrants enrollment of glioblastoma patients in clinical trials offering novel therapeutic strategies.

Gliomatosis Cerebri

Gliomatosis cerebri (WHO grade III) is characterized by widespread infiltration of at least three cerebral lobes, usually with bilateral involvement. The tumor phenotype is usually astrocytic but may be oligodendroglial. MRI shows diffuse T2-weighted hyperintensity of the cerebral hemispheres, without tissue destruction or formation of a focal mass. Prognosis is poor, and treatment of this unresectable neoplasm consists of radiation or chemotherapy.

Optic Pathway Glioma

Optic pathway gliomas are typically low-grade gliomas that usually develop in the optic nerve and chiasm in children. Over half are associated with neurofibromatosis type 1 (in which setting they can be bilateral) and present with visual loss, proptosis, and optic atrophy. The most common histology is pilocytoma astrocytoma. In children, chemotherapy or observation is the management regimen of choice, with radiation reserve for refractory tumors, older children, and adults.

Brainstem Glioma

The brainstem gliomas represent a heterogenous group of neoplasms in children. These include diffuse pontine glioma, cervicomedullary glioma, dorsally exophytic glioma, and tectal glioma. Diffuse pontine gliomas are not usually subjected to biopsy because of the morbidity associated with neurosurgical procedures in this area. Therefore the diagnosis is suggested by the location, imaging features, and malignant behavior. The location is responsible for the poor overall prognosis, with a median survival of 1 year for diffuse pontine glioma.

Oligodendroglial Tumors

The normal oligodendrocyte is a glial cell that forms the myelin sheath of axons in the CNS. Oligodendrogliomas may occur as grade II (low-grade) or grade III (anaplastic) neoplasms. They may occur as pure oligodendroglioma or as a mixed neoplasm with an astrocytic component

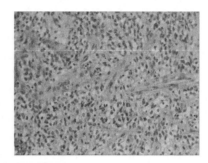

■ **FIGURE 27.2** Histology of oligodendroglioma. Classic fried-egg appearance with chicken-wire vasculature. The fried-egg appearance is due to artifactual clearing of the cytoplasm. (Courtesy of Steven Drexler, MD, Department of Pathology, Winthrop University Hospital, Mineola, New York.)

(oligoastrocytoma). A pure oligodendroglioma may have a better prognosis than a mixed oligoastrocytoma of the same grade. Histologically, oligodendrogliomas are characterized by a "fried-egg" appearance, thin "chicken-wire" capillaries, and microcalcifications (Fig. 27.2). The fried-egg appearance is due to artifactual clearing of the cytoplasm that occurs in paraffin-embedded tumor tissue.

Anaplastic oligodendrogliomas (grade III) are distinguished by significant mitotic activity, microvascular proliferation, or necrosis. The presence of 1p and 19q chromosomal loss is characteristic of oligodendrogliomas and correlates with improved survival and better response to therapy.

KEY POINTS

1. Primary CNS tumors are classified by the WHO as grade I through grade IV.
2. Astrocytomas are an important group of primary CNS brain tumors in adults. Diffuse astrocytomas are classified as low-grade (grade II), anaplastic (grade III), or glioblastoma (grade IV).
3. The median age of diagnosis is older with increasing WHO grade, and median survival is correspondingly shorter.
4. There is class I evidence that survival in glioblastoma can be prolonged by adding temozolomide to radiation therapy, which represents the standard of care for this disease.
5. On microscopy, oligodendrogliomas have a fried-egg appearance.

Ependymal Tumors

Ependymoma and Anaplastic Ependymoma

Ependymomas (WHO grade II) are a type of glioma, with peak incidence in the first and fourth decades of life. They most commonly arise in the fourth ventricle and also represent the most common tumor originating within the spinal cord (intramedullary). Contrast-enhanced MRI reveals well-circumscribed lesions with varying degrees of enhancement. Histologically, perivascular pseudorosettes are notable. More aggressive features (increased mitoses, microvascular proliferation, necrosis) warrant a diagnosis of anaplastic ependymoma (WHO grade III).

Subependymoma

Subependymomas are benign, slow-growing (WHO grade I) neoplasms commonly located in the fourth ventricle (50% to 60%) or lateral ventricles (30% to 40%). As with other intraventricular neoplasms, they often present in middle-aged adults as hydrocephalus, although they can be found incidentally at autopsy.

TABLE 27.5 NEOPLASMS OF THE CONUS MEDULLARIS AND FILUM TERMINALE

Meningioma
Lipoma
Paraganglioma
Myxopapillary ependymoma
Drop metastasis
Leptomeningeal metastasis

Myxopapillary Ependymoma

Myxopapillary ependymoma (WHO grade I) occurs in young adults exclusively in the region of the conus medullaris, cauda equina, and filum terminale. Other neoplasms that can occur in this region are listed in Table 27.5. Myxopapillary ependymomas are slowly progressive tumors characterized by tumor cells arranged, as the name suggests, in a papillary manner around a myxoid stroma. Prognosis is favorable and treatment is surgical resection.

Choroid Plexus Tumors

Choroid plexus papilloma (CPP) and choroid plexus carcinoma (CPC) represent benign and aggressive neoplasms, respectively, of the choroid plexus. These usually present in childhood as hydrocephalus and can arise in the lateral (50%), third (5%), or fourth (40%) ventricle. MRI reveals T2-hyperintense enhancing masses within the ventricles. CPP is usually well demarcated, whereas CPC has irregular margins. Histologically, CPP resembles normal choroid plexus with more crowding of neoplastic cells. CPC shows more aggressive features (frequent mitoses, nuclear pleomorphism, and a degraded papillary pattern).

Neuronal and Mixed Neuronal-Glial Tumors

Dysplastic Gangliocytoma of the Cerebellum (Lhermitte-Duclos Disease)

It is not clear whether these rare, slow-growing lesions of the cerebellum are hamartomas or true neoplasms. When adult-onset, germline phosphatase and tensin (PTEN) mutations are found, pathognomonic for Cowden syndrome. Treatment is surgical resection.

Dysembryoplastic Neuroepithelial Tumor

Dysembryoplastic neuroepithelial tumor (DNET) is a benign tumor that has a peak incidence in the second and third decades of life. DNET is almost always associated with seizures. It is most often found in the medial temporal lobes, with expansion of the cortex and subcortical white matter. Calcification is common. It is treated with surgical resection, and recurrence is rare.

Gangliocytoma and Ganglioglioma

Gangliocytoma and ganglioglioma frequently present in young individuals as seizures and are most commonly located in the temporal lobe. In the case of gangliocytoma, the neoplastic cells have neuronal features, whereas both neuronal and glial (astrocytic) neoplastic elements are found in ganglioglioma. Calcification and cystic changes are common, with areas of nodular enhancement on MRI (Fig. 27.3). Treatment is surgical resection, and prognosis is favorable.

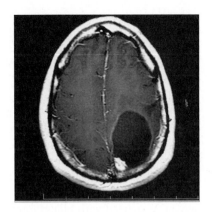

■ **FIGURE 27.3** T1-weighted MRI with contrast shows a cyst with enhancing mural nodule. Differential diagnosis includes several tumors outlined in Table 27.3. In this case, the pathology revealed ganglioglioma. (Courtesy of Jai Grewal, MD, Great Neck, NY.)

Central Neurocytoma

Central neurocytomas are slow-growing intraventricular tumors arising from the region near the foramen of Monro. A differential diagnosis of intraventricular neoplasms is provided in Table 27.6. Average age at diagnosis is 29 years, and hydrocephalus is a common presentation. They are often found near the midline, are histologically indistinguishable from oligodendroglioma, and may be densely calcified.

Paraganglioma of the Filum Terminale

Paraganglioma of the filum terminale is a unique neuroendocrine neoplasm of specialized neural crest cells associated with autonomic ganglia. It arises as an intradural tumor of the caudal equina region and has a peak incidence in the fifth decade. Presentation may include lower back pain, incontinence, and lower extremity sensorimotor deficits. Histologically, these tumors contain chief cells exhibiting neuronal differentiation and forming compact nests known as *zellballen*.

Pineal Parenchymal Tumors

Pineocytoma, pineal parenchymal tumor of intermediate differentiation (PPTID), and pineoblastoma represent the spectrum of neoplasms that arise from the melatonin-producing neuroepithelial cells of the pineal gland, the pinealocytes, or their precursor cells.

Pineocytomas (WHO grade I) are slow-growing well-circumscribed pineal parenchymal tumors (PPTs) representing less than 1% of all intracranial neoplasms, with a median age of diagnosis of 38 years. MRI shows an enhancing pineal region mass. Histologically, a characteristic

TABLE 27.6 INTRAVENTRICULAR TUMORS
Central neurocytoma
Choroid plexus papilloma/carcinoma
Ependymoma
Subependymoma
Subependymal giant cell astrocytoma
Intraventricular meningioma
Choroid glioma of third ventricle

feature is *pineocytomatous rosettes,* which are large zones of fine fibrillary processes surrounded by an oval arrangement of neoplastic cell nuclei. Treatment is neurosurgical resection and shunting for hydrocephalus. Incompletely resected tumors may require radiotherapy.

PPTIDs lack the well-differentiated features seen in pineocytomas, such as pineocytomatous rosettes, and may exhibit necrosis.

Pineoblastomas (WHO grade IV) represent 40% of all PPTs, with most occurring in the first two decades of life. On MRI, they appear as a large, poorly demarcated, heterogeneously enhancing mass. Microscopically, they can resemble other primitive neuroectodermal tumors with small, blue, densely packed cells and possible Homer-Wright and Flexner-Wintersteiner rosettes. Necrosis and hemorrhage are common, and pineocytomatous rosettes are not seen. Pineoblastomas frequently disseminate via CSF pathways. Treatment consists of surgical resection, craniospinal irradiation, and chemotherapy. The 5-year survival rate is 58%. Rarely, they may be associated with bilateral retinoblastomas in children, in which case the pineoblastoma has retinoblastic features; this is known as a trilateral tumor.

Embryonal Tumors

Central Nervous System Primitive Neuroectodermal Tumor

Primitive neuroectodermal tumors (PNETs) are a heterogeneous group of aggressive (WHO grade IV) neoplasms that occur most commonly in children and young adults. They appear as contrast-enhancing lesions on MRI. They are all histologically similar, appearing as small, round blue cells on hematoxylin-eosin staining. Homer-Wright rosettes can be found. These tumors are composed of poorly differentiated neuroepithelial cells with divergent differentiation along neuronal, astrocytic, and ependymal lines. CNS neuroblastoma is characterized by tumor cells with neuronal differentiation; medulloepithelioma cells recreate features of neural tube formation. Ependymoblastoma exhibits ependymoblastic (true) rosettes. PNETs can disseminate via CSF pathways.

Medulloblastoma

Medulloblastoma (WHO grade IV) has been considered to be a type of infratentorial PNET. It is the most common primary brain tumor in children under the age of 10 years and typically occurs near the cerebellum and fourth ventricle. Children under the age of 3 years have a poorer prognosis, and the diagnosis is rarely made over the age of 40. Clinical presentation may consist of hydrocephalus and ataxia; imaging reveals an enhancing mass in the posterior fossa with possible drop metastases to the brainstem and spinal cord. Histology is similar to that of other PNETs, and several subtypes exist.

Atypical Teratoid/Rhabdoid Tumor

Atypical teratoid/rhabdoid tumor (AT/RT-WHO grade IV) is a highly malignant CNS tumor most commonly occurring in young children. AT/RT histologically contains rhabdoid cells and primitive neuroectodermal, mesenchymal, and epithelial elements. It is typically refractory to treatment and uniformly fatal.

Tumors of Cranial and Paraspinal Nerves

Schwanomma

These slow-growing neoplasms of the myelin-producing cells of the peripheral nervous system are most commonly extracranial. When intracranial, they most often develop on the vestibular branch of the eighth (vestibulocochlear) cranial nerve as an enhancing mass in the cerebellopontine angle. Ninety percent are solitary and sporadic; multiple schwanommas are associated with neurofibromatosis type 2 (NF2).

Neurofibroma

Neurofibromas are benign neoplasms arising from the peripheral nerve sheath. Pathology demonstrates hyperplasia of Schwann cells and perineural fibroblasts. They are immunoreactive for S-100 protein. Multiple neurofibromas are the hallmark of neurofibromatosis type 1 (NF1). They arise most commonly from dorsal spinal nerve roots, major nerve trunks, or peripheral nerves; they rarely arise from cranial nerves. Plexiform neurofibromas involve either multiple trunks of a plexus ("bag of worms") or multiple fascicles of a large nerve, such as the sciatic nerve. Clinical presentation may include pain or sensorimotor disturbances. Small asymptomatic tumors are followed with serial imaging; symptomatic ones are treated with microsurgical resection or stereotactic radiosurgery.

Malignant Peripheral Nerve Sheath Tumor

Also associated with NF1, malignant peripheral nerve sheath tumor (MPNST) may arise de novo or via malignant transformation of a plexiform neurofibroma. Clinical presentation includes pain, neurological impairment, and an enlarging mass. Treatment of choice is wide surgical resection followed by radiation therapy for residual disease. These tumors are aggressive, with a high likelihood of recurrence.

Tumors of the Meninges

Meningioma

Meningiomas (WHO grade I) are the most common benign primary brain tumors in adults. These slow-growing, dural-based neoplasms arise from the arachnoid cap cells that form the outer layer of the arachnoid granulations. They may occur over the cerebral convexities, along the falx cerebri (parasagittal), and in the skull base, optic nerve sheath, and dura covering the spine (intraspinal, extramedullary). Incidence increases with age (peak seventh decade) and occurs more commonly in women. Radiation exposure has been known to induce meningiomas, and they have been associated with breast cancer. Presenting symptoms, which may include headaches and seizures, are related to the location of the tumor. On MRI, they are well-circumscribed, homogenously enhancing extra-axial masses with a dural tail. Calcifications are common. Multiple meningiomas may occur in NF2.

There are numerous histological subtypes of meningiomas, as shown in Table 27.7. Typical histological features include a whorled pattern and psammoma bodies. Meningiomas stain positive for vimentin and epithelial membrane antigen (EMA). They typically express progesterone

TABLE 27.7 HISTOLOGICAL MENINGIOMA VARIANTS

WHO GRADE I	WHO GRADE II	WHO GRADE III
Meningothelial	Chordoid	Papillary
Fibrous (fibroblastic)	Clear cell	Rhabdoid
Transitional	Atypical	Anaplastic
Psammomatous		
Angiomatous		
Microcystic		
Secretory		
Lymphoplasmacyte rich		
Metaplastic		

receptors, which may play a role in tumor growth. Mildly increased mitotic activity, increased cellularity, or brain invasion result in a (WHO grade II) diagnosis of atypical meningioma. High mitotic activity is consistent with (WHO grade III) anaplastic meningioma. WHO grades II and III meningiomas have a higher likelihood of recurrence and aggressive behavior.

Treatment of meningiomas is surgical resection when possible, with a possibility of cure with gross total resection, particularly for those overlying the cerebral convexities. Unresectable, recurrent, or high-grade meningiomas are treated with radiation.

Mesenchymal Tumors

Numerous mesenchymal brain tumors are described in the 2007 WHO classification. Only lipomas and hemangiopericytomas will be discussed here.

Lipoma: Lipomas are benign lesions commonly found along the midline, such as the corpus callosum, hypothalamus, sella, and spinal cord. They are usually incidental and may be associated with other congenital anomalies, such as agenesis of the corpus callosum. They are well-demarcated lesions containing adipose tissue. Similar to the MRI signal characteristics of fat, they are hyperintense on T1-weighted imaging and hypointense on T2-weighted imaging. They are hypodense on CT. Surgical excision is rarely required, and they should be observed clinically.

Hemangiopericytoma: Hemangiopericytomas (WHO grade II) are rare meningeal neoplasms that can be confused with meningiomas. They arise from the dura, and are densely cellular and highly vascular. On MRI they appear as solitary, well-demarcated masses with dural attachment and are isointense on T1-weighted images and hyperintense on T2-weighted images with intense contrast enhancement. In contrast to meningiomas, they are devoid of calcifications. Histological evaluation shows sheets of uniform cells within a network of reticulin fibers and slit-like branching vascular channels, known as staghorn sinusoids. They are vimentin-positive but have only weak EMA-reactivity. They may metastasize to bone, lung, and liver and after surgical resection, local recurrence is typical. Following resection, radiation therapy reduces local recurrence and prolongs survival. Median survival at first recurrence is 4 to 5 years.

Hemangioblastoma

Hemangioblastomas usually appear as cysts with enhancing nodules on MRI and are typically found in the posterior fossa or spinal cord. They are postulated to have an angio-mesenchymal origin. They are WHO grade I neoplasms with favorable prognosis following gross total resection. Multiple hemangioblastomas are associated with Von-Hippel Lindau syndrome (Table 27.8).

Primary Central Nervous System Lymphoma

Primary central nervous system lymphoma (PCNSL) may be associated with HIV, in which case it would be considered an AIDS-defining illness. However, it can also occur in the absence of HIV. Most PCNSLs are B-cell lymphomas with peak incidence in the sixth decade of life. Like diffuse astrocytomas, they are quite infiltrative. They are homogenously enhancing, with evidence of mass effect and cerebral edema, and they favor deep cerebral and periventricular areas. The eyes and spinal cord may be involved and should be evaluated by slit-lamp examination and MRI, respectively. PCNSL is usually a mass lesion of the brain parenchyma and usually remains confined to the CNS. However, systemic lymphomas can metastasize to the CNS, in which case they typically seed the CSF fluid pathways (leptomeningeal metastasis or lymphocytic meningitis).

Diagnosis is established by stereotactic biopsy, and extensive surgical resection should be avoided. If PCNSL is suspected, corticosteroids should be avoided before biopsy, if neurologically feasible, because steroids can cause normalization of imaging and lessens the likelihood of

TABLE 27.8 GENETIC SYNDROMES ASSOCIATED WITH NERVOUS SYSTEM TUMORS

SYNDROME	NERVOUS SYSTEM	SKIN	OTHER	LOCUS	GENE	PROTEIN	FUNCTION
Neurofibromatosis type 1	Neurofibroma, MPNST, optic nerve glioma, astrocytoma	Café-au-lait, axillary freckling	Iris hamartomas, osseous lesions, pheochromocytoma, leukemia	17q11	NF1	Neurofibromin	Tumor suppressor gene *ras* GTPase-activating protein regulating cell proliferation and differentiation
Neurofibromatosis type 2	Bilateral vestibular schwannomas, peripheral schwannoma, meningiomas, meningioangiomatosis, spinal ependymoma, astrocytoma, glial hamartias, cerebral calcifications	None	Posterior lens opacities, retinal hamartoma	22q12	NF2	Merlin or schwannomin	Tumor suppressor gene, binds to actin, regulating membrane cytoskeleton
Tuberous sclerosis	Subependymal giant cell astrocytoma, cortical glioneuronal hamartomas (tubers), ependymal hamartomas (candle gutterings)	Angiofibroma (adenoma sebaceum), subungual fibromas	Cardiac rhabdomyoma, renal angiomyolipoma, pulmonary lymphangiomatosis	9q34 (TSC1), 16p13 (TSC 2) 60% sporadic	TSC1, TSC2	Hamartin (TSC 1), tuberin (TSC 2)	Tumor suppressor genes, tuberin-hamartin complex suppresses activation of the mTOR pathway (which increases proliferation and cell growth)
von Hippel-Lindau	Cerebellar and spinal cord hemangioblastoma	None	Renal cell carcinoma, pheochromocytoma, renal angiomatosis, cysts of kidney and pancreas, cyst adenoma of epididymis	3p25	VHL	pVHL	Tumor suppressor gene, role in protein degradation and angiogenesis
Li-Fraumeni	Diffuse astrocytoma, medulloblastoma, supratentorial PNET	None	Bone and soft tissue sarcoma, breast cancer	17p13	TP53	p53	Tumor suppressor gene, promotes apoptosis in cells with DNA damage
Cowden	Dysplastic gangliocytoma of the cerebellum (Lhermitte-Duclos)	Multiple trichilemmoma, fibroma	Oral mucosa fibroma, hamartomatous colon polyps, thyroid tumors, breast cancer	10q23	PTEN	PTEN	Tumor suppressor gene, expression causes cell cycle arrest and apoptosis, regulates PI3K/Akt pathway
Turcot	Medulloblastoma, glioblastoma	Café-au-lait	Colorectal polyps or carcinoma	5q21, 3p21, 7p22	APC, hMLH1, hPMS2	APC, hMLH1, hPMS2	APC tumor suppressor gene regulating β-catenin, hMLH1, hPMS2-mismatch repair proteins
Gorlin	Medulloblastoma (desmoplastic)	Nevoid basal cell carcinomas, palmar and plantar pits	Jaw keratocysts, ovarian fibroma	9q22	PTCH1	Ptc1	Tumor suppressor, suppresses smoothened-mediated cell proliferation

APC, adenomatous polyposis coli; hPMS2, human postmeiotic segregation increased 2; hMLH1, human mutL homolog; mTOR-mammalian; PTCH, *Drosophila* patched homologue 1; PI3K, phosphoinositol-3-kinase, target of rapamycin; PTEN, phosphatase and tensin homolog.

an accurate diagnosis. In the setting of HIV, treatment consists of whole-brain radiation therapy and prognosis is poor. Treatment of non–HIV-associated PCNSL consists of a chemotherapy regimen based on high-dose methotrexate and radiation therapy to the brain. Prognosis of individuals younger than 50 is better than that of older individuals.

Germ Cell Tumors

Germinoma

Germinoma is the most common type of CNS germ cell tumor. It typically presents around the time of puberty near midline structures (pituitary or pineal gland). Pineal region germinomas are much more common in boys. On imaging, they may be isointense to normal brain, but are typically contrast-enhancing. Histologically, germinomas are characterized by large, undifferentiated cells in monomorphous sheets or lobules, with reactive (nonneoplastic) lymphocytes. CSF markers (alpha-fetoprotein, beta–human chorionic gonadotrophin) may be helpful in diagnosis and in monitoring tumor growth (Table 27.9). Germinomas are sensitive to radiation and chemotherapy.

Teratoma

Teratomas contain tissue of all three embryonic cell lines: ectodermal, mesodermal, and endodermal. They can be divided into mature and immature variants. Mature teratomas contain well-differentiated adult tissue, and the immature teratomas are poorly differentiated. Successful surgical excision of mature teratomas yields an excellent prognosis; immature teratomas are treated with chemotherapy and radiation and have an intermediate prognosis.

Choriocarcinoma

Choriocarcinoma is a tumor usually occurring extracranially, but it can develop, rarely, in the brain. The tumor tissue is differentiated along trophoblastic lines and contains cytotrophoblastic and syncytiotrophoblastic elements. The syncytiotrophoblasts produce beta–human chorionic gonadotrophin, which can be measured in CSF. Choriocarcinoma has a high risk of hemorrhage. It has a poor prognosis and is aggressively treated with chemotherapy.

Tumors of the Sellar Region

Craniopharyngioma

Craniopharyngiomas (CPs) originate from Rathke's pouch epithelium and are the most common supratentorial primary brain tumors in children. The incidence has a bimodal distribution with one peak at age 10, and a second peak between the fifth and sixth decade. They are

TABLE 27.9 USEFUL TUMOR MARKERS IN CEREBROSPINAL FLUID

TUMOR	MARKER
Yolk sac tumors	AFP, PLAP
Choriocarcinoma	Beta-HCG
Germinoma	c-*kit*, PLAP, beta-hCG
Teratoma	AFP

AFP, alpha-fetoprotein; hCG, human chorionic gonadotrophin; PLAP, placental alkaline phosphatase.

most commonly located in the suprasellar region, where they may compress the optic chiasm from the superior and posterior direction, resulting in bitemporal inferior quadrantanopia. In addition to visual field defects, they may also cause hydrocephalus and endocrinopathy from compression of the pituitary axis. CP is a well-circumscribed tumor with solid and cystic components. The cystic component contains dark, viscous, cholesterol-rich fluid that may spill into the subarachnoid space, causing chemical meningitis. Pathology shows squamous cell aggregates, foci of anuclear keratinocytes (wet keratin) with calcifications, and cholesterol clefts.

Pituitary Adenoma

These slow-growing neoplasms of the adenohypophysis represent the most common tumors of the sellar region. They are considered microadenomas if less than 10 mm in diameter; larger tumors are denoted as macroadenomas. Microadenomas usually present with endocrine dysfunction, whereas macroadenomas usually do not secrete hormones and produce symptoms by compression of parasellar structures.

Pituitary adenomas can be classified by both their hormonal products and their tinctorial properties. Secreted hormones may include prolactin, growth hormone, adrenocorticotrophic hormone (ACTH), thyroid-stimulating hormone (TSH), luteinizing hormone, or follicle-stimulating hormone (FSH). The most common hormonal abnormality is hyperprolactinemia, which occurs as a result of primary hypersecretion or compression of the pituitary stalk. The latter causes reduced flow of dopamine (prolactin-inhibiting factor) to the prolactin-producing cells. The tinctorial classification divides adenomas based on their staining properties into acidophilic, basophilic, and chromophobic categories.

On MRI, adenomas appear as a hypointense lesion on T1-weighted images and enhance less than the normal gland. On touch preparation, pituitary adenomas shed cells more copiously than normal pituitary tissue. Microscopically, there is degradation of the normal acinar arrangement. Hemorrhage or infarction of the tumor may produce pituitary apoplexy.

The treatment of macroadenoma is surgical resection, preferably via a transsphenoidal approach. For unresectable or partially resected lesions, radiation may be considered. The majority of treated patients need pituitary hormone replacement therapy. Prolactinomas may be treated with dopamine-agonists, such as bromocriptine, which may reduce the tumor size and improve symptoms.

KEY POINTS

1. Perivascular pseudorosettes are the histological hallmark of ependymoma; Homer-Wright rosettes are characteristic of PNET and medulloblastoma.
2. PCNSL is treated with chemotherapy and radiation. Surgical resection should be avoided, and corticosteroids impair the pathological diagnosis.
3. Meningiomas are characterized by EMA positivity and exhibit a dural tail on MRI.
4. Germinomas, the most common pineal region tumors, are much more common in boys.
5. Neurofibromas and MPNSTs are associated with NF1; multiple schwannomas are associated with NF2.

Familial Tumor Syndromes Involving the Nervous System

Several inheritable syndromes that involve tumors of the central or peripheral nervous system have been described, as outlined in Table 27.8. These are autosomal dominant syndromes involving tumor suppressor genes. However, over half of tuberous sclerosis cases occur as spontaneous mutations.

■ CYSTS OF THE CENTRAL NERVOUS SYSTEM

Colloid Cyst

Colloid cysts are rare. They are filled with proteinaceous or cholesterol-containing fluid and may occur in the anterior third ventricle. They may present with hydrocephalus or even sudden death if a ball-valve effect causes the ventricle to become acutely obstructed.

Epidermoid Cyst

An epidermoid cyst is formed from inclusion of nonneoplastic ectodermal tissue at the time of neural tube closure. It occurs in the cerebellopontine angle and parasellar locations, presenting during adulthood as cranial nerve dysfunction, aseptic meningitis, or seizures. On MRI, signal characteristics on T1- and T2-weighted images are identical to those in the CSF. A distinguishing feature is the presence of hyperintense signal on diffusion-weighted imaging. Microscopically, the cyst wall shows keratinizing stratified squamous epithelium with degenerating keratinocytes forming the central eosinophilic material. Treatment, if necessary, is surgical resection.

Dermoid Cyst

Dermoid cysts have a predilection for the lumbosacral spine and conus medullaris. They can also occur in the region of the fontanelle and fourth ventricle. The cyst content is similar to that found in epidermoid cysts plus secretions from sebaceous glands and the presence of hair follicles. These result in heterogenous signal on MRI. This benign lesion can be resected, but may recur.

Arachnoid Cyst

These cysts are lined by meningothelial cells and may be multilocular. Entrapment of CSF may result in symptoms of a mass lesion. Common locations include the temporal operculum, cerebellopontine angle, and cisterna magna. They have been associated with areas of inflammation and hemorrhage.

■ METASTATIC TUMORS

Brain Metastasis

Metastases to the brain parenchyma are more common than primary brain tumors and are found in approximately 15% of patients with advanced cancer. Metastases typically occur in patients with advanced systemic cancer, but may occasionally be the presenting lesion. In patients not known to have cancer, metastasis should be considered in the differential diagnosis of a newly discovered brain mass. A search for a primary cancer should be considered.

The most common site is the gray-white cortical junction. The abrupt narrowing of the vasculature at this site allows the hematogenously disseminated tumor emboli to lodge. Central necrosis develops as the tumor outgrows its blood supply. Metastases are well demarcated and provoke substantial vasogenic edema.

Lung cancer is the most common primary, accounting for approximately 50% of all brain metastases. Of these, non–small-cell lung cancer (NSCLC) accounts for two-thirds of brain metastases from lung cancer. Breast cancer is the next most frequent primary site (15%), followed by melanoma, gastrointestinal cancer, and renal cell carcinoma (5% to 10% each). The most common etiologies of brain metastases and those likely to bleed are described in Table 27.10. Eighty percent of metastases are supratentorial, which reflects the relative proportion of cerebral blood flow. However, pelvic and GI tumors are more likely to metastasize to the posterior fossa.

In 50% of patients, metastases are multiple. Lung and melanoma primaries are more likely to produce multiple metastases, whereas renal cell, breast, and colon cancer tend to produce

TABLE 27.10 CHARACTERISTICS OF BRAIN METASTASIS

MOST COMMON HISTOLOGIES METASTASIZING TO THE BRAIN	BRAIN METASTASES WITH HIGH RISK OF HEMORRHAGE
Lung (male and female)	Melanoma
Breast (female)	Renal cell carcinoma
Melanoma	Choriocarcinoma
Gastrointestinal	

solitary metastasis. Metastases from melanoma, renal cell carcinoma, and choriocarcinoma have a particularly high likelihood of hemorrhage.

The treatment of brain metastasis consists of whole-brain radiation therapy, although surgical excision or stereotactic radiosurgery may be warranted for solitary or symptomatic lesions.

Spinal or Vertebral Metastasis

Spinal metastasis should be considered in a patient known to have cancer presenting with back pain, leg weakness, bowel or bladder incontinence, or other signs of spinal cord compression. The most common site of metastasis is the vertebral body with tumor cells seeding this area hematogenously via the valveless venous Batson's plexus. As the tumor grows, it forms an epidural mass compressing the spinal cord. Myelopathy occurs via demyelination and venous infarction. Associated back pain may be worsened by cough. MRI shows extrinsic compression of the thecal sac. Neurological function can deteriorate rapidly and permanently, and acute management includes high-dose corticosteroids. Radiation therapy can result in tumor shrinkage, particularly for radiosensitive tumors, such as lymphoma, myeloma, and prostate cancer. Renal cell carcinoma and NSCLC are typically radioresistant. The most important prognostic factor is the pretreatment neurological function. Breast, lung, and prostate cancer each account for approximately 20% of epidural cord compression.

Intramedullary spinal cord metastasis is relatively rare. Lung cancer, particularly the small cell type, accounts for about half of these cases. Other etiologies include melanoma, lymphoma, and renal cell carcinoma.

Dural and Skull Metastasis

Skull metastases usually occur in the setting of bony metastases elsewhere in the body. The majority are asymptomatic. However, they may present with localized pain, headache, seizures, or focal neurological deficits or as a superficial mass. They occur as a result of hematogenous spread via the arterial system, Batson's plexus, or direct extension from a skull base tumor. The most common primary tumors are breast, lung, and prostate.

Cancer may metastasize to the dura, producing compression or invasion of the underlying brain. Tumor cells may obstruct the venous sinuses or produce subdural fluid collections and hematomas. Management includes surgery and radiation therapy.

Leptomeningeal Metastasis

Also known as neoplastic or carcinomatous meningitis, leptomeningeal metastasis (LM) involves metastases to the pial surface and subarachnoid spaces. LM is associated with several aggressive primary brain tumors (medulloblastoma, PNET, ependymoma, and high-grade gliomas), as well as with advanced systemic cancer. LM often occurs in patients with coexisting parenchymal brain metastasis. The primary malignancy may spread to the leptomeninges hematogenously, via direct extension from brain parenchymal or epidural metastases or via growth along cranial and spinal nerves. Tumor cells disseminate via CSF pathways; therefore symptoms may occur along the entire neuraxis. If tumor cells obstruct CSF flow, hydrocephalus may result. Multiple cranial neuropathies and multiple levels of spinal cord and spinal root dysfunction are suggestive of the diagnosis. On MRI, there may be diffuse meningeal enhancement and enhancement of cranial nerves and spinal nerve roots. Nodular disease may be evident. Normal MRI results, however, do not exclude the diagnosis, and CSF cytology demonstrating malignant cells is considered the diagnostic gold standard. Serial CSF samples may be needed. The prognosis for LM is usually poor, with survival measured in weeks, although longer survival has been observed in patients with LM from breast cancer. The systemic cancer is usually advanced; thus systemic chemotherapy is the mainstay of treatment with intrathecal chemotherapy used palliatively.

■ PARANEOPLASTIC SYNDROMES

Paraneoplastic syndromes are a group of disorders resulting from remote effects of a systemic malignancy. Many of these syndromes affect the nervous system and are presumably immune-mediated. The tumor expresses neural proteins, which provokes an immune response against both the tumor and the nervous system. Both humoral and cell-mediated immunity may be involved in neurological dysfunction. These syndromes are diagnosed by the presence of high titers of specific antibodies in the blood and CSF. Paraneoplastic syndromes may precede the diagnosis of a systemic cancer. Therefore a thorough search for malignancy is warranted when a paraneoplastic syndrome is diagnosed. The course of the underlying neoplasm may be indolent, possibly because of antitumor immune surveillance. These syndromes usually result in significant neurological disability, and response to treatment is often poor. Treatment modalities include intravenous immunoglobulin, plasmapheresis, and immunosuppression with corticosteroids and cytotoxic agents. Specific syndromes are outlined in Table 27.11.

TABLE 27.11 PARANEOPLASTIC SYNDROMES INVOLVING THE NERVOUS SYSTEM

SYNDROME	CLINICAL FEATURES	ASSOCIATED CANCERS	ANTIBODIES
Cerebellar degeneration	Subacute truncal and appendicular ataxia, dysarthria, diplopia, vertigo, nystagmus	Breast, ovarian, Hodgkin's lymphoma, SCLC, thymoma, testicular germ cell	Anti-Yo, anti-Ri, anti-Tr, anti-Hu, anti-CV2, anti-CV2, anti-Ma1
Encephalomyelitis limbic, cortical, brainstem, cerebellar	Subacute confusion, memory loss, seizures, myelitis	SCLC, thymoma, testicular germ cell	Anti-Hu, anti-CV2, anti-CV2, anti-Ma
Subacute sensory neuronopathy	Sensory loss, paresthesia, dysesthesia, sensory ataxia	SCLC	Anti-Hu, anti-CV2
Opsoclonus-myoclonus	Subacute opsoclonus, myoclonus, and ataxia	Neuroblastoma, breast, SCLC	Anti-Hu, anti-Ri, anti-Hu, anti-Ma
Cancer-associated retinopathy	Scotomatous visual field loss, decreased visual acuity, photosensitivity	SCLC, gynecologic tumors	Antirecoverin
Melanoma-associated retinopathy	Progressive visual loss	Melanoma	Antibody against retinal bipolar cells

(continued)

TABLE 27.11 PARANEOPLASTIC SYNDROMES INVOLVING THE NERVOUS SYSTEM (Continued)

SYNDROME	CLINICAL FEATURES	ASSOCIATED CANCERS	ANTIBODIES
Optic neuritis	Central vision loss	SCLC	May be associated with paraneoplastic encephalomyelitis
Necrotizing myelopathy	Rapidly progressing Ascending sensory deficit, sphincter dysfunction, paraplegia	Several carcinomas and lymphomas	Unknown
Motor neuron syndrome, subacute motor neuronopathy	Progressive lower motor neuron weakness	HL and non-Hodgkin lymphoma (NHL)	Unknown
Stiff person syndrome[a]	Muscle stiffness, rigidity, spasms	Breast, lung, HL non-paraneoplastic	Anti-amphiphysin anti-GAD
Chronic sensorimotor neuropathy	Distal symmetric sensorimotor deficits	Plasma cell dyscrasias	Unknown
Pandysautonomia	Hypothermia, hypoventilation, cardiac arrhythmia, sympathetic hyperactivity	SCLC, pancreas, thyroid, rectum, HL, carcinoid of lung	Anti-Hu against nicotinic acetylcholine receptors
Peripheral nerve vasculitis	Painful, asymmetric, sensorimotor deficits or MNM	SCLC, NHL	Unknown
Myasthenia gravis	Marked fatigability and fluctuating weakness	Thymus, thyroid, breast, SCLC, lymphoma	Anti-Ach, antititin
Lambert-Eaton myasthenic syndrome	Weakness, autonomic dysfunction	SCLC	Anti-VGCC (P/Q type)
Dermatomyositis	Proximal muscle weakness, heliotropic rash	Breast, lung, ovary, GI	Anti-Jo1
Neuromyotonia	Cramps, undulating muscle twitching at rest (myokymia)	Thymus, SCLC, HL	Anti-VGKC
Acute necrotizing myopathy	Painful proximal weakness	Lung, breast, GI	Unknown

[a]May also occur as a nonparaneoplastic syndrome, which is associated with anti-GAD rather than antiamphiphysin antibodies.

Alternative terminology for autoantibodies: anti-Hu ↔ type 1 anti-neuronal nuclear antibody (ANNA1); anti-CV2 ↔ collapsin response mediator protein 5 (CRMP5); anti-Yo ↔ anti-Purkinje cell antibody (APCA); anti-Ri ↔ type 2 anti-neuronal nuclear antibody (ANNA2); anti-Jo1 ↔ anti-histidyl t-RNA synthetase.

Ach, acetylcholine; HL, Hodgkin lymphoma; NHL, non-Hodgkin lymphoma; VGCC, voltage-gated calcium channel; VGKC, voltage-gated potassium channel.

■ NEUROLOGICAL COMPLICATIONS OF RADIATION THERAPY

Toxicity from radiation therapy can be divided into three types based on the amount of time that has elapsed since the completion of radiation. *Acute* toxicity manifests as encephalopathy within days to weeks of therapy. The risk increases with higher dose, larger volume of brain irradiated, and poorer baseline cognitive status. The pathogenesis may involve breakdown of the blood-brain barrier, leading to cerebral edema. Corticosteroids may be used to prevent and manage acute toxicity. *Early delayed* toxicity usually occurs within a few weeks of treatment and is usually reversible. It may present as somnolence and neurological deterioration. It usually resolves spontaneously and may be managed with corticosteroids. *Late radiation injury* occurs months to years following therapy and is often irreversible. Radiation necrosis may be difficult distinguish from tumor on imaging and can similarly progress over time. If corticosteroids fail to control the necrotic process, surgical resection may be warranted. Cognitive impairment is one of the most frequent complications in long-term survivors and can range in severity. Deficits may involve attention, learning, memory, processing speed, ability to multitask, and word-finding ability. This is clinically a subcortical dementia and may or may not be associated with corresponding hyperintensity on T2-weighted images. Psychostimulants (e.g., methylphenidate) in conjunction with serial neuropsychological evaluations have been used to help patients remain functionally active.

■ ELECTROCONVULSIVE THERAPY IN PATIENTS WITH BRAIN TUMORS

Although considered high risk in patients with brain tumors, electroconvulsive therapy (ECT) has been performed in this patient population. ECT is associated with increased cerebral blood flow and possible breakdown of the blood-brain barrier and may risk herniation in patients with elevated ICP. However, there may be a role for ECT in treating refractory depression in patients with small, solitary brain masses without any evidence of elevated ICP. In carefully selected patients with brain tumors who are closely monitored, the risk of performing ECT is not necessarily much higher than the usual risk.

KEY POINTS

1. The most common metastatic solid tumors to the brain include lung and breast cancer.
2. LM occurs when tumor cells spread via CSF pathways, and may be treated with intrathecal chemotherapy.
3. Paraneoplastic syndromes are immune mediated and may precede the diagnosis of a malignancy.
4. *Late toxicity* from radiation therapy may be irreversible; *acute* and *early delayed* toxicity may improve spontaneously or with corticosteroids.
5. Brain tumors are a relative contraindication to ECT; however, the procedure has been performed safely in patients with small, solitary lesions devoid of significant mass effect.

■ SUGGESTED READINGS

Bradley WG, Daroff RB, Fenichel GM, et al, eds. *Neurology in Clinical Practice.* 4th ed. Philadelphia: Butterworth-Heinemann; 2004.

Ellison D, Love S, Chimelli L, et al. *Neuropathology: A Reference Text of CNS Pathology.* 2nd ed. Philadelphia: Elsevier; 2004.

Flemming KD, eds. *Neurology Board Review.* Florence: Informa Healthcare; 2007.

Fuller GN, Goodman JC. Tumors. In: Fuller GN, Goodman JC, eds. *Practical Review of Neuropathology.* Philadelphia: Lippincott Williams & Wilkins; 2001.

Gilio P, Gilbert MR. Cerebral radiation necrosis. *Neurologist* 2003;9:180–188.

Grewal J, Grewal HK, Forman AD. Seizures and epilepsy in cancer: etiologies, evaluation, and management. *Curr Oncol Rep* 2008;10:63–71.

Kesari S, Wen PY. Neuro-oncology. In: Samuels MA, ed. *Manual of Neurologic Therapeutics.* 7th ed. Philadelphia: Lippincott Williams & Wilkins; 2004.

Louis DN, Ohgaki H, Wiestler OD, et al, eds. *WHO Classification of Tumors of the Central Nervous System.* 4th ed. Lyons: IARC; 2007.

Mowzoon N, Vernino S. Neoplasms of the nervous system and related topics. In: Mowzoon N, Norden AD, Kesari S. Cancer neurology: Primary and metastatic brain tumors. In: Atri A, Milligan TA, eds. *Hospital Physician Neurology Board Review Manual.* Wayne, PA: Turner White Communications; 2006.

Rasmussen KG, Perry CL, Sutor B, et al. ECT in patients with intracranial masses. *J Neuropsychiatry Clin Neurosci* 2007;19:191–193.

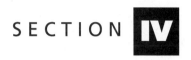
Neurochemistry and Neurogenetics

CHAPTER 28

Behavioral Neurochemistry and Pharmacology

Alan C. Swann

■ INTRODUCTION

Brain function is simultaneously organized across three spheres—spatial, neurochemical, and temporal. In this chapter we will explore the chemical organization of the brain and its relationship to spatial and temporal organization. First, we will describe the basis of neural excitability and the action potential, because these phenomena underlie chemical effects on neural activity. Next, we will describe the main transmitter systems. Finally, we will discuss integration of these systems in relation to the regulation of behavior and its disorders. Basic principles of this review include the following: (a) systems of transmitters in the brain vary in their distribution and in their chemical specificity, but have common underlying characteristics; (b) beliefs once considered axiomatic repeatedly have been disproved, and there is no reason that current views are any more immune to refutation than older ones were; (c) there are many layers of regulation of neuronal function and of interactions among transmitter systems; and (d) as a result, regulation of basic aspects of behavior that are necessary to survive overlap and involve combinations of each major type of system. These areas of overlap may be most susceptible to the subtle but pervasive disturbances underlying serious neuropsychiatric disorders.

■ THE NEUROCHEMISTRY OF ELECTRICAL ACTIVITY AND NEURAL EXCITABILITY

The Action Potential and Neuronal Excitability

Brain function is based on the ability of groups of neurons to communicate by propagation of action potentials. To understand how specific treatments influence brain function, we will first briefly review the mechanisms regulating neural activity. These mechanisms are the ultimate targets of drug action. Figure 28.1 summarizes ionic gradients across the neuronal membrane that contribute to membrane potentials, along with three voltage-dependent cation channels prominently associated with action potentials. In summary, they are as follows:

1. A *negative charge gradient,* with the inside of the cell negative compared to the outside.
2. A *negative concentration gradient for Na$^+$* ions, producing potential energy that can be linked to electrical activity or transport of neurotransmitters, their precursors, and metabolites across the cell membrane.
3. A strongly *negative concentration gradient for Ca^{2+}*, positive gradient for K$^+$, and negative gradient for Cl$^-$. The Cl$^-$ gradient is the basis for gamma-aminobutyric acid (GABA)-mediated inhibition.
4. *Ion channels* are pores that selectively allow ions to cross the cell membrane, increasing or decreasing the electrical potential across the membrane. *Voltage-gated* channels are opened

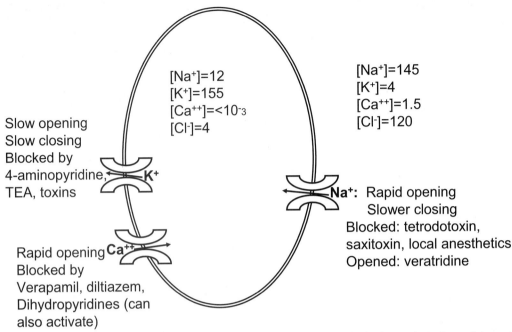

■ **FIGURE 28.1** Principal ion concentrations and fluxes in the action potential. The figure shows intracellular and extracellular ion concentrations in mM, with salient properties of voltage-dependent Na^+, K^+, and Ca^{2+} channels. TEA, tetraethylammonium.

by changes in the membrane potential. *Ligand-gated* channels are opened by the binding of transmitters to receptor sites that can be either physically part of the ion channel or coupled to it by G proteins or other second messengers. They make the more subtle changes in potentials that, in turn, can activate voltage-gated channels.

The action potential is based on the collapse of the Na^+ gradient. The normal resting membrane potential in excitable cells ranges from −60 to −90 mV. Excitatory potentials (e.g., from activation of ligand-gated ion channels by transmitters) or metabolic conditions can lower and raise the membrane potential locally. These postsynaptic excitatory or inhibitory potentials (also called receptor potentials) are summed over the time that the relevant channels are open. As the membrane potential decreases, the fast-activating Na^+ channel has an increasing probability of being open. Sodium ions flood through this channel and down their electrochemical gradient, temporarily reversing the direction of the membrane potential. The voltage-dependent K^+ channel opens and closes more slowly than the Na^+ channel. As it opens, it allows K^+ ions to leave the cell down the chemical and (temporary) electrical gradient, repolarizing the cell. The action potential is propagated along the cell surface, except where it is insulated by myelin, which speeds the spread of the action potential along axons. Between action potentials the gradients are restored by diffusion and Na^+,K^+-ATPase.

Energy Metabolism and Neuronal Activity: Relationship to Neuroimaging

Functional neuroimaging largely measures, indirectly, changes in the activity of Na^+,K^+-ATPase, which is triggered by high intracellular Na^+ and acts to restore the resting ionic gradients. This process is the main source of activity-dependent energy utilization in both neurons and glia. Established methods of functional neuroimaging include positron emission tomography (PET), single photon emission computed tomography (SPECT), and functional magnetic resonance imaging (fMRI).

PET scanning with deoxyglucose measures increased glucose uptake to meet the metabolic demand of Na^+,K^+-ATPase activity. The brain normally relies on glucose as its energy source.

Local blood flow is generally coupled to chemical conditions associated with metabolic activity, leading to increased blood flow to electrically active areas. This is measured by PET scanning with labeled water, with SPECT, or fMRI, which uses endogenous oxygenated hemoglobin as a contrast agent.

Any condition that alters relationships between energy metabolism and electrical activity or between energy metabolism and blood flow can lead to spurious effects.

KEY POINTS

1. Neurons have a negative resting membrane potential with large gradients of Na^+, K^+, Ca^{2+}, and Cl^-.
2. The electrochemical Na^+ gradient provides the potential energy to drive many transmembrane transport systems.
3. Receptor potentials open ion channels that increase (hyperpolarize; inhibitory) or decrease (depolarize; excitatory) the resting membrane potential.
4. If the resting membrane potential reaches a critical value, voltage-dependent Na^+ channels open rapidly and allow Na^+ to enter the cell, resulting in an action potential.
5. Restoration of cation gradients by Na^+,K^+-ATPase is the largest component of activity-dependent neuronal energy metabolism and is measured indirectly by functional neuroimaging.

■ PROPERTIES OF MAJOR TRANSMITTER SYSTEMS

General

This section describes basic dimensions of neurotransmitter economy. Each is a potential target for pathophysiology or drug action.

Spatial Organization

Transmitter systems range from specific pathways to diffuse distribution throughout the brain. The monoamine systems are characterized by well-defined clusters of neurons in the midbrain, pons, and medulla that integrate environmental and internal stimuli to project throughout the brain. These projections can be wide projections from a compact source, as in norepinephrine, or more specifically defined, as with dopamine. Other transmitter systems, such as amino acids, are more diffusely organized.

Transmitter Economy

The function of neurotransmitter systems is affected by the synthesis, storage, release, and breakdown of the transmitters. Synthesis, in turn, is potentially sensitive to availability of precursors and regulation of synthetic enzymes. These interactions are summarized in Figure 28.2. Processes in transmitter economy have varying degrees of specificity relative to other areas of cell function. Monoaminergic systems, including catecholamines and indoleamines, have a relatively high degree of specificity, generally resulting in production of stable and useless metabolites that must be excreted, and which provide indices of transmitter utilization. Other systems, especially amino acids, are more integrated into cell metabolic pathways. Acetylcholine is an example of a monoaminergic system that is integrated into cell metabolism, with both precursors and products being integrally related to energy and phospholipid metabolism.

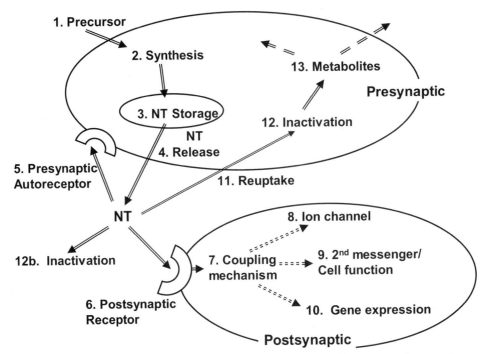

■ **FIGURE 28.2** Regulation and expression of neurotransmitter function. (*1*) Precursors of monoamines or acetylcholine have Na^+-dependent uptake. (*2*) Synthesis is regulated by neural activity and product concentrations. (*3*) Storage in vesicles, usually with ATP and other modulators, is Na^+-dependent and protects transmitters from metabolic breakdown. (*4*) Release occurs with depolarization and is Ca^{2+}-dependent. (*5*) Presynaptic autoreceptors usually inhibit transmitter release or cell firing. They have coupling mechanisms analogous to those of postsynaptic receptors. (*6*) Postsynaptic receptors are coupled to effector mechanisms by coupling proteins. (*7*) Coupling mechanisms often involve GTP-dependent G proteins, which can stimulate or inhibit second messenger or effector systems. (*8*) Some receptors are coupled to ion channels via coupling proteins; for others, the ion channel is intrinsic to the receptor. (*9*) Via coupling proteins, receptor occupation can stimulate or inhibit adenyl or guanyl cyclase, phospholipase C and phosphatidylinositol hydrolysis, phospholipid or protein methylation, Ca^{2+} mobilization, phospholipase A2–related arachidonic acid cascades, and other mechanisms. (*10*) Compounds produced or released by receptor binding can diffuse into the nucleus and alter gene expression. (*11*) Monoamines and gamma-aminobutyric acid are removed from the synapse by Na^+-dependent transport systems. (*12*) Monoamines are inactivated via oxidative deamination or O-methylation by specific enzymes; amino acids re-enter cellular metabolic cycles.

Regulation of Receptor Function

The availability and function of receptors is regulated by exposure to their ligands, as well as by conditions in the cell. These will be discussed with specific receptors, and include the following:

1. *Negative feedback regulation* increased exposure to ligand results in reduction of the density or function of receptors in the cell membrane.
2. *Autoreceptors* can carry out negative or positive feedback regulation.
3. *Genetic regulation* of receptors can be complex, including the presence of several protein subunits, potentially regulated by different genes, and processes such as gene splicing, RNA editing, and posttranslational processing.
4. *Receptors* can form oligomers of the same or different receptors in the membrane, changing receptor function or membrane localization.

Use-Dependent Modulation

Negative feedback control characterizes physiological systems in which recognition of a signal is crucial. Examples are regulation of monoamine receptor density and sensitivity by exposure to ligand, regulation of firing rate by autoreceptors in response to synaptic availability of transmitter, and inhibition of firing by excessive stimulation of a system with a complementary behavioral role.

Positive feedback control characterizes systems that have to increase capacity to meet demand. Skeletal muscle is a good example. Think how bizarre life would be if muscle mass and function were regulated by negative feedback control. In excitatory amino acid systems, increased electrical activity can result in increased synaptic capacity. These mechanisms are central to learning and memory. A cellular example is posttetanic potentiation, a neurophysiological example is kindling, and sensitization of motor responses to stressors or stimulants is a behavioral example. These mechanisms all require the function of excitatory amino acid systems, increased cell calcium, and modification of presynaptic function by diffusion transmission.

Properties of Transmitter Receptors

The two main structural and functional receptor categories are G protein–coupled (metabotropic) receptors and ligand-gated ion channels. These receptors are coupled by GTPase-dependent proteins (G proteins) to second messenger, or effector, systems. Examples are alpha- and beta-noradrenergic receptors; D1, D2, D3, D4, and D5 dopaminergic receptors; most serotonin receptor types; M1 and M3 muscarinic receptors; metabotropic glutamate receptors; GABA-B receptors; most peptide receptors; purinergic adenosine and P2Y receptors; and endocannabinoid receptors.

With ligand-gated ion channels (ionotrophic receptors), the binding of agonist directly alters the function of an ion channel. Examples are muscarinic M2 receptors, GABA-A and GABA-C receptors, N-methyl-D-aspartate (NMDA) and alpha-amino-3-hydroxy-5-methyl-4-isoxazolepropionate (AMPA) glutamate receptors, and purinergic P2X receptors.

Drug Interactions with Receptors

Agonists bind to the receptor and have the same effect as its endogenous ligands. A partial agonist binds to the receptor and does the same thing as the endogenous ligand, but less effectively. The intrinsic activity of a partial agonist is the percentage of optimal effect when the receptor is fully occupied by the drug. A partial agonist with low intrinsic activity can stabilize the function of a system, because full occupation of the receptor with the partial agonist has less activity than with the endogenous agonist, but at least has some preserved function, rather than loss of function, with an antagonist.

Antagonists bind to the receptor, but binding does not have the effect of the endogenous ligand. The antagonist inactivates the receptor by preventing agonist binding.

The effectiveness of agonists and antagonists depends on their concentration and affinity for the receptor compared to those of the endogenous ligand. PET scanning with labeled receptor ligands can measure receptor effects of a drug on receptor occupancy in vivo, showing how effectively a drug competes with an endogenous transmitter.

Functions of Transmitter Receptors

Hundreds of receptor types in the brain bind scores of transmitters, activating or inhibiting dozens of effector systems. Some compounds rapidly activate or inhibit cells (generally amino acids), whereas others have slower effects that provide the background for more rapid signaling. Effects of receptor binding, whether inotropic or metabotropic, include the following:

- *Activating ion channels,* which alter the membrane potential and therefore the probability of an action potential. Stimuli that increase the membrane potential (hyperpolarizing) are inhibitory, and stimuli that reduce the membrane potential (depolarizing) are excitatory.
- *Activating* or *inhibiting second messenger systems,* which orchestrate processes relative to excitability, metabolic activity, or synthesis or storage of transmitters.

- *Altering transmitter release* through Ca^{2+} channels or effects on transmitter economy.
- *Regulating receptor function* or membrane availability, for the same (autoreceptor) or a different (heteroceptor) transmitter.
- *Binding to nuclear or genomic receptors* or causing release of substances that bind to nuclear receptors or that interact directly with the genome.

Interactions Among Transmitter Systems

No system in the brain works alone. Interactions are described later in detail. Heterosynaptic autoreceptors alter the activity or release of other transmitters. Transmitter systems can stimulate or inhibit cells releasing other transmitters. Heterodimers or other oligomers can form with different transmitters.

KEY POINTS

1. Interacting systems of transmitters can directly influence neuronal excitability through rapid depolarization or hyperpolarization or can influence the ionic and metabolic background of neural activity.
2. Transmitter systems may be dispersed throughout the brain, may be limited to discrete areas, or may consist of systems in which discrete collections of cells project to large areas of the brain by long fiber tracts.
3. Precursors are taken up, usually by Na^+-dependent mechanisms, and converted to the transmitter, which is released into the cytoplasm or stored in vesicles. Once released, the compound may diffuse away or may be taken back up into the presynaptic cell and inactivated.
4. The effectors bind to receptors that generally fall into two classes—inotropic receptors linked to ion channels and metabotropic receptors linked via coupling proteins to second messenger systems.
5. Receptor density and function are generally regulated by negative feedback; systems of functional capacity are regulated by positive feedback mechanisms that govern neural plasticity.

Monoamines

The monoamine transmitters consist of the catecholamines (dopamine, norepinephrine, and epinephrine), the indoleamines (serotonin and melatonin), histamine, and acetylcholine. These compounds share Na^+-dependent uptake of precursors, synthesis that is inhibited by high product concentrations and increased with high electrical activity, Na^+-dependent vesicular storage, Ca^{2+}-dependent release from vesicular and cytoplasmic pools, multiple receptor subtypes with both excitatory and inhibitory properties, and a modulatory role in synaptic function. The pharmacology of these processes is summarized in Table 28.1. Norepinephrine, dopamine, and serotonin share additional features and have been referred to as the trimonoamine modulatory system. They are formed from essential amino acids, have stable inactive metabolites, and exercise relatively slow modulatory effects superimposed on fast transmission mediated by amino acid transmitters.

Catecholamines

This description of catecholamine system regulation is based on the diagram in Figure 28.2 and information summarized briefly in Table 28.1.

TABLE 28.1 REGULATION OF MONOAMINE AND CHOLINERGIC NEUROTRANSMITTER SYSTEMS

FUNCTION	DOPAMINE	NOREPINEPHRINE	SEROTONIN	ACETYLCHOLINE
Precursor	L-Tyrosine	L-Tyrosine	L-Tryptophan	Choline Acetyl Co-A
Sensitive to exogenous precursor	++	+	+++	++
Rate-limiting enzyme	Tyrosine hydroxylase	Tyrosine hydroxylase	Tryptophan hydroxylase	Choline acetyltransferase
Immediate precursor	L-DOPA	Dopamine	5-Hydroxy tryptophan	–
Immediate synthetic enzyme	DOPA decarboxylase	Dopamine beta-hydroxylase	Decarboxylase	–
Reuptake inhibitor	Amantidine	Desipramine	Fluoxetine	HC-3[a]
Degradative enzymes	MAO-A or B (i) COMT (e)	MAO-A (i) COMT (e)	MAO-A	Cholinesterase
Location of cell bodies	Substantia nigra Ventral tegmental area	Locus coeruleus Lateral tegmentum	Midbrain raphe nuclei	Diffuse

[a] Inhibits choline uptake; there is no high-affinity acetylcholine reuptake.

Transmitter Economy:

Synthesis: Epinephrine, norepinephrine, and dopamine are synthesized from the amino acid L-tyrosine. Uptake of L-tyrosine into neurons is sodium dependent, requiring energy from the extracellular-intracellular sodium gradient. The rate-limiting enzyme tyrosine hydroxylase is regulated by product inhibition (negative feedback). Increased enzyme synthesis is induced by prolonged increases in neuronal activity. The product, L-DOPA, is a common precursor of all catecholamines, but exogenous L-DOPA increases synthesis of dopamine more than norepinephrine. Dopamine beta-hydroxylase (DBH) converts dopamine to norepinephrine. Norepinephrine is converted to epinephrine by phenylethylamine N-methyltransferase.

Storage and Release: Catecholamines are stored in vesicles that also contain adenosine triphosphate (ATP) and (in the case of norepinephrine) DBH and released in a calcium-dependent process when cells are depolarized. Norepinephrine and dopamine also have a more immediately available cytoplasmic pool. Reserpine-like drugs deplete vesicular catecholamines. Stimulants increase catecholamine release; cocaine acts primarily on vesicular pools, and amphetamines act more on cytoplasmic pools. Cytoplasmic catecholamines that are not released are quickly metabolized (see later discussion).

Reuptake: Once released into the synaptic cleft, catecholamines can be taken back up into the presynaptic cell and inactivated. Inhibition of catecholamine reuptake increases synaptic availability of catecholamines and is a common mechanism in antidepressants (tricyclic, serotonin-reuptake inhibitors, serotonin-norepinephrine reuptake inhibitors) and antiparkinsonian drugs (dopamine reuptake inhibitors).

Inactivation: Catecholamines are oxidized to useless metabolites that diffuse into cerebrospinal fluid (CSF) and plasma and are eventually excreted in the urine so they can be measured by biological psychiatrists. Catecholamine breakdown starts with monoamine oxidase (MAO), a mitochondrial enzyme. There are two common forms of MAO—MAO-A (inhibited by clorgyline) and MAO-B (inhibited by deprenyl). Norepinephrine is metabolized preferentially by MAO-A, eventually forming 3-methoxy-4-hydroxyphenylglycol (MHPG), while dopamine is metabolized equally by MAO-A and MAO-B, eventually forming homovanillic acid (HVA). Transmitter that is not taken up into the presynaptic cell is inactivated initially by catechol O-methyltransferase (COMT).

Clinical Correlates: The more active the system is, the more effect an exogenously administered precursor (e.g., L-tyrosine or L-DOPA) can have on transmitter synthesis. Inhibition of MAOe is a mechanism of action for a class of antidepressive agents (most of which are nonselective between types A and B), but their clinical usefulness is limited by interactions with other drugs and dietary amines. Measurement of catecholamine metabolite production can measure transmitter utilization and turnover. MHPG and HVA cross the blood-brain barrier. They can be measured in plasma, are excreted in the urine, and provide a measure of utilization of the parent amine in the central nervous system (CNS). Levels of these metabolites do not always reflect functional activity because direct inactivation of reuptake or degradative enzymes can result in increased transmitter availability in the face of decreased metabolite concentrations. Further, MHPG and HVA in peripheral body fluids is not all from the brain, because approximately half of MHPG and a greater proportion of HVA are formed peripherally. MHPG and HVA (blood, urine, or CSF) are elevated in mania.

Roles in Behavior and Brain Function: Norepinephrine has an important role in vigilance, attention, and responses to novelty. Stimulation of alpha-1 receptors (alpha-1A, B, and C) activates the protein kinase C-phospholipase C second messenger system and generally has a net stimulating effect on the postsynaptic cell. Beta-receptors (beta-1, 2, and 3) activate the adenylate cyclase system and usually have an inhibitory effect on the postsynaptic cell. In addition to neuronal effects, norepinephrine has prominent effects on cerebral blood flow via cerebral microvessels.

Clinical Effects of Norepinephrine: Stimulation of norepinephrine release results in subjective activation and anxiety in normal humans, panic or severe anxiety in individuals with anxiety or depressive disorders, and risk for hypomania in individuals with bipolar disorder. Norepinephrine is believed to be involved in anxiety, mania, and psychotic states. Drugs that enhance norepinephrine availability, including MAO inhibitors (MAOIs) and norepinephrine reuptake blockers, can be effective antidepressive agents, although direct norepinephrine receptor agonists or precursors do not seem to have this effect.

Dopamine acts through discrete systems, in contrast to the more diffuse effects of norepinephrine. Dopamine is substantially more abundant in the brain than is norepinephrine. D1 receptors are generally excitatory and stimulate adenylate cyclase; D2 receptors are more often inhibitory and inhibit adenylate cyclase. Many behavioral effects of dopamine require stimulation of both D1 and D2 receptors. D5 receptors resemble D1; D3 and D4 receptors resemble D2. Receptor blockade results in protection against overstimulation, improvement in delusions, and organization of speech and (presumably) thought, impairment of motivation, and Parkinsonian motor disorders.

Epinephrine is substantially less abundant than norepinephrine and dopamine in the CNS. It inhibits firing of the locus coeruleus.

Spatial Organization of Catecholamine Systems: Norepinephrine in the CNS has two major sources. The larger and more widespread consists of projections from the locus coeruleus, involved in regulation of attention and stimulus orientation. The locus coeruleus projects diffusely from the pons to the cerebral cortex, hippocampus, limbic system, spinal cord, and cerebellum. The locus coeruleus is activated by novel or noxious stimuli. Locus coeruleus firing is inhibited by mu opioid receptors, epinephrine, noradrenergic alpha-2 receptors, and GABA-A receptors. The locus coeruleus is activated by cholinergic and excitatory amino acid receptors. A second noradrenergic system projects from the lateral tegmentum to the hypothalamus, amygdala, and septum and to many of the projection areas of the locus coeruleus and is involved in neuroendocrine effects of norepinephrine.

Dopamine acts through several more discrete systems. These differ in terms of their regulation by autoreceptors and in terms of peptides co-released with dopamine, and include the following:

- The *nigrostriatal system,* projecting from the substantia nigra to the corpus striatum, with prominent autoreceptor regulation, involved in the accessory motor system.
- The *mesocortical system* projecting from the ventral tegmental area to the prefrontal, cingulate, and entorhinal cortices, without prominent autoreceptors, and involved in the initiation of action. This system has the highest firing rate and is most sensitive to precursor.
- The *mesolimbic system* projecting from the ventral tegmental area to limbic structures such as the nucleus accumbens and amygdala, without prominent autoreceptors, involved in anticipating and responding to rewards.
- The *tuberoinfundibular system* projecting from arcuate and paraventricular hypothalamus to the intermediate lobe of the pituitary and to the median eminence, inhibiting prolactin release.
- Other medium-length systems involved in endocrine regulation, including the incertohypothalamic system and the medullary system, involving the tractus solitarius.
- Short-fiber systems, including retinal amacrine cells and periglomerular cells in olfactory bulb.

Epinephrine neurons are primarily in the lateral tegmentum and medulla; they inhibit firing of the locus coeruleus and project to the spinal cord and paraventricular nucleus of the vagus nerve.

Regulation and Plasticity of Catecholamine Systems: Postsynaptic receptors are regulated by several layers of negative feedback control. Excessive exposure to agonist down-regulates receptor number and uncouples receptors from cellular effectors. Similarly, denervation or drugs that block receptors result in increased numbers of receptors in the membrane.

Noradrenergic systems are regulated by inhibitory alpha-2 autoreceptors on nerve endings or cell bodies. Blockade of norepinephrine reuptake or breakdown results in reduced noradrenergic firing rate as a result of activation of alpha-2 receptors by synaptic norepinephrine.

Dopaminergic D2 autoreceptors have a prominent role in the nigrostriatal system but not in mesocortical, mesolimbic, or tuberoinfundibular systems. Systems lacking autoreceptors are less likely to develop tolerance in response to increased dopaminergic activity.

Inhibitory postsynaptic alpha-2 and D2 receptors are activated at higher neurotransmitter or agonist concentrations. These heterosynaptic receptors regulate other transmitter systems (see later discussion of Figure 28.3). For example, heterosynaptic alpha-2 receptors can reduce firing of dopaminergic, serotonergic, and cholinergic neurons (see later discussion).

Sensitization: Dopaminergic and noradrenergic systems are susceptible to sensitization by exposure to stressors and pharmacological stimulation. Optimal sensitization appears to require activation of D2 dopamine receptors and alpha-1 noradrenergic receptors. Sensitization may be related to development of substance-dependence and recurrence in affective disorders.

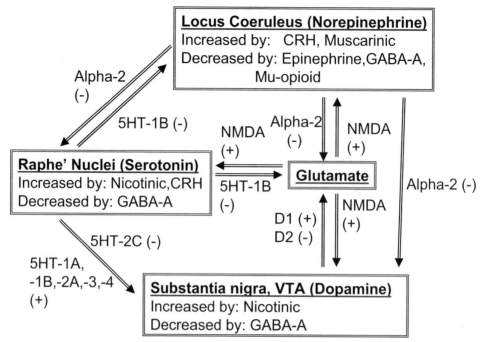

■ **FIGURE 28.3** Interactions among monoaminergic systems and glutamate. Diagram of the main inhibitory (−) and excitatory (+) links among norepinephrine, serotonin, dopamine, and glutamate systems.

KEY POINTS

1. Catecholamines are synthesized from L-tyrosine. The rate-limiting step is production of L-DOPA by tyrosine hydroxylase. DBH catalyzes formation of norepinephrine from dopamine.
2. Catecholamines are stored in vesicles and can be released from either vesicles or cytoplasm.
3. Catecholamines are taken up by Na^+-dependent carriers and metabolized by MAO or COMT.
4. Firing rates of catecholaminergic neurons are under feedback control by autoreceptors.
5. Norepinephrine projects diffusely and is involved in alertness, orientation, and novelty or stress.
6. Dopamine has several relatively discrete systems and is involved in motor activity, motivation, and reward systems.

Serotonin

Transmitter Economy: See Figure 28.2 and Table 28.1.

Synthesis: L-Tryptophan is the amino acid precursor of serotonin. L-Tryptophan is converted to 5-hydroxytryptophan, by tryptophan hydroxylase, the rate-limiting enzyme of serotonin synthesis. With increased activity, administration of precursor becomes more effective in increasing serotonin synthesis. Tryptophan hydroxylase is sensitive to product inhibition and is induced by prolonged activation.

Storage and Release: Serotonin is stored in vesicles and released in a Ca^{2+}-dependent manner resembling that of catecholamines. Newly synthesized cytoplasmic serotonin is preferentially released and, if not released, is promptly metabolized. Vesicular serotonin, like catecholamines, can be depleted by reserpine and cocaine.

Reuptake: Serotonin, like catecholamines, is removed from synapses by a sodium-dependent reuptake system. Inhibition of serotonin reuptake increases synaptic availability of serotonin and is a common mechanism of antidepressive drugs. Reuptake blockade results in stimulation of autoreceptors and a resulting compensatory reduction in firing rate.

Inactivation: As with catecholamines, the most important enzyme in serotonin inactivation is MAO, especially type A. The main metabolite of serotonin is 5-hydroxyindoleacetic acid (5-HIAA), which can be measured in CSF, plasma, and urine.

Clinical Correlates: The more active that serotonergic neurons are, the more effectively administration of precursor (L-tryptophan) can increase serotonin synthesis. Most 5-HIAA in peripheral body fluids is from peripheral sources (primarily the gastrointestinal tract) rather than brain. 5-HIAA in CSF is low in patients with aggressive or impulsive behavior and with violent or severe suicidal behavior.

Roles in Behavior and Brain Function: Serotonin has prominent roles in behavior and in motor regulation. In the regulation of goal-directed, drive-related behavior, it appears complementary to dopamine, acting to inhibit many drive-related and consummatory behaviors, to inhibit aggressive behavior, and to reduce impulsive behavior. Destruction of serotonergic systems increases impulsive behavior in animals, but only if the dopaminergic system is intact. Serotonin interacts with dopamine in the accessory motor system and is important in regulating sleep and neuroendocrine function.

Spatial Organization: The midbrain raphe nuclei project widely to the cerebral cortex, limbic system, hypothalamus, basal ganglia, and spinal cord.

KEY POINTS

1. Serotonin regulation is largely analogous to that of catecholamines.
2. Serotonin is synthesized from its precursor, L-tryptophan, by tryptophan hydroxylase. Serotonin is released from cytoplasmic or vesicular pools, is retrieved from the synapse by an Na^+-dependent reuptake system, and is inactivated in the cell by MAO-A.
3. Serotonin has prominent behavioral roles that often are complementary to those of dopamine, reducing consummatory or drive-related behavior, aggression, and impulsivity. Low serotonin function is associated with impulsivity, aggression, and suicide risk.

Acetylcholine

Transmitter Economy: See Figure 28.2 and Table 28.1.

Synthesis: Acetylcholine is synthesized from acetyl coenzyme A and choline, catalyzed by choline acetyltransferase. Both precursors have prominent metabolic roles other than acetylcholine synthesis. Acetyl coenzyme A comes mostly from glycolysis, followed by oxidation of pyruvate or from the citric acid cycle. Choline is derived from phospholipids or can enter cells through Na^+-dependent uptake. Availability of choline can limit the rate of acetylcholine synthesis when the cell is active. About half of the choline required for acetylcholine synthesis is recycled after synaptic hydrolysis of acetylcholine.

Storage and Release: Vesicular storage is Na^+-dependent, with Ca^{2+}-dependent release.

Reuptake and Inactivation: Acetylcholine is broken down in the synapse to choline and acetate by acetylcholinesterase. Approximately half of the resulting choline is taken back up into the presynaptic cell. This choline is used preferentially for acetylcholine synthesis. Unlike in catecholamines or serotonin, there is no high-affinity reuptake system for acetylcholine itself. Also unlike in catecholamines and serotonin, there are no useless stable metabolites—acetate and choline are recycled or disappear into cell metabolism.

Roles in Behavior and Brain Function: Muscarinic M1 and M2 receptors are involved in regulation of alertness and arousal, selective attention and memory, and motor function. Exposure to drugs that activate muscarinic receptors can cause depression in humans, and antagonists can cause delirium.

Nicotinic acetylcholine receptors are modulatory, fast-acting, ligand-gated ion channels that depolarize cells directly through Na^+ and Ca^{2+} fluxes and indirectly by stimulating excitatory amino acid release. Nicotine is involved in regulation of motivation and reward (partially by increasing dopamine release) and in enhancing working memory. Nicotinic receptors are also involved in response inhibition. Nicotinic stimulation increases serotonin and dopamine release. Overall, stimulation of nicotinic receptors increases cognitive and sensory efficiency and reduces impulsivity. Cognitive deficits reported in schizophrenia appear related in part to nicotinic function; the high rate of smoking in schizophrenia may be an attempt at self-treatment.

Spatial Organization: Unlike catecholamines or serotonin, no discrete structures project throughout the CNS in the way the noradrenergic locus coeruleus does. Instead, cholinergic systems are more widely distributed, being prominent in the reticular activating system, which regulates alertness, and in the accessory motor system, but also widely distributed in cortical and subcortical structures.

Plasticity of Cholinergic Systems: Cholinergic receptors undergo use-dependent regulation by up-regulation or down-regulation in response to changes in ligand exposure. Muscarinic M1 to M3 receptors form homodimers and heterodimers that vary in their sensitivity to use-dependent regulation.

KEY POINTS

1. Cholinergic systems are diffusely organized throughout cortex, brainstem, and basal ganglia, with prominent effects on memory, attention, and motivation.
2. The precursor choline is taken up in a Na^+-dependent process that is potentially rate limiting for acetylcholine synthesis or derived from phospholipids. Acetylcoenzyme A comes from energy metabolism. The rate-limiting synthetic enzyme choline acetyltransferase is regulated by product concentration and neural activity.
4. Unlike catecholamines and serotonin, acetylcholine is hydrolyzed in the synapse and choline is recycled.
5. Acetylcholine has presynaptic and postsynaptic receptors and is regulated by heterosynaptic alpha-2 noradrenergic receptors.
6. Acetylcholine has largely metabotropic muscarinic receptors and inotropic nicotinic receptors. Both types are important in attention and cognitive function.

Amino Acid Systems

Excitatory Amino Acids

Transmitter Economy: The main excitatory amino acid transmitters in the CNS are glutamate, aspartate, and glycine. The immediate source of these compounds for neuronal function, as well as their main site of metabolic inactivation or conversion, is the Krebs cycle. Therefore regulation of excitatory amino acid systems interacts with energy metabolism and protein synthesis. Only a small fraction of the relevant amino acids is involved in neurotransmission. Amino acids can be stored in vesicles; the structure of these vesicles differs from that of monoamine storage vesicles.

Roles in Behavior and Brain Function: Excitatory amino acids are the primary neural activators, causing rapid depolarization in addition to other, more modulatory effects. They are important in learning and memory, and in processes of neuronal plasticity, including sensitization and kindling. They increase firing of monoaminergic cells. Via the amygdala, they translate CNS arousal to autonomic nervous system activity. An appropriate level of amino acid transmission is required for maintenance of the activity of neural pathways, but excessive stimulation results in neurotoxicity, or, at the level of larger groups of cells, seizure activity. Glutaminergic receptors fall into three broad classes—NMDA receptors, AMPA receptors, and metabotropic receptors. NMDA receptors, generally excitatory, are coupled to a Ca^{2+} channel and are important in neuronal plasticity, both adaptive (memory and associational learning) and maladaptive (excitotoxicity and apoptosis). A binding site for glycine strongly facilitates NMDA receptor function; D-serine may be the physiological ligand for this site. In addition, these receptors are regulated by neuregulins (whose genetic regulation may be implicated in schizophrenia and bipolar disorder) and tyrosine protein kinases. AMPA receptors are coupled to ion channels and mediate fast excitatory transmission. They have a wide variety of subunit structures. Metabotrophic receptors are a family of G protein–coupled receptors.

Spatial Organization: Excitatory amino acids are spread diffusely throughout the brain, in many cases as interneurons. They do not have the coherent pathway structure of monoaminergic systems.

Plasticity of Excitatory Amino Acid Function: Excitatory amino acid systems have a central role in use-dependent regulation of neuronal activity and the cellular processes that underlie memory and learning. Stimulation of these systems is required for posttetanic potentiation (or posttetanic depression), behavioral sensitization, kindling, and memory. Excessive stimulation, however, leads to seizure activity, neurotoxicity, and cell death.

Inhibitory Amino Acids

Transmitter Economy: As with excitatory amino acids, inhibitory amino acid systems blend into other metabolic systems. GABA is synthesized from glutamate by glutamic acid decarboxylase (GAD), which is specific to the CNS. It is broken down by GABA transaminase (GABA-T), producing succinic acid semi-aldehyde, which is metabolized by succinic acid dehydrogenase to succinate, re-entering the Krebs cycle. Therefore GABA synthesis and breakdown short-circuits part of the Krebs cycle, with a slight energy disadvantage, producing three molecules of ATP rather than three molecules of ATP plus one of GTP in the corresponding part of the unmodified Krebs cycle. As with monoamines, GABA has Ca^{2+}-dependent release and Na^{+}-dependent reuptake.

Roles in Behavior and Brain Function: GABA is the most abundant neurotransmitter in the brain. Through GABA-A receptors, GABA is the primary inhibitory neurotransmitter in the brain. GABA-A receptors function by increasing the probability that a chloride channel will open, enabling chloride ions to enter via a strong concentration gradient, hyperpolarizing the cell. Stimulation of GABA-A receptors results in sedation and impaired concentration and memory and raises thresholds for seizure activity. Potential properties of drugs that activate the GABA-chloride ionophore system include anticonvulsant activity, reduced anxiety, and sedation. Some have abuse potential, including alcohol, benzodiazepines, and barbiturates. Direct agonists include muscimol and 3-aminopropane sulfonate. Antagonists include biculline and picrotoxin.

GABA-B receptors are G protein–coupled receptors that activate guanyl cyclase. Baclofen is a GABA-B receptor agonist. Most antidepressive treatments up-regulate GABA-B receptors in animals, but baclofen, a GABA-B agonist, is not an effective antidepressive agent in humans.

Glycine is an inhibitory transmitter in the spinal cord and brainstem, as well as being a potential positive effector at NMDA receptors.

Spatial Organization: As is the case with excitatory amino acids, GABA neurons are widespread throughout the brain, often acting as inhibitory interneurons.

KEY POINTS

1. Amino acids are the most abundant transmitters in the brain and are primarily involved in fast neuronal signaling, complementary to the slower, more modulatory effects of monoamines.
2. Amino acids have both G protein–coupled (metabotropic) and ion channel-coupled (inotropic) receptors.
3. The main excitatory amino acid is glutamate. Activation of glutamate receptors is required for use-dependent regulation of neuronal systems, underlying learning and other forms of behavioral plasticity. Excessive stimulation, however, can result in seizures or cell death.
4. The main inhibitory transmitter (and most abundant neurotransmitter in the brain) is GABA. GABA activity protects against seizures, but excessive GABA activity results in impairment of concentration, memory, and motor coordination.

Neuropeptides

Transmitter Economy

Neuropeptides range in size from tripeptides such as thyrotropin-releasing hormone (TRH) to larger proteins, such as brain-derived neurotropic factor (BDNF). They are synthesized de novo or from precursor peptides such as pro-opiomelanocortin or pro-TRH. Conversion from precursors is mediated by prohormone convertases, which are themselves regulated by other peptides. Like other transmitters, they are stored in vesicles, which protect them from breakdown by proteases. The morphology and appearance of neuropeptide vesicles differ from those of monoamine vesicles. Release of neuropeptides, like that of other transmitters, is Ca^{2+}-dependent, but a stronger Ca^{2+} current is required for neuropeptide release than for monoamine or amino acid release. Therefore a single action potential may release vesicle-stored monoamines, but release of neuropeptides from the same presynaptic nerve ending may require repeated stimulation.

Major Peptidergic Systems

Neuropeptide receptors include both presynaptic and postsynaptic G protein–coupled receptors. Table 28.2 summarizes peptide systems that appear to have prominent roles in behavior. This is a general introduction rather than a comprehensive account of this expanding field. Many neuropeptides also have roles as hypothalamic-releasing factors. This review will focus on the roles of peptides in the brain and on behavior and will not address their roles as releasing factors.

Neuropeptide Y (NPY), the most abundant neuropeptide in the brain, has five classes of G protein–coupled receptors (Y1 to Y5). NPY appears to be an important compensatory anti-stress (anxiolytic) peptide released by stressful stimuli. NPY is co-released with NE in the locus

TABLE 28.2 SOME GENERAL ROLES OF PEPTIDE SYSTEMS

PEPTIDE	FUNCTION	REMARKS
Neuropeptide Y	Energy balance Response to stressors Reproductive Autonomic Sleep (+)	Reduces anxiety-like behavior May integrate stress, energy balance, and reproductive function
Corticotrophin-releasing hormone	Response to stressors Autonomic	Activates locus coeruleus Increases anxiety-like behavior Possibly complementary to NPY effects Possible involvement in drug craving
Thyrotropin-releasing hormone	Integrates energy metabolism Response to stressors	Alters food intake Reduces anxiety-like behavior Increased locomotion Increased arousal
Brain-derived neurotrophic factor	Protects against neurotoxicity and promotes neurogenesis Responses to stressors Energy balance Cognitive function	Promotes behavioral plasticity by increasing glutamate release Synthesis induced by estrogen Induces NPY synthesis
Galanin	Response to stressors Sleep (+)	Stress buffer effect
Leptin	Energy balance	Acts as adiposity signal Redirects reward away from food Facilitates TRH release
Angiotensin II	Autonomic Response to stressors	
Endorphins	Pain, nociception Response to stressors Memory	
Substance P	Nociception Response to stressors	
Melanocortins, orexins	Energy balance	Increase food intake
Somatostatin	Sleep (−) Energy balance	
Vasopressin	Memory Response to reward Aggression	Increases aggression Enhances rewarding stimuli
Oxytocin	Social attachment Reinforcement	Reduces drug effects Reduces food intake

coeruleus and sympathetic nervous system in response to stressors or to physical activity. NPY modulates release of transmitters, including GABA, dopamine, serotonin, nitric oxide, and corticotrophin-releasing hormone (CRH). NPY can be neuroprotective by inhibiting the toxic release of glutamate and nitric oxide.

Galanin, co-released with norepinephrine or acetylcholine, also appears to have a stress-buffering effect. NPY and galanin both increase sleep.

CRH has a partially complementary role to NPY, also being released by stressful stimuli, and having many opposing behavioral effects, including anxiety, behavioral activation, wakefulness, and decreased eating. CRH activates the locus coeruleus in response to stressors. TRH has a wide range of roles in regulation of energy balance, in addition to its control of thyrotropin and thyroid hormone release. The prohormone convertase that produces TRH from pro-TRH is stimulated by leptin, a peptide that, in general, reduces energy intake and increases energy utilization in response to fat. Release of TRH is increased by stressors and by changes in energy balance. It has been reported to increase locomotion and arousal. TRH has variable effects on food intake.

Opioid peptide systems (including enkephalins, endorphins, and dynorphins) are important in modulating response to rewarding and stressful stimuli and inhibiting the indirect pain pathway. Mu endorphin receptors inhibit locus coeruleus firing. Enkephalins modulate responses to dopamine and regulate the balance between GABA and glutamate in the corpus striatum, important in motivation and initiation of action.

BDNF promotes neurogenesis and protects against neurotoxicity. Its primary receptor, tyrosine kinase receptor B (TrkB), activates second messenger systems, including protein kinase C-gamma and phosphatidylinositol kinase. It is involved in many aspects of behavior, including inhibition of food intake and responses to stressors. BDNF may be involved in adaptive and neuroprotective effects of physical activity. There are tantalizing relationships between BDNF and affective disorders and schizophrenia. Two large meta-analyses found no evidence for a relationship, but smaller studies found possible relationships to subgroups with early onset or rapid cycling of illness.

Co-release of Peptides and Monoamines

For years it was considered axiomatic that each neuron, or certainly each synapse, released a single neurotransmitter. The discovery of widespread co-release of neuropeptides and classical neurotransmitters has revealed a new dimension of synaptic flexibility.

Some of the more prominent systems of co-release between peptides and classical transmitters are summarized in Table 28.3. These systems have the following characteristics:

- For the same transmitter, different subsystems may co-release different peptides.
- The peptide may inhibit or stimulate release of the transmitter and vice versa.
  - The peptide may inhibit or enhance effects of the transmitter and vice versa.
  - Peptide co-release may change, as during normal development.
  - Peptide co-release may be a function of the frequency or strength of stimulation, generally requiring more stimulation than monoamine release.

TABLE 28.3 EXAMPLES OF CO-RELEASE OF MONOAMINE AND PEPTIDE NEUROTRANSMITTERS

MONOAMINE	PEPTIDE	BRAIN AREA
Dopamine	Neurotensin	Ventral tegmental area
	Cholecystokinin	Ventral tegmental area
Norepinephrine	Enkephalin	Locus coeruleus
	Neuropeptide Y	Medulla, locus coeruleus
	Galanin	Locus coeruleus, amygdalae
Epinephrine	Neurotensin	Medulla
	Neuropeptide Y	Medulla
Serotonin	Substance P	Medulla
	Thyrotropin-releasing hormone	Medulla
	Enkephalin	Medulla, pons
Acetylcholine	Vasoactive intestinal peptide	Cortex
	Enkephalin	Cortex
	Substance P	Pons
Gamma-aminobutyric acid	Somatostatin	Thalamus, cortex
	Cholecystokinin	Cortex
	Neuropeptide Y	Cortex

KEY POINTS

1. Neuropeptides have integrative roles in complex aspects of behavior and integrate brain function with metabolic and environmental conditions. They are important in regulation responses to stressors, energy metabolism, sleep and alertness, pain, and reproductive function.
2. Neuropeptides that were originally identified as hypothalamic-releasing factors for pituitary hormones often have prominent roles in brain beyond releasing hypothalamic hormones.
3. Neuropeptides are widely co-released with monoamine and amino acid transmitters, often modifying or regulating the transmitter effect.

Other Systems

Purinergic Receptors

Neuronal Roles of Adenosine Triphosphate: ATP is a neuroeffector that acts at the junction of energy metabolism and neuronal activity. It is the substrate for ion transport ATPases, for adenylate cyclases, and for protein kinases. It is the precursor for purinergic transmitters. The high concentrations of ATP in monoamine transmitter vesicles may, in part, have a role as a co-transmitter.

There are two major classes of purinergic receptors. P1 receptors are coupled to G proteins and include adenosine A1, A2A, A2B, and A3 receptors. There are two groups of P2 receptors. P2X are ligand-gated ion channels; P2Y receptors are G protein-coupled receptors. Purinergic receptors extensively form heterodimers with other purinergic receptor types or with receptors from other transmitter classes. Formation of A2A-D2 heterodimers in the corpus striatum has been perhaps the most widely studied. Heterodimerization increases D2 receptor function and may be involved in behavioral sensitization to drugs of abuse and in schizophrenia.

Endocannabinoids

Marijuana, like many herbal drugs, activates a specific receptor system in the brain. Endogenous cannabinoids, through G protein–coupled CB-1 and CB-2 receptors, have many roles in brain function, including memory, motivation, motor activity, pain, appetite, and thermoregulation. Endogenous cannabinoid systems appear to be neuroprotective, reducing toxic release of glutamate and nitric oxide.

Endogenous cannabinoids have many functions outside the brain, including immunomodulation and vasodilation, resembling those of nitric oxide (see later discussion).

KEY POINTS

1. Many neuroeffector systems fall outside the established categories of monoamines, amino acids, and peptides.
2. Purinergic receptors use ATP as a transmitter precursor and interact extensively with monoamines through formation of heterodimers.
3. Endocannabinoids have prominent motivation, cognitive, and neuroprotective effects.

Diffusion Transmission: Nitric Oxide

Nitric oxide is the best studied of a new class of compounds that acts by diffusion. Postsynaptic activity modulates presynaptic cells through release of nitric oxide, which diffuses into the presynaptic cell and initiates changes resulting in increased synaptic efficacy. Nitric oxide also diffuses into other cells in the vicinity, facilitating function in these cells. The nearer the cell is to the active postsynaptic cell, the stronger is the effect.

Transmitter Economy

L-Arginine, the precursor of nitric oxide, is taken up by glia in a Na^+-dependent mechanism. It is then released into the synapse and taken up by neurons. Within the neuron, it is converted by nitric oxide by nitric oxide synthase (NOS). Inhibitors of NOS, such as N(G)-nitro-L-arginine methyl ester (L-NAME), can be used as probes to study roles of nitric oxide.

Roles of Nitric Oxide

Nitric oxide diffuses across cells and within cell compartments. It activates soluble cytoplasmic guanyl cyclase and inhibits mitochondrial cytochrome c oxidase. The mitochondrial effect influences energy metabolism and the balance between glycolysis and the pentose phosphate pathway in glucose metabolism. Stimulation of guanyl cyclase activates cellular cascades that are important in the adaptation to increased electrical activity. Accordingly, inhibition of NOS by L-NAME prevents posttetanic potentiation and interferes with behavioral sensitization and learning.

Nitric oxide is involved in use-dependent regulation of neuronal activity, including posttetanic potentiation, behavioral sensitization, and kindling. In addition to behavioral sensitization to cocaine, amphetamine, methylphenidate, nicotine, alcohol, and morphine, it also promotes rewarding and conditioned effects of these compounds. At physiological concentrations, nitric oxide has a neuroprotective effect, but it is neurotoxic at high concentrations.

Non–Central Nervous System Roles: Nitric oxide is involved in regulation of the circulatory and immune systems. In the circulatory system it protects against atherogenesis and reduces blood pressure. Inhibition of nitric oxide synthesis potentiates norepinephrine-induced vasoconstriction. The antihypertensive drug nitroprusside and the cardiac vasodilator nitroglycerine were widely used long before the mechanism of their action through nitric oxide was understood.

KEY POINTS

1. Nitric oxide, derived from L-ariginine, is the most widespread example of neuroeffectors that diffuse readily across cells and compartments and do not interact with classical receptors.
2. By activating soluble guanyl cyclases, nitric oxide is involved in neuronal plasticity and adaptation to high levels of electrical activity, leading to its prominent role in cellular aspects of memory, behavioral sensitization, and posttetanic potentiation.
3. Nitric oxide regulates neuronal energy metabolism by inhibiting cytochrome c oxidase.

Transmitter Interactions

Transmitter systems can interact via heteroceptors that alter transmitter release or firing rate, postsynaptic receptors that alter firing rate or that alter sensitivity to cellular effects of the transmitter, and regulation of expression or coupling of receptors in the neuronal membrane through formation of heterodimers or other oligomers.

Regulation and Interactions of Monoaminergic Systems

Figure 28.3 summarizes major transmitter effects on monoaminergic systems, including interactions among dopamine, norepinephrine, and serotonin.

Norepinephrine: Norepinephrine has inhibitory interactions with serotonin and dopamine via noradrenergic alpha-2 and serotonergic 1B receptors. Serotonin modulates activity of each of the three long-tract dopaminergic systems. Serotonin 1A, 1B, 2A, 3, and 4 receptors all increase dopamine release; 5HT-2C receptors inhibit dopamine release. Serotonin and dopamine have strong positive correlations in turnover rates, consistent with their complementary behavioral roles.

Monoamine Effects on Other Systems: Serotonin 5HT-1B receptors also inhibit acetylcholine, GABA, and glutamate release; dopamine stimulates glutamate release via D1 receptors and inhibits glutamate release via D2 receptors; and norepinephrine inhibits acetylcholine release via alpha-2 receptors and increases glutamate release via beta-1 receptors.

Peptide and Amino Acid Effects on Monoamines: Effects of neuropeptides and amino acid transmitters are generally consistent with their relationships to motivation and responses to stressors. For example, mu opiate receptors inhibit locus coeruleus firing. CRH increases firing rates of noradrenergic neurons in the locus coeruleus and serotonergic neurons in the dorsal raphe. Via NMDA receptors, glutamate stimulates release of norepinephrine, dopamine, and serotonin. GABA-A receptors inhibit firing of the locus coeruleus. Release of GABA in the locus coeruleus is increased by elevated blood pressure and inhibited by low blood pressure.

Receptor Aggregation

Formation of receptor aggregates is a relatively recently recognized mechanism of transmitter interaction. Examples include heterodimers between A2A and D2 receptors, which increase D2 function, and between A1 and A2A receptors, which result in switching between inhibition and stimulation of glutamate release. Receptor aggregation can affect (a) ligand binding, including increased or decreased affinity or cooperativity; (b) coupling to second messenger systems; (c) up-regulation or down-regulation in response to ligand exposure; and (d) receptor localization.

KEY POINTS

1. Interactions among neurotransmitter systems richly increase the range for adaptation and variability in neuronal function.
2. The most prominent mechanisms include presynaptic heteroceptors, activation of complementary groups of neurons, and receptor aggregation.
3. Monoaminergic systems are activated by NMDA receptors, inhibited by GABA-A receptors, and have reciprocal activation and inhibition by heterosynaptic autoreceptors.

■ INTEGRATED BEHAVIORAL AND PHYSIOLOGICAL MECHANISMS

Pharmacological Aspects of Motor Regulation

Mechanisms of motor control overlap with other aspects of behavior, especially motivation, and with mechanisms of psychotropic drugs. These interactions underlie many side effects of psychotropic treatments. Relevant properties of psychotropic drugs are summarized in Table 28.4.

The Supplementary Motor Cortex

The supplementary or accessory motor system integrates motor activity with the regulation of motivation and timing. The corpus striatum receives excitatory glutamatergic inputs from the cerebral cortex and excitatory D1 and inhibitory D2 inputs from the substantia nigra, and it has

TABLE 28.4 SOME TRANSMITTER EFFECTS OF PSYCHOTROPIC DRUG CLASSES

CLASS	ILLNESS/SYMPTOM TARGETS[a]	EFFECT[a]
Antipsychotic	Overstimulation Psychotic states Schizophrenia Mania	Dopamine D1, D2 blockade Serotonin 5HT2 blockade Cholinergic M1 blockade Noradrenergic alpha-1 blockade Histaminergic H1 blockade
Antidepressant	Depressive episodes Anxiety disorders Stress-related disorders Chronic pain Impulse control disorders	Norepinephrine, dopamine, 5HT reuptake blockade Monamine oxidase inhibition Serotonergic 5HT1a agonism, 5HT2 blockade Noradrenergic alpha-1, alpha-2 blockade Cholinergic M1 blockade Histaminergic H1 blockade
Anticonvulsant	Seizure disorders Mania Depressive episodes Neuropathic pain Impulsive aggression	Enhance GABA receptor function or GABA turnover Inhibit excitatory amino acid function or turnover Interfere with sodium or calcium channel function Potential neuroprotective actions
Lithium	Mania Depression Impulsive aggression	Interfere with many processes involving calcium or magnesium Increase serotonin turnover or synthetic capacity Inhibit transmitter-coupled cAMP synthesis (dopamine, norepinephrine) Inhibit or stabilize phospholipase C/phosphatidylinositol systems Potential neuroprotective actions through inhibition of bcl-2, glycogen synthase B kinase, and other systems

[a] This is not intended to be a complete list but to show representative effects within each class. Effects of individual drugs vary within classes; not all drugs in a class share the same effects.
cAMP, cyclic adenosine monophosphate; GABA, gamma-aminobutyric acid.

inhibitory cholinergic interneurons. There are inhibitory GABA outputs to the substantia nigra and globus pallidus. Two circuits regulate the supplementary motor cortex—the direct pathway and the indirect pathway.

The direct pathway is stimulatory. The striatum receives excitatory D1 inputs and projects to the supplementary motor cortex via substance P and GABA. GABA acts via GABA-A and presynaptic inhibitory GABA-B receptors to regulate dopamine release. The net effect of dopaminergic activity in this system is stimulation.

The indirect pathway is inhibitory, with inhibitory D2 inputs to striatum and outputs that are GABAergic and enkephalinergic. Adenosine A2A receptors have a reciprocal interaction with D2 receptors through heterodimerization and effects on second messenger systems. Presynaptic A2A receptors on glutamatergic neurons increase the effectiveness of glutamate release. Dopaminergic activity has a net stimulatory effect in this pathway (by inhibiting inhibitory neurons). Therefore dopaminergic stimulation activates the supplementary motor cortex by stimulating the direct pathway and inhibiting the indirect pathway.

Motor Effects of Antipsychotic Drugs

Antipsychotic drugs block D2 dopamine and HT2 serotonin receptors; the potency with which they block these receptors and their ability to block other monoamine receptors varies widely. They have marked effects on motor activity and its relationship to motivation.

Acute Effects: The acute effects of D2 receptor blockade on motor control include dystonias, Parkinsonism, and akathisia and correlate with D2 affinity. Akathisia is a state of severe motor restlessness that can cause substantial distress and has led to suicide attempts. The proposed mechanism of akathisia is imbalance between dopaminergic and serotonergic activity.

Chronic Effects: Long-term motor effects of antipsychotic drugs can emerge during treatment or on withdrawal of treatment, especially if rapid. These effects include tardive dystonia, tardive Parkinsonism, and tardive dyskinesia.

Tardive dyskinesia, characterized by involuntary movements of the mouth, tongue, and/or extremities, was originally thought to be caused by dopamine supersensitivity, but this model is inconsistent with its time course, persistence, and treatment response characteristics. It appears to be related to excitatory amino acid dysregulation and oxidative stress. Animal models require stimulation of NMDA receptors and can be prevented or reduced by ritanserin (5HT2 antagonist), vitamin E, valproic acid (enhances GABA function), and NMDA antagonists. Nonpharmacological tardive dyskinesia may also occur. Elevated movement disorder rating scores were reported in 12% of one sample of treatment-naïve adolescents; 6% met tardive dyskinesia clinical criteria. One study found dyskinesias in 15% of first-episode patients. This underscores the importance of motor dysregulation in the pathophysiology of schizophrenia.

Atypical or Second-Generation Antipsychotics: Because of movement and motivational side effects of conventional antipsychotics, second-generation or "atypical" antipsychotics were developed. This heterogeneous group of drugs generally has lower affinity for D2 receptors, higher affinity for 5HT-2 receptors, and similar clinical efficacy compared to that of conventional antipsychotics. Extrapyramidal side effects and tardive dyskinesia appear less prominent than with conventional antipsychotics, but these problems have all been reported for all of the atypical antipsychotic drugs. Clozapine has the lowest incidence, and risperidone and aripiprazole have the highest incidence, with quetiapine, olanzapine, and ziprasidone having intermediate levels.

Serotonergic Drugs

Serotonergic drugs can have prominent motor effects. Lithium treatment can be associated with tremors (usually increased on intention and improved by beta-noradrenergic antagonists), parkinsonism, dystonias, akathisia, and tardive dyskinesia (one report found new onset in 9% of subjects who had not had antipsychotic treatment for at least 6 months). These effects may be related in part to serotonergic-dopaminergic interactions. It has been suggested that concomitant lithium treatment could increase vulnerability for tardive dyskinesia in patients receiving antipsychotic treatments. Serotonin reuptake inhibitors have been associated with akathisia, dystonia, dyskinesia, parkinsonism, and tardive dyskinesia.

KEY POINTS

1. The accessory motor system involves connections between the basal ganglia and motor cortex, involved in initiation and coordination of action and linking motor and motivational systems. Antipsychotic drugs have strong effects on regulation of the accessory motor system.
2. Short-term effects of antipsychotic drugs associated with imbalances between dopamine and acetylcholine or serotonin can result in drug-induced parkinsonism, dystonias, or akathisia.
3. Long-term effects also may involve neurotoxicity, resulting potentially in tardive dyskinesia, dystonia, parkinsonism, or akathisia.
4. These drugs can be valuable treatments, and with vigilant management severe effects can be detected early and treated or prevented.

Systems That Regulate Physiology and Behavior

Table 28.5 summarizes neurobehavioral mechanisms that cut across psychiatric diagnostic categories. Regulation of these aspects of behavior is important in pathophysiology of major psychiatric illnesses. As understanding of the brain progresses, it will be possible to understand psychiatric and neurological illnesses in terms of underlying mechanisms of brain function rather than as the current descriptive syndromes. Table 28.5 shows that physiologically important aspects of behavior, such as energy intake and arousal, are regulated by multiple interacting systems. Effects on a single system, such as BDNF, can have far-reaching effects but will mobilize compensatory mechanisms, making it potentially difficult to identify a primary disturbance. These interacting systems have several salient properties, as follows:

- Each is regulated by a balance of positive and negative effectors.
- Regulation of each involves each of the basic types of transmitter system acting in concert—monoamines acting via long fiber tracts, amino acids, and neuropeptides.
- The same transmitters are involved in many systems.
- The systems have multiple interactions.

TABLE 28.5 SOME TRANSMITTER MECHANISMS IN BEHAVIOR

FUNCTION	FACILITATE	INHIBIT	REMARKS
Motivation/reward	Dopamine, endorphins Endocannabinoids	Serotonin	Substance use disorders Affective disorders
Aggression	Dopamine Vasopressin	Serotonin	
Eating	Orexins Dopamine Neuropeptide Y Endocannabinoids	Leptins (circulating) Serotonin Melanocortins BDNF Alpha-MSH CRH	Integration: dorsal vagal complex, hypothalamus Also reduced by cocaine-amphetamine–related transcript (CART)
Cognitive: attention, working memory, executive function	Catecholamines Acetylcholine (muscarinic and nicotinic) Vasopressin Nitric oxide	GABA	Schizophrenia, Affective disorders
Sleep (total)	Serotonin, galanin GABA-A, neuropeptide Y Ghrelin Gonadotropin-releasing hormone Adenosine A1	Acetylcholine CRH Somatostatin Glutamate	Melatonin affects timing
Sleep (REM)	Acetylcholine (REM-ON in tegmentum)	Norepinephrine (REM-OFF in locus coeruleus)	On-and-off systems fire reciprocally
Behavioral sensitization to stressors and stimulants	Excitatory amino acids (NMDA, AMPA) Dopamine Norepinephrine? Nicotine Nitric oxide	GABA Serotonin?	Substance use disorders Affective disorders

AMPA, alpha-amino-3-hydroxy-5-methyl-4-isoxazolepropionate; BDNF, brain-derived neuropathic factor; CRH, corticotropin-releasing hormone; GABA, gamma-aminobutyric acid; NMDA, *N*-methyl-*D*-aspartate; REM, rapid eye movement.

Energy intake, for example, is regulated by several neuropeptides and interacts with mechanisms of motivation and responses to stress. Satiety signals from the gastrointestinal tract, including peptide YY and cholecystokinin, stimulate the vagus nerve and nucleus tractus solitarius (NTS). Inputs from the NTS are integrated with adiposity signals (leptins, insulin) in the arcuate nucleus of the hypothalamus. These inputs are integrated with peptides that increase food intake (including neuropeptide Y and agouti-related protein) and that reduce food intake (including CRH, pro-opiomelanocortin, TRH, and oxytocin).

Disorders in regulation of these interlocking aspects of behavior and physiology result in disturbances of brain function that are prominent in psychiatry and neurology.

KEY POINTS

1. Regulation of behaviors that are basic to survival cuts across psychiatric diagnostic syndromes.
2. These mechanisms include energy balance, arousal, attention, responses to stress, motivation, reinforcement, and regulation of motor activity.
3. These mechanisms are regulated by interacting neuropeptide, amino acid, and monoamine systems.

■ MAJOR PSYCHIATRIC ILLNESSES AND THEIR TREATMENTS

Mechanisms and Examples of Drugs

Table 28.6 summarizes examples of treatment agents acting on the areas of transmitter regulation that were summarized previously and shown in Figure 28.2. Problems related to tolerance and dependence may develop more readily with drugs acting directly on receptors, though they are certainly not absent in drugs acting on transmitter release or uptake. In fact, the latter group includes widely used drugs of abuse, including most stimulants. Some treatments, such as lithium and anticonvulsants, have multiple mechanisms and lend themselves less readily to this kind of classification. Primary mechanisms for lithium action, for example, may lie in areas of metabolic or ionic regulation that are not directly related to any specific neurotransmitter. Drugs classified as anticonvulsants have multiple mechanisms of anticonvulsant action, as well as other cellular effects that are not directly related to the seizure threshold.

Evolving Models for Neuropsychiatric Illnesses

Advances in understanding brain function have worked in tandem with understanding neuropsychiatric disorders, but not generally according to the plans or expectations of investigators. Essentially all currently used treatments were developed serendipitously rather than derived from physiological models of the relevant illness. Studies of these drugs' mechanisms spurred research in neuropharmacology and neurochemistry. For example, investigations based on monoamine reuptake blockade have yielded rich benefits in terms of understanding synaptic regulation in monoaminergic cells. In addition, attempts were made to reason backward from mechanisms of treatments to hypothetical mechanisms of illness. These endeavors have been less successful. As would be expected from the information summarized earlier, perhaps especially in Table 28.4, models based on transmitter regulation can become increasingly complex without really changing conceptually.

Table 28.7 summarizes behavioral abnormalities, drug effects, and classically proposed mechanisms for four major neuropsychiatric disorders. Mechanisms of action of old treatments have helped to change formulations of illnesses. For example, the course of illness in bipolar disorder is consistent with a prominent role for kindling/sensitization effects, which would

TABLE 28.6 EXAMPLES OF MECHANISMS OF WIDELY-USED TREATMENTS[a]

TYPE OF ACTION	MECHANISM	EXAMPLE	APPLICATION
Transmitter economy	Dopamine precursor	L-DOPA	Antiparkinson
	5HT synthesis (L-tryptophan uptake)	Lithium	Antimanic ?Mood stabilizing
	Release	Amphetamine	Stimulant
	Reuptake inhibitor	Cocaine	Stimulant
		Serotonin	Antidepressive Antianxiety
		Norepinephrine	Antidepressive
		Dopamine	Antiparkinson
	Degradation inhibitor	Monoamine oxidase inhibitor	Antidepressive
Presynaptic receptor	Agonist	Clonidine	Antihypertensive Opiate withdrawal
Postsynaptic receptor	Antagonist	Dopamine D2	Antipsychotic
	Agonist	Benzodiazepine, gamma-aminobutyric acid	Sedative/anxiolytic
Ion channel	Inhibitor	Voltage-gated Ca^{2+}	Antihypertensive ?Antimanic
	Mixed effects	Ligand-gated Na^+, Cl^-	Anticonvulsant Antimanic ?Mood stabilizing
Postreceptor	Protein kinase C system	Lithium	Antimanic ?Mood stabilizing

[a]This is not intended to be a complete listing but to show examples of drugs acting on each of the aspects of transmitter regulation described in this chapter.

TABLE 28.7 MECHANISMS AND CLASSICAL TREATMENTS FOR MAJOR PSYCHIATRIC DISORDERS

DISEASE ENTITY	BEHAVIORAL MECHANISMS	ORIGINAL PROPOSED MECHANISMS	CLASSICAL TREATMENTS
Schizophrenia	Motivation Screening of stimuli Social attachment	Dopamine excess	Dopamine antagonists
Depression	Motivation/reward Cognitive function	Catecholamine deficit Serotonin deficit	MA uptake inhibitors Monamine oxidase inhibitors
Bipolar disorder	Motivation/reward Behavioral sensitization	Excess norepinephrine/ reduced Acetylcholine Excess norepinephrine/ reduced 5HT	Lithium Anticonvulsants Dopamine-5HT2 antagonists
Addictive disorders	Motivation/reward Behavioral sensitization Drug-specific actions	Abnormal dopamine (reward deficiency) 5HT deficit	Replacements or antagonists of abused drugs Inhibition of rewarding effects

favor the use of anticonvulsive agents in this illness. However, the first use of carbamazepine and valproate preceded, and basically caused, the ascendancy of kindling-like ideas in this illness. Similarly, many treatments, most notably lithium, have complex effects on cellular and behavioral plasticity. These effects have led to formulations in which mechanisms of cellular plasticity and neuroprotection were important, but the treatments were originally instituted decades before the interesting effects, which have not yet been linked definitely to mechanisms of illness or drug response, were discovered.

Treatments for Psychiatric Disorders

Based on the principles discussed in this review, we will briefly summarize current treatments in major affective, psychotic, and addictive disorders. This is not intended to be a comprehensive review of psychopharmacology. We hope, in fact, that this section will be the first to become obsolete. We will organize the review by diagnosis, allowing for considerable overlap in treatments and their clinical and neural targets.

Bipolar Disorder

Neural and Syndromal Targets: Bipolar disorder is marked by depressive and manic episodes, a recurrent course, and interepisode neurocognitive and behavioral problems. Most treatments have been aimed at treating episodes, but arguably the most important aim of treatment is prevention of episodes. Physiologically, patients with bipolar disorder have increased sensitivity to catecholamines and an apparent imbalance between subcortical and prefrontal cortex activity. The recurrent nature of bipolar disorder, the association of severe stressors with a more severe course, and mutual susceptibility between bipolar disorder and addictive disorders suggests a prominent role of behavioral sensitization in this illness.

Treatment Strategies: Table 28.8 summarizes treatments and their targets for bipolar disorder. Response to treatments for episodes is influenced by severity of the course of illness. Lithium is one of the few treatments with evidence for efficacy in manic episodes, depressive episodes, and episode prevention, but it appears substantially less effective in patients with a severe course of illness. Anticonvulsive agents vary in their effectiveness for either depression or mania, possibly related in part to their ability to combine GABA facilitation with excitatory amino acid inhibition, because drugs such as lamotrigine that are less effective inhibitors of GABA function are relatively more effective for depression than for mania. Similarly, there is an apparent class effect for antipsychotic agents for mania, but apparent variability in their antidepressive effects. Antidepressive agents can reduce acute depressive symptoms (though this is controversial because a large National Institute of Mental Health–funded add-on study was negative) but have never been shown to be effective in preventing depressive episodes and may destabilize the course of some patients. Many, perhaps most, patients require multiple treatments with complementary effects.

Major Depressive Illness

Physiological Targets: Once thought to be related to deficits in noradrenergic and/or serotonergic function, current ideas on pathophysiology of depression are more related to stress-related systems, including CRH and BDNF. However, most or all currently effective antidepressive agents enhance function of serotonergic and/or noradrenergic systems.

Treatment Strategies: Evidence for clinical predictors of response is highly variable, ranging from motor slowing or low norepinephrine metabolite levels predicting relative response to norepinephrine reuptake blockers, to atypical features predicting response to MAOIs. In general, treatments that were effective for the acute episode appear to prevent recurrence. One

TABLE 28.8 TREATMENTS AND TARGETS IN BIPOLAR DISORDER[a]

DRUG CLASS	DRUG	KEY EFFECTS	CLINICAL TARGET	REMARKS
Lithium	Lithium	Second messenger, 5HT synthesis, ?neuroprotection	Acute mania Acute depression Prevention	?Genetic response; worse response if unstable course
Anticonvulsive	Valproate	Increase gamma-aminobutyric acid ?Neuroprotection	Acute mania ?Acute depression ?Prevention	?Also if substance use disorder
	Carbamazepine	Ion channel	Acute mania	
	Lamotrigine	Inhibit excitatory amino acid	?Acute depression Prevention	Prevents depression > mania
Atypical antipsychotic	Aripiprazole	D2, 5HT-2 partial agonist	Acute mania Prevent mania	Strongest akathisia
	Olanzapine	D2, 5HT-2 antagonist	Acute mania Prevention	Strongest metabolic effects
	Quetiapine	D2, 5HT-2 antagonist	Acute mania Acute depression Prevention	Prevention only as add-on Moderate metabolic effects
	Risperidone	D2, 5HT-2 antagonist	Acute mania	Strongest extrapyramidal symptoms of atypical agents Moderate metabolic effects
	Ziprasidone	D2, 5HT-2 antagonist	Acute mania	
Conventional antipsychotic	Haloperidol	D2 antagonist	Acute mania	Stronger extrapyramidal symptoms than atypical agents

[a] Clinical targets are based on evidence from placebo-controlled clinical trials. Note that, in general, antipsychotic drugs are also antagonists at other receptors including alpha-1 noradrenergic, H1 histaminergic, and M1 muscarinic receptors.

prominent characteristic of antidepressive (and also antipsychotic and mood-stabilizing treatments) is the gradual onset of action. This suggests that, rather than the immediate direct effect of the drug, treatment response may be dependent on an adaptation to drug exposure. For example, norepinephrine reuptake blockade would result in long-term stabilization of noradrenergic function by down-regulation of postsynaptic receptors and reduction in firing rate by presynaptic receptors.

A substantial minority of patients in depressive episodes do not respond to their initial treatment. Strategies for inadequate response include addition of a drug with a different mechanism; change to a different drug; addition of an augmenting agent, such as lithium or thyroid hormone; or use of a nonpharmacological treatment, such as electroconvulsive treatment, transcranial magnetic stimulation, or vagal nerve stimulation.

Treatment of anxiety disorders (generalized anxiety disorder, panic disorder) and stress-related disorders (posttraumatic stress disorder) tends to resemble that for depressive disorders. These conditions also widely coexist with bipolar disorder, however.

Schizophrenia

Physiological Targets: Most treatment strategies for schizophrenia have focused on psychosis proneness, which in turn is related to overstimulation. Antipsychotic agents that block D2 receptors address this target, but can impair motivation and motor regulation.

Other targets include neurocognitive impairment, affective disturbances, and recurrence. Genetic and animal studies suggest that nicotinic and glutamate receptor systems may be important in schizophrenia. For example, cognitive disturbances, including impairment of sensory gating, may be related to impaired nicotinic functioning. The fact that nicotine restores sensory gating and increases dopamine and serotonin release may contribute to the high rate of cigarette smoking in schizophrenia. There is much less current evidence about treatment effectiveness in these domains.

As discussed in the section on motor function, there is substantial overlap between treatments used in schizophrenia and regulation of the accessory motor system. This illustrates how important the regulation of motivation is in schizophrenia. Treatments that block dopaminergic systems potentially interfere further with mechanisms of motivation, creating a treatment dilemma that may be only partially resolved by second-generation antipsychotic treatments.

Treatment Strategies: Conventional and atypical antipsychotic agents are similarly effective in treating psychotic symptoms but vary in their effects on motor regulation and, additionally, in metabolic and other potentially severe side effects (see Tables 28.4, 28.7, and the antipsychotic section of Table 28.8). The jury is still out in terms of neurocognitive effects, potentially an important aspect of treatment. Other problems in schizophrenia, including affective symptoms, behavioral problems such as aggression, and substance use, may require adjunctive treatments. Candidates include agents with anticonvulsive properties that could enhance GABA and/or stabilize excitatory amino acid function or agents with antidepressive properties that might enhance motivation.

Addictive Disorders

Physiological Targets: Targets and treatment strategies are summarized in Table 28.9. Treatments for addictive disorders may be aimed at blocking or replacing responses to the target drug. Alternatively, treatments may be aimed directly at mechanisms of reward, motivation, or impulsivity that are involved in addictions. Potential targets include dopaminergic, opioid, serotonergic, and amino acid systems. Relatively successful treatments have been directed at opiate systems, at replacing rewarding effects of abused drugs, and at reducing impulsivity or other behaviors predisposing to drug use. Behavioral sensitization may be involved in the transition to problematic drug use.

TABLE 28.9 PHARMACOLOGICAL TREATMENTS FOR SUBSTANCE USE DISORDERS

POTENTIAL TREATMENT	TARGET DRUG	MECHANISM	REMARKS
Disulfiram	Alcohol	Acute discomfort ?Dopamine beta-hydroxylase inhibition	Dopamine beta-hydroxylase inhibition may also be effective for other drugs
Acamprosate	Alcohol	Excitatory amino acid antagonist	
Naltrexone	Alcohol, opiate	Mu opioid antagonist	Other opiate antagonists or mixed agonist-antagonists also effective
Topiramate	Alcohol, stimulant	Excitatory amino acid antagonist	
Selective serotonin reuptake inhibiters	Stimulant	Serotonin reuptake blockade	Only effective with behavioral treatment
Antipsychotic agents	Stimulant	D2 blockade	Consistently ineffective

Treatment Strategies: Treatments aimed at reducing rewarding or motivating effects of abused drugs by blocking dopamine receptors have had only limited success. Treatments that block opioid receptors have had more success, being effective in treating alcohol and stimulant use disorders in addition to opiate use. Treatments that enhance serotonergic function also appear effective when combined with specific behavioral treatments. Treatments including topiramate (an anticonvulsant acting primarily on excitatory amino acid function), which has been reported to reduce alcohol and stimulant use, may work by reducing behaviors such as impulsivity that predispose to drug use. Some treatments may have multiple mechanisms. For example, disulfiram is used to treat alcohol use disorders because it interferes with breakdown of acetaldehyde. However, disulfiram also inhibits DBH, preventing conversion of dopamine to norepinephrine. This may also contribute to the effectiveness of disulfiram and may suggest that it or other DBH inhibitors could be effective in treating stimulant addictions. There are as yet no treatments directed (at least intentionally) at mechanisms related to behavioral sensitization. Virtually all successful pharmacological agents require nonpharmacological treatments as well. When addictive disorders coexist with affective disorders or schizophrenia, both the addictive and the other disorder must be treated.

KEY POINTS

1. Major psychiatric disorders, including bipolar disorder, major depressive illness, schizophrenia, and addictive disorders, are related to the aspects of brain function that integrate behavior and physiology.
2. Targets for treatment of symptoms of acute exacerbations, impairment between episodes, and recurrence or change over time. Most treatments are currently based on acute symptoms.
3. Treatments for bipolar disorder include lithium, valproate, lamotrigine, and antipsychotic agents.
4. Current treatments for major depressive illness, including monoamine reuptake blockers and monoamine oxidase inhibitors, enhance or stabilize monoaminergic function, although the source of their effectiveness may lie in stress-related systems.
5. Current treatments for schizophrenia, antipsychotic agents, generally have D2 and 5HT2 blockade in addition to a complex array of other possible effects.
6. Treatments for additions can focus on (a) blocking the actions of specific drugs, (b) blocking rewarding effects, (c) enhancing reward-like effects to reduce drug craving and/or substitute a less-harmful drug, (d) reducing behaviors such as impulsivity that may predispose to drug use, or (e) preventing mechanisms, related to behavioral sensitization, that may underlie the transition from casual to problematic use.

■ CONCLUSION

Brain function is organized by multiple interacting systems. The basis of these systems is the regulation of the membrane potential, leading to increased or decreased probability of firing. However, this mechanism is not binary, because the consequences of neuronal firing may depend on its pattern and frequency. Basic neuroeffector systems that work together to integrate physiology and behavior include the following:

- Monoamine neurotransmitters, with modulatory effects on cell function, highly specific systems of synthesis and degradation, and far-reaching neuronal systems based on long tracts projecting from relatively discrete brainstem sites
- Amino acid systems, combining modulatory effects with rapid stimulation or inhibition of firing and diffuse distribution

- Peptidergic systems, often co-released with monoamines or amino acids, with prominent roles in stress responses and integration of behavior and metabolism
- Diffusion systems, using dissolved gases, most commonly nitric oxide, providing a local signal of neuronal activity and triggering adaptive responses to it
- Other, often integrative systems, such as the purinergic system, whose precursor, ATP, is also central to energy metabolism and second-messenger systems

These systems work together to regulate behavioral and physiological functions, including vigilance and attention, sleep, motivation, and energy balance. The systems have many layers of regulation and interaction that, if disrupted, can result in severe neuropsychiatric disorders. As we understand their regulation better, we will be able to devise pathophysiology-based diagnosis and treatment for severe neuropsychiatric illnesses.

CHAPTER 29

Neurogenetics

Patricia E. Greenstein

■ INTRODUCTION

This chapter will outline the importance of history taking, and pedigree construction and analysis when suspecting a genetic component to a neurological disease. It will emphasize some of the genetic components of neurological diseases important to neurologists and psychiatrists. Genetic diseases cover a vast area that exceeds the scope of this chapter. Neuromuscular disorders have been covered in other chapters.

Genetics plays a very important role in the pathophysiology of human disease. In neurological disorders, it is widely accepted that mendelian inheritance can account for 5% to 10% of these diseases. Mendelian traits represent the most basic and simple patterns of inheritance. Nonmendelian traits represent some complexity in their mode of inheritance, in which the classic pattern may not always apply and epigenetic factors are associated with disease mechanisms. Regardless of the mode of inheritance, defining specific genetic factors that are associated with certain neurological diseases and their functional role are very important in patient management and genetic counseling, as well as understanding the mechanism of the disease to ultimately develop new therapeutics.

It is estimated that there are approximately 20,000 to 30,000 genes in the human genome. Approximately one third of these genes are expressed in the nervous system, and thus a phenotype with neurological features is common.

■ TAKING A GENETIC HISTORY

Looking for neurological disease genes in a patient or the family begins with a clear description of the phenotype. This is the observable expression of the genetic information (genotype) as a structural, clinical, and cellular or biochemical trait.

What then follows is a detailed family history. When taking the history, it is useful to draw a detailed pedigree of the first-degree relatives (e.g., parents, siblings, and children), because they share 50% of genes with the patient.

The family history should include information about ethnic background, age, health status, consanguinity, and (infant) deaths. Next, the physician should explore whether there is a family history or illnesses related to the current problem. Because of the possibility of age-dependent expressivity and penetrance, the family history will need intermittent updating. If the findings suggest a genetic disorder, the clinician will have to assess whether some of the patient's relatives may be at risk for carrying or transmitting the disease. In this circumstance, it is useful to confirm and extend the pedigree based on input from several family members. This information may form the basis for carrier detection, genetic counseling, early intervention, and prevention of a disease in relatives of the index patient.

The patterns shown by single-gene disorders in pedigrees depends on two factors: the chromosomal location of the gene locus, which may be autosomal (located on an autosome or nonsex chromosome), and whether the phenotype is dominant (expressed when only one

TABLE 29.1 PATTERNS OF MENDELIAN INHERITANCE

INHERITANCE	DOMINANT	RECESSIVE
Autosomal	Autosomal dominant	Autosomal recessive
X-linked	X-linked dominant	X-linked recessive

chromosome of a pair carries the mutant allele, despite the normal allele expressed on the other chromosome of the pair) or recessive (expressed only when both chromosomes of a pair carry a mutant allele).

Thus there are four basic patterns of mendelian inheritance (Table 29.1).

■ MENDELIAN INHERITANCE

Autosomal Dominant Inheritance

A phenotype expressed in the same way in both homozygotes and heterozygotes is dominant, that is, if only one of the two alleles is mutated. Males and females are equally affected. Looking at a pedigree, there is male-male transmission. There is a 50% risk to each child of an affected parent. Multiple generations are affected, and expression of the phenotype can be highly variable (Fig. 29.1).

Some examples of diseases with autosomal dominant inheritance include Huntington's disease, spinocerebellar ataxia, myotonic dystrophy, and inherited forms of Alzheimer's disease.

Autosomal Recessive Inheritance

Autosomal recessive disease occurs only in homozygotes, individuals with two mutant alleles and no normal alleles. In these diseases, one normal gene copy in a heterozygote is able to compensate for the mutant allele and prevent the disease from occurring. A typical pedigree is shown in Figure 29.2.

In this typical pedigree, in which males and females are equally affected, there is a 25% risk of homozygosity to children of carrier parents. There is a single generation affected, and consanguinity is sometimes present. Consanguineous marriages occur in people related by descent from a common ancestor. This increases the chance that both parents are carriers of a mutant allele at the same locus.

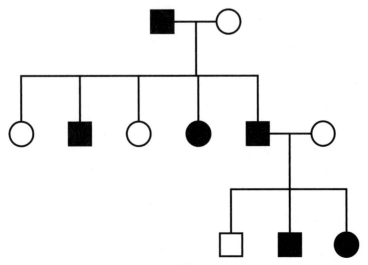

■ **FIGURE 29.1** Autosomal dominant inheritance.

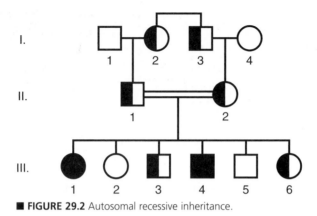

■ **FIGURE 29.2** Autosomal recessive inheritance.

Some examples of neurological diseases that are inherited in an autosomal recessive fashion are Friedreich's ataxia, Tay Sach's disease, and Canavan's disease.

X-Linked Recessive Inheritance

The inheritance of X-linked recessive phenotypes follows a defined pattern and is typically expressed in all males who receive it, but only in those females who are homozygous for the mutation. Thus X-linked recessive diseases are generally restricted to males, with the exception of rare manifesting female carriers, who are generally more mildly affected, as determined by the pattern of X-inactivation. The gene responsible for the condition is transmitted from an affected man through all of his daughters. The gene is ordinarily never transmitted directly from father to son. Isolated cases are usually the result of a new mutation.

A typical pedigree is illustrated in Figure 29.3. Examples of such diseases are Duchenne's and Becker's muscular dystrophy.

X-linked Recessive Inheritance

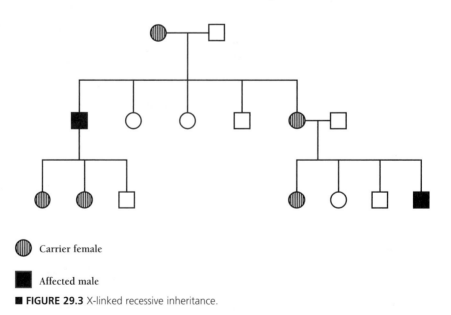

◍ Carrier female

■ Affected male

■ **FIGURE 29.3** X-linked recessive inheritance.

Mitochondrial Inheritance

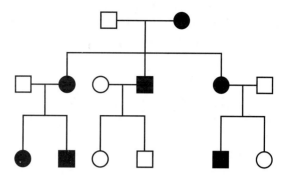

■ **FIGURE 29.4** Mitochondrial inheritance.

X-Linked Dominant Inheritance

As noted previously, an X-linked phenotype is described as dominant if it is regularly expressed in heterozygotes. The distinguishing feature of a fully penetrant X-linked dominant pedigree is that *all* the daughters and *none* of the sons of affected males are affected. If any daughter is unaffected or any son is affected, the inheritance must be autosomal and not x-linked.

Examples of this that are important to neurologists and psychiatrists are Rett's syndrome, incontinentia pigmenti, and fragile X syndrome.

■ MITOCHONDRIAL PATTERNS OF INHERITANCE

The mitochondrial chromosome is an approximately 16.5-kb circular DNA molecule (mtDNA) located outside the nucleus of the cell in the mitochondrial organelle (Fig. 29.4). The ovum and not the sperm supplies the zygote with all of its mitochondria. Therefore a mother carrying a mutation in mtDNA will pass the mutation on to all of her offspring, whereas a father carrying the mutation passes it to none. Defects in mtDNA demonstrate maternal inheritance. The other unique feature of mitochondrial inheritance is that there is passive segregation of mitochondria at cell division. In other words, the mtDNA replicates and sorts randomly among newly synthesized mitochondria, which are then distributed between the two daughter cells. This results in variation in proportion of mutant and wild-type mitochondria, a concept known as "heteroplasmy." Mitochondrial function is essential to nearly all cells, and the phenotypic expression of a mutation in mtDNA depends on the relative proportions of normal and mutant mtDNA making up different tissues. This balance between "wild-type" and "mutant" mtDNA accounts for reduced penetrance, pleiotropy, and variable expression within a pedigree.

KEY POINTS (MITOCHONDRIAL INHERITANCE)

1. Transmission is along the maternal germline.
2. All children are at risk.
3. None of an affected male's children are affected.
4. Highly variable expression and severity.
5. Cytoplasmic inheritance.
6. Heteroplasmy (mixing of wild-type and mutant mtDNA).

■ POLYGENIC INHERITANCE

Some syndromes are presumed to be the result of the additive effect of a small number of multiple genes. This is still speculative, but could include some forms of mental retardation, hypertension, epilepsy, or nonmendelian dementias.

■ MULTIFACTORIAL INHERITANCE

Multifactorial inheritance refers to disorders that result from the combination of an inherited genetic disposition acting in concert with an environmental insult, for example, acute intermittent porphyria following phenobarbital administration.

This concept has clinical relevance. It is important in the management of patients with seizure disorders who are fast or slow metabolizers. Another example is multiple sclerosis, in which there is a presumed immunological predisposition to some unknown environmental trigger. Most common neurodevelopmental disorders have complex inheritance, as do autism and most dementias. The key aspects to understanding complex genetic traits include the following:

- Many genes contribute to the phenotype.
- Each gene contributes only a portion to the genetic risk.
- Variants commonly present in the general population may contribute.
- Environmental influences may also contribute.

The disease status itself may be an arbitrary cutoff of what is a continuous distribution of a phenotype.

■ CHROMOSOMAL DISORDERS

Abnormalities of chromosomes may be either numerical or structural and may involve one or more autosomes, sex chromosomes, or both. The most common type of chromosomal abnormality is aneuploidy, an abnormal chromosomal number resulting from an extra or missing chromosome.

Clinical phenotypic features that are important to recognize when considering a chromosomal disorder include the following:

1. Multiple birth defects
2. Involvement of midline structures: brain, heart, kidneys, gastrointestinal system
3. Bilateral inguinal hernias
4. Mental retardation
5. Dysmorphic facial features

The chromosomal disorders that are important for neurologists and psychiatrists to recognize include trisomies 21 (Down's syndrome), 13, 18, and 47,XXY (Klinefelter's syndrome).

■ ATYPICAL PATTERNS OF INHERITANCE

Exceptions to Mendelian inheritance do occur in unusual single-gene disorders and must therefore be considered when evaluating a patient.

The two disorders relevant to neurologists and psychiatrists are Prader-Willi syndrome (PWS) and Angelman syndrome (AS). They are two contiguous-gene deletion syndromes in which multiple genes are deleted from a specific region of chromosome 15q11–q13. The diagnosis can be made on a high-resolution karyotype (analysis of the chromosomes), but more definitively by fluorescence in situ hybridization (FISH) analysis of the Prader-Willi critical region. In this analysis a fluorescent probe is hybridized to some genomic DNA from 15q11–q13. The hybridized probe fluoresces when the chromosomes are viewed with a wavelength of light that excites the fluorescent dye. If there is a deletion on one of the chromosomes, it will be visible under a microscope.

PWS is a relatively common dysmorphic syndrome with the following phenotypic features: severe hypotonia at birth, obesity, short stature, hypogonadism, and mental retardation. In 70% of cases, there is a detectable cytogenetic deletion on the long arm of chromosome 15 inherited from the patient's father. Thus the genomes of these patients have genetic information in 15q11–q13 derived entirely from their mothers. By contrast, in AS there is a deletion of approximately the same region, but on the chromosome 15 inherited from their mother. Patients therefore have their entire 15q11–q13 information derived only from their fathers. The phenotype of these patients is also very different and includes short stature, severe mental retardation, seizures, and spasticity ("the happy puppet").

KEY POINTS

1. Diagnosis of a contiguous-gene deletion syndrome is usually by karyotype analysis and FISH.
2. These disorders have well-described phenotypes.
3. Multiple genes are deleted, and usually patients have mental retardation.

■ GENETIC COUNSELING AND ETHICAL ISSUES

Genetic counseling is a process by which a trained medical professional explains the genetic contribution of a disorder to a patient. When a disorder is suspected of being heritable, however, there is an added dimension—the need to inform other family members of their risk and the means available to them to modify their risk.

Just as the unique feature of genetic disease is its tendency to recur within families, the unique aspect of genetic counseling is its focus, not only on the original patient (proband) but also on the patient's family, both present and future.

The medical professionals trained to provide genetic counseling include physicians, those who have doctorate-level training in medical genetics, certified genetics counselors, and nurses with special training in medical genetics.

During the process of genetic counseling, patients are not told what decisions to make with regard to the various testing and management options, but, instead, are provided information and support. This approach to counseling, referred to as nondirective counseling, has been adopted widely as the standard of practice in the field. Genetic counseling is not limited to giving information and calculating risk for disease, but it is rather a communication process that requires understanding of the complex psychosocial issues associated with a genetic disorder in a family.

There are many potential pitfalls in interpreting genetic test results. Most tests have a high degree of reliability, but there are opportunities for misinterpretation. These are most specifically related to linkage-based indirect tests or detection of benign polymorphisms (variants) in direct testing. Patients found to carry specific mutations may be perceived as "different" by themselves, members of their families, or members of society. There can be a great deal of guilt and altered self-image and self-blame, particularly if the gene they carry is transmitted to a child or other members of their family.

Unlike many medical tests, genetic test results may have implications for many members of a family. At all times the privacy of individuals within the family must be respected and the risks of discovery of information about others in the family discussed before testing.

This particularly applies to presymptomatic counseling of family members at risk for diseases, in particular, Huntington's disease (HD). The counseling is particularly complex given that HD is a progressive degenerative disease for which there is no treatment or cure. Fewer than 10% of at-risk people seek testing, and concerns have been raised that predictive testing may lead to an increase in deaths by suicide among identified carriers. However, there is evidence to suggest from looking at large centers who offer presymptomatic testing that people who choose to be tested are psychologically selected for a favorable response to testing. It is recommended, however, that presymptomatic counseling be offered only in established centers with good psychiatric or psychological support services. People with high levels of depression or hopelessness should be referred for psychiatric counseling before decision making about genetic testing.

■ GENETICS OF ALZHEIMER'S DISEASE AND DEMENTIA

Genetic factors play an important role in many types of dementia. The most common form of dementia is Alzheimer's disease (AD). AD is frequently divided into early onset and late onset, with the dividing line being 60 to 65 years of age.

Three genes are known to cause early-onset AD. The first is the amyloid precursor protein or APP gene. APP is normally cleaved at the beta and gamma secretase sites to produce a 40–42 amino acid, the beta-peptide. It is this peptide that is deposited in excess in the brains of persons with AD. The most common mutation in this gene is at position 717 and leads to the increased production of the Abeta peptide. The importance of this peptide in AD pathogenesis is further highlighted by the associated plaques and tangles in people with Down's syndrome (trisomy 21) with three copies of the APP gene.

Mutations in *presenilin-1*, a gene on chromosome 14, are also a rare cause of autosomal dominant, young-onset AD. The families with mutations in APP and PS-1 typically have onset in their 40s and live for 6 to 10 years.

Presenilin-2 is a homolog of PS-1 on chromosome 1. Mutations in PS-2 also cause early-onset autosomal dominant AD in rare families. There is a wider range of age of onset from 40 to 75 years. Of these three genes, PS-1 is by far the most common. Even so, all mutations in these three genes represent less than 2% of all AD.

Late-onset AD is by far the most common type of dementia. It is generally accepted that there must be several genetic factors playing a role. The only factor recognized and confirmed is Apo E. Apo E is an important lipid and cholesterol transporter. There are 3 alleles: E2, E3, and E4. One form is inherited from each parent. The E4 allele is a significant AD risk factor. The role for APOE as a major susceptibility locus in AD was suggested by four independent lines of evidence: linkage analyses in late-onset families with an aggregation of AD, increased association of the E4 allele with AD patients compared with controls, the discovery that the Apo E protein is a component of the AD amyloid plaque, and the finding that Apo E binds to the Abeta peptide. Normal function in neurons is not known, but, as mentioned, is a component of an amyloid plaque. That being said, it is neither necessary nor sufficient for the disease.

Determining a patient's Apo E genotype does not add much value to making a diagnosis of AD. Furthermore, it is not clear that the Apo E genotyping of asymptomatic individuals will provide useful information about risk for developing AD.

Other Alzheimer's Disease Genes

Statistical analysis suggests that an additional four to eight genes may significantly modify the risk for AD. The identity of these genes remains unknown. In addition, case control association studies have implicated a long list of candidate genes (>100) in AD, and their roles in the genetic specification of risk for AD is unclear.

KEY POINTS

1. Sporadic AD (~75%).
2. AD associated with Down's syndrome (<1%).
3. Familial (~25%).
4. Late-onset familial (AD2) (15% to 25%): Apo E risk factor.
5. Early-onset familial AD (AD1, 3, 4) (<5%); AD1—*presenilin 1*, AD2—APP, AD4—*presenilin 2*.

TABLE 29.2 FRONTOTEMPORAL DEMENTIA–RELATED DISORDERS

Frontotemporal dementia

Frontal lobe dementia

Frontal dementia with motor neuron disease

Pick's disease

Pick complex

Primary progressive aphasia

Semantic dementia

Corticobasal degeneration

■ FRONTOTEMPORAL DEMENTIA

A second form of dementia is frontotemporal dementia (FTD). Classic Pick's disease is considered a subtype. The age of onset is typically from the 40 to 60 years age range, with a prominent behavioral disorder usually with frontal network dysfunction, sometimes a language disturbance, and relatively spared memory. There is selective degeneration in the orbitofrontal lobes or temporal lobes. The pathology is quite variable and ranges from discrete deposits of tau protein to nonspecific neuronal loss. FTD with excessive tau deposition is often referred to as a tauopathy. Most of the familial autosomal dominantly inherited cases have been caused by a variety of mutations in the tau gene. These mutations can alter the function of microtubules and sometimes change the normal 1:1 ratio of 3 repeat to 4 repeat tau. A subtype of FTD that is sometimes associated with motor neuron disease has neuronal tau negative inclusions but is ubiquitin positive. These patients do not have mutations in tau, but have been found to have mutations in a progranulin gene. Mutations in tau and progranulin each represent 10% of all FTD cases (Table 29.2).

■ AUTOSOMAL DOMINANT ARTERIOPATHY WITH SUBCORTICAL INFARCTS AND LEUKOENCEPHALOPATHY

Cerebral autosomal dominant arteriopathy with subcortical infarcts and leukoencephalopathy (CADASIL) is an autosomal dominant disorder associated with dementia, early-onset multiple strokes, and history of migraine. The pathological lesions occur in the white matter, and the changes seen on magnetic resonance imaging (MRI) can be confused with multiple sclerosis plaques. On electron microscopy, there are osmophilic granules deposited in the media of the vessels. The disease is caused by point mutations in the *Notch-3* gene.

■ GENETICS OF TRIPLET REPEAT DISEASES

In all types of mendelian inheritance, a reliable assumption is that mutations are stably transmitted from generation to generation; that is, all affected members of a family share the identical inherited mutation. By contrast, a new class of genetic disease has been recognized—diseases resulting from unstable dynamic mutations. These dynamic mutations can involve anything from a series of trinucleotides to a complex sequence of dodecamer repeats. The triplet repeat disorders are the most common in this group (Fig. 29.5).

These diseases are caused by expansion of a normally polymorphic number of trinucleotide repeats within a gene. Most of the diseases are predominantly neurological disorders. Many of these disorders exhibit anticipation, which is defined as earlier age of onset and increasing severity of disease in subsequent generations of a family. There is variability of the degree of

Genetics of triplet repeat diseases:

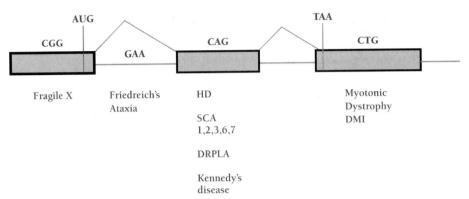

■ **FIGURE 29.5** Triplet repeat diseases.

the expansion of the repeat in each disease and a greater tendency for the repeat to expand than to contract. The risk for expansion may vary depending on the sex of the transmitting allele. Diseases with expansion include the following:

Autosomal dominant with expansion in a coding exon:
    Huntington's disease
    All of the dominant spinocerebellar ataxias
Autosomal dominant with expansion in the 3' untranslated portion of the gene:
    Myotonic dystrophy
Autosomal recessive with a CGG repeat expansion in an intron and purported mechanisms:
    Friedreich's ataxia
X-linked recessive:
    Kennedy's disease
X-linked dominant:
    Fragile X syndrome

Fragile X syndrome (MIM 309550) is the most common inherited form of mental retardation and occurs in about 1:1500 males. It is an X-linked dominant disorder with reduced penetrance. This was the first disorder ascribed to a triplet repeat expansion. The *FMR1* gene (fragile X mental retardation gene) was discovered to contain a CGG repeat located in the 5' UTR. The full mutation is caused by more than 200 CGG repeats. These full-mutation expansions are generally accompanied by complete or partial silencing of the *FMR1* gene, with subsequent deficiency of absence of the FMR1 protein, which leads to fragile X syndrome.

Fragile X mental retardation is characterized phenotypically by moderate to severe mental retardation, macroorchidism, and distinct facial features, including long face, large ears, and prominent jaw. Most show unusual behavior, with alternating anxiety and hilarity, disordered hyperactivity, and aggressiveness. The cognitive phenotype ranges from a general intelligence corresponding to mild to moderately severe mental retardation. Other psychiatric syndromes include attention-deficit hyperactivity disorder, oppositional defiant disorder, enuresis, and encopresis.

Males with Full Mutation Alleles

The phenotypic features of males with a full mutation and, hence, the fragile X syndrome, vary in relation to puberty. Prepubertal males tend to have normal growth but large occipitofrontal head circumference (>50th percentile). Other physical features that are not readily recognizable in the preschool-age child become more obvious with age. These involve the craniofacies (long face, prominent forehead, large ears, and prominent jaw) and genitalia (macro-orchidism), delayed attainment of motor milestones and speech, and abnormal temperament (hyperactivity, hand flapping, hand biting, temper tantrums, and occasionally autism). Behaviors in postpubertal males with fragile X syndrome often include tactile defensiveness, poor eye contact, perseverative speech, problems in impulse control, and distractibility. Ophthalmologic, orthopedic, cardiac, and cutaneous abnormalities have also been noted

The fragile X-associated tremor/ataxia syndrome (FXTAS) is characterized by late-onset progressive cerebellar ataxia and intention tremor in men who have a premutation (55–200 CGG repeats). Other neurological findings include short-term memory loss, executive function deficits, cognitive decline, Parkinsonism, peripheral neuropathy, lower limb proximal muscle weakness, and autonomic dysfunction. Penetrance is age related; symptoms are seen in 17% of men ages 50 to 59 years, in 38% of ages 60 to 69 years, in 47% of ages 70 to 79 years, and in 75% of age 80 years or older. Some female permutation carriers may also develop tremor and ataxia. Symmetrical regions of increased T2 signal intensity has been seen in the middle cerebellar peduncles and adjacent cerebellar white matter.

■ HUNTINGTON'S DISEASE

Huntington disease (HD) is a progressive disorder of motor, cognitive, and psychiatric disturbances. The disease is inherited as an autosomal dominant trait and is due to a CAG repeat expansion in the open reading frame that encodes a polyglutamine tract. Normal alleles have 9 to 30 repeats, and patients affected with HD have more than 40 repeats. The HD protein is termed huntingtin, and as yet its function is unknown.

HD displays anticipation, which is a phenomenon that occurs with increasing severity and younger age of onset when transmitted through the pedigree. Expansion occurs when the transmitting allele is paternal, which is why the severe early-onset juvenile form of the disease, seen with the largest expansions (70–121 repeats), is always paternally inherited.

Because HD most commonly presents after the end of the reproductive years, it is likely to be passed on by persons who carry the mutant gene and are unaware that they are at risk. Since the gene has been cloned, an area of presymptomatic testing has evolved. The complexity of this problem arises because there is no treatment or cure for HD and the disease carries such a serious prognosis. The ethical issues are beyond the scope of this review but are highlighted here to underscore the complexities of genetic testing and its consequences.

■ MYOTONIC DYSTROPHY

Myotonic dystrophy (DM) is an autosomal dominant multisystem disease characterized by dystrophic muscular weakness, with myotonia and distal muscle wasting. It is the most common form of an inherited myopathy, with an incidence of 1 in 8000. The clinical phenotype is highly variable, and patients often exhibit additional signs of cataracts, premature frontal balding, cardiac conduction abnormalities, and diabetes mellitus. The pattern of weakness is also characteristic—there is ptosis, neck flexor weakness, and bifacial weakness. There is proximal shoulder and hip girdle myopathic weakness, and there can also be distal wasting with myotonia at the thenar eminences. The disease is notorious for lack of penetrance and its variable expressivity even within the same generation. This disease also displays anticipation, sometimes leading to a congenital form of the disease that is associated with a very high neonatal mortality rate. Curiously, babies born with congenital myotonic dystrophy (CMD) are born almost always to affected mothers and not to affected fathers. These affected mothers may have only a mild phenotype and are often first diagnosed only in the newborn nursery when their baby is found to be severely affected. The disease is associated with a CTG expansion in the 3′ untranslated region of a protein kinase gene (DMPK) on chromosome 19. This gene encodes a serine/threonine kinase. The normal range for repeats in *DMPK* is 5 to 30. Mildly affected individuals (cataracts or frontal balding as a phenotype) have 50 to 80 repeats, and bifacial weakness and myopathy are seen when the repeat size is greater than 99. When the repeat size approximates the several hundreds range, diabetes and cardiac conduction abnormalities are present. Severely affected neonates can have up to 2000 copies. The disease displays somatic mosaicism (differing number of CTG repeats within different tissues of the same person, particularly with CMD). The DM phenotype is reproduced in a mouse model, in which the expanded CUG repeat is placed within a transgene encoding human skeletal actin, which is unrelated to *DMPK*. Toxic gain of function at the RNA level may be a general mechanism resulting in this phenotype.

■ FRIEDREICH'S ATAXIA

Friedreich's ataxia (FRDA), a spinocerebellar ataxia, constitutes a fourth category of trinucleotide repeat diseases. The disease is autosomal recessive and to date is the only known triplet repeat disease inherited in this manner. In most cases the expansion is a GAA repeat in an intron of a gene that encodes a mitochondrial protein called frataxin, which is involved in iron metabolism in the mitochondrion. The disorder usually presents before adolescence, but patients with this disorder have now been identified in their later 20s and 30s. Phenotypically, it is characterized by axial and appendicular ataxia, dysarthria, posterior column dysfunction, and the triad of pes cavus, areflexia, and extensor plantar responses. There is often associated scoliosis. The larger the GAA expansion, the more likely a patient is to develop diabetes and dilated cardiomyopathy. Repeat expansions are typically between the 100 and 1200 range. Expansion within the intron interferes with normal expression of the frataxin protein; because FRDA is recessive, loss of expression of both alleles is required to produce the clinical disease.

Genetics of Spinocerebellar Ataxia

We have discussed Friedreich's ataxia as an example of the only triplet repeat syndrome that is inherited as an autosomal recessive trait.

Autosomal dominant SCA syndromes have many more overlapping signs. They can be difficult to distinguish on clinical grounds. Common features to all include gait ataxia and dysarthria. Phenotypic features in some ataxias that may help define the syndrome include ocular dysmetria, extrapyramidal signs, peripheral nerve disease, intellectual decline, and seizures. These are features with some predictive value for specific gene defects (Fig. 29.6).

Autosomal Dominant Spinocerebellar Ataxias

- Now 28 syndromes and still accumulating
- 10 easily testable

Disease	Locus	Mutation
SCA1	6p22.3	CAG poly Q
SCA2	12q24.12	CAG poly Q
SCA3	14q32.21	CAG poly Q
SCA6	19p13.2	CAG poly Q
SCA7	3p14.1	CAG poly Q
SCA8	13q21.33	CTG/CAG
SCA10	22q13	ATTCT
SCA12	5q32	CAG
SCA14	19q13.4	Various mut
SCA17	6q27	CAG poly Q

■ **FIGURE 29.6** Autosomal dominant spinocerebellar ataxias.

■ GENETICS OF BASAL GANGLIA DISORDERS

Parkinson's disease (PD) can be inherited in an autosomal dominant or autosomal recessive manner; however, most cases of PD are thought to result from the effects of multiple genes and environmental risk factors.

To date, 10 monogenic Parkinson genes have been linked to a chromosome and 5 genes have been identified. The autosomal recessive PD with genes implicated include *parkin* (50% of all autosomal recessive disease), *PINK1*, and *DJ1*.

Mutations in three known genes *SCNA* (PARK1), *UCHL1* (PARK5), and *LRRK2* (PARK8) result in autosomal dominant PD. PARK1 (alpha-synuclein) was the first family described in the Italian families from Contursi and later found in some Greek kindreds. Phenotypically, this is younger age of onset PD, with a mean age onset of 46 years. This type of PD does have the presence of Lewy bodies and is levodopa responsive. Because of the paucity of mutations of *SCNA* identified in a large number of affected individuals who have been screened, it is now recognized that the mutation is not a common cause of familial PD.

The *UCHL1* gene (PARK5) has been identified in a single sibling pair in a German kindred, with a mean age of onset of approximately 50 years. There are conflicting results in the literature that this mutation may just represent a common polymorphism in the gene.

By far the most interesting is PARK8 or the *LRRK2* gene (leucine-rich repeat kinase 2), which encodes a protein kinase named dardarin (from *dardara,* the Basque word for tremor). The phenotype is late-onset, autosomal dominant, dopa responsive PD. A recent finding is the frequency of the G2019S *LRRK2* mutation, which accounts for 3% to 41% of familial late-onset PD.

In a letter published in the *New England Journal of Medicine* (January 2006 354;4:424–425), the authors mention that this mutation is responsible for autosomal dominant PD in 3% to 6% of cases with European ancestry. Among Ashkenazi Jews with PD, the frequency of this G2019S mutation was 18.3%. Among normal controls, the frequency of the allele was 1.3%. Most importantly, the mutation was present in nearly 30% of subjects defined as having an affected first-, second-, or third-degree relative. A very important issue to discuss, which is not as yet resolved, is the penetrance of this mutation in Ashkenazi families. The studies to date give estimates of 25% to 31%. Clinically, this has important consequences in counseling.

■ WILSON'S DISEASE

Wilson's disease (WD) is an autosomal recessive disorder of copper metabolism that can present with hepatic, neurological, or psychiatric disturbances, or a combination of these, in individuals ranging in age from 3 years to over 50 years; symptoms vary among and within families—a phenomenon known as phenotypic heterogeneity.

Neurological presentations include movement disorders (tremors, poor coordination, loss of fine-motor control, chorea, choreoathetosis) and rigid dystonia (mask-like facies, rigidity, gait disturbance, pseudobulbar involvement). Psychiatric disturbance includes depression, neurotic behaviors, disorganization of personality, and, occasionally, intellectual deterioration. Kayser-Fleischer rings result from copper deposition in Descemet's membrane of the cornea and reflect a high degree of copper storage in the body. The diagnosis of WD depends on the detection of low serum copper and ceruloplasmin concentrations, increased urinary copper excretion, the presence of Kayser-Fleisher rings in the cornea, and/or increased hepatic copper concentration. *ATP7B*, a copper-transporting P-type ATPase, is the only gene known to be associated with WD. Molecular genetic testing of the *ATP7B* gene is clinically available. The mutation detection rate varies depending on the test method and the individual's ethnicity. Molecular genetic testing is playing an increasingly important role in diagnosis because copper studies are frequently equivocal. Molecular genetic testing is important for determining the genetic status of at-risk siblings, so that copper chelation therapy may be offered before the onset of organ injury.

■ GENETICS OF ISCHEMIC STROKE

By far the majority of strokes that occur are nongenetic, that is, they result from cardiac risk factors such as hypertension. In the future, we will be able to identify individuals with polymorphisms in the genome that may function as risk factors for stroke, coupled with other gene-gene interactions, or gene-environment interactions. This is an ongoing work in progress. This section will review a few important mendelian and mitochondrial disorders that can cause ischemic stroke.

Fabry's Disease

Fabry's disease (FD) is an X-linked recessive lysosomal storage disorder caused by mutations in the alpha-galactosidase A gene. With a prevalence of 1 case per 117,000 live births, FD is the second most prevalent metabolic storage disorder after Gaucher disease. Affected males are unable to metabolize globotiaosylceramide (Gb3) normally, resulting in progressive lysosomal accumulation of Gb3 in vascular endothelial cells and smooth muscle cells. Organs involved include the brain, kidney, small unmyelinated nerve fibers in the skin, myocardium, dorsal root ganglion, and autonomic nervous system.

Clinical diagnosis is based on the presence of skin angiokeratomas, renal disease, and painful small fiber neuropathy. Stroke in patients with FD occurs in the third or fourth decade of life and usually involves the small vessels. Both small and large artery strokes can occur by the fifth decade of life and appear to be related to in-situ thrombosis of a small-caliber blood vessel with Gb3 deposits. However, this is not the only mechanism of stroke, because these patients get cardiac disease with left ventricular hypertrophy and hypertension. Replacement therapy with alpha-galactosidase A (Fabrazyme) has been shown to be of benefit in preventing renal disease and stroke, and there appears to be some benefit in the reduction of neuropathic pain.

Mitochondrial Encephalopathy, Lactic Acidosis, and Stroke-like Episodes

The mitochondrial DNA mutations that result in mitochondrial encephalopathy, lactic acidosis, and stroke-like episodes (MELAS) cause defects in the respiratory chain enzymes in complex I of the oxidation phosphorylation pathway. There is an A-G substitution at nucleotide position 3243 in the gene encoding tRNA leucine. Phenotypically, patients with MELAS present with stroke-like episodes, seizures, migraines, and severe lactic acidotic episodes. The stroke-like episodes have a predilection for the occipital lobes. The diagnosis of mitochondrial disease can also be made on muscle biopsy with ragged red fibers, which are pathognomonic.

Cerebral Autosomal Dominant Arteriopathy with Subcortical Infarcts and Leukoencephalopathy

Cerebral autosomal dominant arteriopathy with subcortical infarcts and leukoencephalopathy (CADASIL) is an autosomal dominant disorder associated with dementia, early-onset multiple strokes, and a history of migraine. The pathology is primarily in the white matter, and the changes seen on MRI can be confused with multiple sclerosis plaques. On electron microscopy, there are osmophilic granules deposited in the media of the vessels. The disease is caused by point mutations in the *Notch-3* gene. Stroke, dementia, psychiatric disease, and migraine are common features of CADASIL. The diagnosis can be approached pathologically, with the presence of vascular osmophilic granules seen on electron microscopy of the skin, muscles, and peripheral nerves.

Sickle Cell Disease

Sickle cell disease is an autosomal recessive disorder in which valine is substituted for glutamic acid at position 6 of the beta-polypeptide chain of hemoglobin. This is an important cause of stroke in children of African and African American descent. The mutation causes polymerization of aggregation of abnormal hemoglobin within red blood cells. In addition, they have compensated hemolytic anemia, mild jaundice, and vaso-occlusive pain crises. This is an important cause of stroke in young children and has been successfully treated with blood transfusions, intended to reduce the concentration of hemoglobin S levels to less than 30% of total hemoglobin.

KEY POINTS

Causes of stroke can be categorized as follows:
Mendelian
Cardioembolic:
   Familial atrial myxoma
   Familial dysrhythmias
   Cardiomyopathies
Thromboembolic:
   Homocystinuria
   Dyslipidemias
   Hemoglobinopathies
Prothrombotic states:
   Protein C/S/ATIII
   Prothrombin gene mutation
Small vessel diseases:
   CADASIL
   Fabry's disease
   Sickle cell disease
Mitochondrial disease:
   MELAS
Heart dissection:
   Marfan's
   Ehler's Danlos IV
Channelopathies:
   Familial hemiplegic migraine
Nonmendelian
Stroke as a multifactorial disorder
Complex trait (hypertension, diabetes, etc.)

■ GENETICS OF EPILEPSIES

Genetic factors have been recognized to play a role in epileptogenesis. Evidence comes from both animal studies and human data. In human studies, the information about the genetic contribution comes from twin studies, association studies, and some gene identification studies in mendelian forms of epilepsy with seizures as part of the phenotype.

Family studies show an increased risk of epilepsy (2.5%) in relatives of patients with epilepsy compared with the general population. The risk is greater for relatives of probands with generalized epilepsies than for relatives of probands with partial seizures.

Twin studies have shown concordance rates for epilepsy of 50% to 60% in monozygotic twins and 15% in dizygotic twins. Concordance rates are higher in the generalized seizure disorders than in partial epilepsies.

What is important to remember is that although the identification of genes involved in monogenic epilepsies has given important insights into the pathophysiology of the disease, these monogenic epilepsies account for only 1% to 2% of all human epilepsies, with the large majority being complex multifactorial disorders (Fig. 29.7).

Some of the genetic syndromes associated with single gene disorders are outlined in Table 29.3.

Genetics of Epilepsy Summary

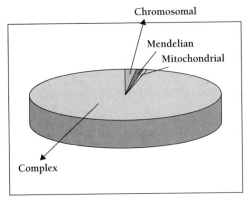

■ **FIGURE 29.7** Genetics of epilepsy.

TABLE 29.3 GENETIC SYNDROMES ASSOCIATED WITH SINGLE GENE DISORDERS

Genetic disorders that cause epilepsy as a major manifestation (symptomatic causes of epilepsy)

Malformations

    Tuberous sclerosis

    Subcortical band heterotopia

Degenerative conditions

Childhood degenerative diseases

    Progressive myoclonic epilepsy

    Unverricht-Lundborg

    Neuronal ceroid lipofuscinoses

    Lafora body disease

Mitochondrial disorders

Single gene epilepsies: Individually rare, usually clinically distinctive, usually autosomal dominant

    Benign familial neonatal convulsions

    Two genes, potassium channel mutations

    Autosomal dominant nocturnal frontal lobe epilepsy

    Acetylcholine receptor subunit mutation

    Generalized epilepsy/febrile seizures syndrome

    Several loci; heterogeneous clinical syndromes may be common

        Gamma-aminobutyric acid (GABA) receptor mutations in two pedigrees

    Sodium channel mutation (SCN1)

    Mendelian forms of focal seizures

    Temporal lobe epilepsy with auditory features mapping to chromosome 10q but not cloned yet

    Other single-gene syndromes

    Epilepsy with more complex genetic characteristics

    Juvenile myoclonic epilepsy predisposition mapping to chromosome 6

    Childhood absence epilepsy

    Juvenile absence epilepsy

    Rolandic epilepsy

■ GENETICS OF MITOCHONDRIA

Mitochondria are unique organelles with their own genome, which is a 16.6-kb circular molecule with no introns. There are three important functions of mitochondria within a cell. The first critical function is the production of adenosine triphosphate via an intricate series of oxidative phosphorylation pathways mediated by five complexes. During this process, the mitochondria produce reactive oxygen species, which function as important antioxidants. The third important function of the oxidative phosphorylation pathway is to activate genes that induce apoptosis within a cell.

Mechanisms of mitochondrial inheritance have been explained earlier in the chapter. The most important principles to underscore are heteroplasmy, which is the mixing of wild-type and mutant mitochondria within a cell, explaining the heterogeneity of the phenotype, and strict maternal inheritance. Mitochondrial DNA is particularly susceptible to mutations and has 10-fold the mutation rate of nuclear DNA. This is thought to be due to the fact that there are no histones in mitochondria and there is a less effective DNA repair mechanism.

Virtually all tissues and organ systems depend on oxidative metabolism and may therefore be affected in these disorders. Highly oxidative tissues, such as the nervous system and eye, are most prominently affected. These include the following:

Central nervous system: Seizures, myoclonus, ataxia, stroke-like episodes (MELAS), dementia, Leigh's disease, some migraines, Leber's hereditary optic neuropathy, chronic progressive external ophthalmoplegia, Kearn-Sayer syndrome
Peripheral nervous system: Myopathy (myoclonus epilepsy with ragged red fibers [MERRF]), neuropathy (axonal and demyelinating)
Somatic: Endocrine (diabetes mellitus, thyroid disease), cardiac (heart block, cardiomyopathy), deafness, renal disease, short stature

There are sensitive and specific tests for many of the mitochondrial diseases. Most mtDNA point mutation–mediated diseases can be diagnosed noninvasively by blood test. mtDNA deletion–mediated disease requires skeletal muscle biopsy as the source of DNA for molecular genetic testing. This testing provides a rational basis for genetic counseling. The counseling issues are complex. There are marked intrafamilial and interfamilial variability with diseases such as MELAS and MERRF, making counseling difficult because some single mtDNA deletions are nearly always sporadic.

■ FUTURE OF GENETIC MEDICINE

The last half of the 20th century began with the discovery of Mendel's laws of inheritance and their application to human biology and medicine and culminated in the Human Genome Project. For the first time in history, *Homo sapiens* has a complete inventory of its genes, which will allow expanding knowledge in which various diseases and disease predispositions will be attributed to each variation within the genome.

■ GENERAL WEBSITE REFERENCES

McKusick VA. Online mendelian inheritance in man. Available at: http://www3.ncbi.nlm.nih.gov: A complete catalog of autosomal dominant, recessive and X-linked phenotypes.
University of Washington: Gene Tests. Available at: http://www.genetests.org: Good site for review articles; lists laboratories that offer genetic testing for both clinical and research purposes.

■ GENERAL REFERENCE

Nussbaum RL, McInnes RR, Willard HF, eds. *Thompson and Thompson Genetics in Medicine.* 7th ed. Philadelphia: WB Saunders; 2007.

■ **REFERENCES SPECIFIC TO PARTICULAR TOPICS**

Berkovic SF, Howell RA, Hay DA, et al. Epilepsies in twins: genetics of the major epilepsy syndromes. *Ann Neurol* 1998;43:435–445.

Bird TD. Gene clinics. Available at: http://www.geneclinics.org/profiles/alzheimer/details.html.

Campuzano V, Montermini L, Moltò MD, et al. Friedreich's ataxia: autosomal recessive disease caused by an intronic GAA triplet repeat expansion. *Science* 1996;271:1423–1427.

DiMauro S, Moraes CT. Mitochondrial encephalomyopathies. *Arch Neurol* 1993;50:1197–1208.

Dürr A, Cossee M, Agid Y, et al. Clinical and genetic abnormalities in patients with Friedreich's ataxia. *N Engl J Med* 1996;335:1169–1175.

Hassan A, Markus HS. Genetics and ischaemic stroke. *Brain* 2000;123:1784–1812.

Joseph JT, Richards CS, Anthony DC, et al. Congenital myotonic dystrophy pathology and somatic mosaicism. *Neurology* 1997;49:1457–1460.

Joutel A, Corpechot C, Ducros A, et al. *Notch*3 mutations in CADASIL, a hereditary adult-onset condition causing stroke and dementia. *Nature* 1996;383:707–710.

Hagerman RJ, Leavitt BR, Farzin F, et al. Fragile-X-associated tremor/ataxia syndrome (FXTAS) in females with the FMR1 premutation. *Am J Hum Genet* 2004;74:1051–1056.

The Huntington's Disease Collaborative Research Group. A novel gene containing a trinucleotide repeat that is expanded and unstable on Huntington's disease chromosomes. *Cell* 1993;72:971–983.

Kamboh MI. Molecular genetics of late-onset Alzheimer's disease. *Ann Hum Genet* 2004;68(Pt4):381–404.

Lucking CB, Dürr A, Bonnet AM, et al. Association between early-onset Parkinson's disease and mutations in the *parkin* gene. *N Engl J Med* 2000;342:1560–1567.

Morris HR, Khan MN, Janssen JC, et al. The genetic and pathological classification of familial frontotemporal dementia. *Arch Neurol* 2001;58:1813–1816.

Selkoe D. The genetics and molecular pathology of Alzheimer's disease. *Neurol Clin* 2000;18:903–921.

Tiraboshi P, Hansen LA, Masliah E, et al. Impact of APOE genotype on neuropathologic and neurochemical markers of Alzheimer's disease. *Neurology* 2004;62:1977–1983.

Tsuang DW, Bird TD. Genetics of dementia. *Med Clin North Am* 2002;86:591–614.

Neurological Complications of Systemic Disease

■ CARDIOLOGY

Rheumatic valvular disease	Embolism
Infective endocarditis	Septic embolism
	Hemorrhage
	Mycotic aneurysm
	Meningitis
	Abscess
	Encephalopathy
Coronary artery disease	Embolism
Myocardial infarction	
Aortic stenosis	Syncope
Nonbacterial endocarditis	Embolism
Libman-Sacks endocarditis	Embolism
Arrhythmia	Syncope

■ AORTIC DISORDERS

Aneurysm	Recurrent laryngeal palsy
	Cord/cauda ischemia
Dissection	Cord/cauda ischemia
Aortitis	Central nervous system vasculitis

■ HYPERTENSION

Hypertension is a risk factor	Cerebral hemorrhage
	Large vessel atheroma
	Small vessel ischemia (lacunae)
Hypertensive encephalopathy	Encephalopathy
	Focal deficit ischemia or hemorrhage

■ HEMATOLOGY

Red Blood Cells

Polycythemia	Headache
	Vertigo
	Chorea
	Cerebral infarction

Anemia	
Iron deficiency	Restless legs
	Pica
	Papilledema/retinal hemorrhages
Megaloblastic	Peripheral neuropathy
	Subacute combined degeneration
	Encephalopathy
Hemoglobinopathies	
Extramedullary hematopoiesis	Cord compression
	Cranial neuropathy
	Ischemic stroke

White Blood Cells

Neutropenia	Infection
Leukemia	Hemorrhage
	Hyperviscosity
	Meningitis
	Neuropathy
Lymphoma	Mass lesion
	Meningitis
	Intravascular lymphoma with small strokes
	Compressive neuropathies
	Infection
Hypereosinophilia (idiopathic)	Encephalopathy
	Peripheral neuropathy
	Focal lesions
	Myalgia
Plasma cell dyscrasias	
Myeloma	Spinal fracture
	Cranial neuropathy
	Peripheral neuropathy
Waldenström	Hemorrhage/ischemia
	Encephalopathy
	Myelopathy
	Peripheral neuropathy
	Hyperviscocity
Amyloid	Peripheral neuropathy
Paraproteinemia/MGUS	Peripheral neuropathy
POEMS	Polyneuropathy
	Organomegaly
	Endocrinopathy
	M protein
	Skin rash
Cryoglobulinemia	Stroke/stroke-like
	Peripheral neuropathy
Coagulopathy	Hemorrhage
Disseminated intravascular coagulation	Encephalopathy
	Hemorrhage

■ RESPIRATORY DYSFUNCTION

Hypoventilation	Hypoxic encephalopathy
	Headache
	Papilledema
Hyperventilation	Dizziness
	Paresthesias
	Tetany

■ RENAL FAILURE

All causes	Encephalopathy
	Asterixis/myoclonus
	Seizures
	Coma

■ RHEMATOLOGICAL DISORDERS

Ankylosing spondylitis	Spinal fracture
	Cord/cauda compression
Disseminated lupus	Psychiatric changes
	Seizure
	Encephalopathy
	Stroke
	Chorea
	Myelitis
	Peripheral neuropathy
	Cerebellar ataxia
	Cranial neuropathy
Rheumatoid arthritis	Peripheral neuropathy
	Entrapment syndromes
Scleroderma	Myopathy
	Peripheral neuropathy
	Myelopathy
	Cerebrovascular disease
	Encephalopathy
Sjögren disease	Focal brain lesions (white matter)
	Encephalopathy
	Meningoencephalitis
	Psychiatric—usually affective
Vasculitides (e.g., polyarteritis, Churg Strauss)	Encephalopathy
	Stroke
	Headache
	Mononeuritis multiplex
Wegener granulomatosus	Visual loss
	Ocular palsy
	Arthralgia/myalgia
	Stroke

Giant cell arteritis

Headache
Visual loss
Stroke
Psychiatric changes

Behçet disease

Headache
Psychiatric changes
Focal deficits
Meningitis
Seizure

■ SARCOIDOSIS

Cranial Neuropathy
Aseptic meningitis
Hydrocephalus
Focal brain lesions
Myelopathy
Neuropathy
Myopathy

■ ONCOLOGY

Metastases

Focal brain lesions
Meningitis
Seizure
Myelopathy
Plexopathy
Neuropathy

Paraneoplastic syndromes

Encephalopathy
Peripheral neuropathy
Cerebellar ataxia
Opsoclonus/myoclonus
Lambert-Eaton syndrome
Polymyositis
Vasculitis
Limbic encephalitis
Motor neuron disease
Necrotizing myelitis

■ ENDOCRINE DISORDERS

Thyroid
    Hyperthyroidism

Myopathy
Periodic paralysis
Tremor
Chorea
Neuropathy
Exophthalmos
Seizure
Psychiatric changes
Atrial fibrillation with embolism
Myasthenia

Hypothyroidism	Encephalopathy (pseudodementia)
	Coma
	Seizure
	Ataxia
	Psychosis
	Peripheral neuropathy
	Carpal tunnel syndrome
Hashimoto disease	Encephalopathy

Parathyroid

Hyperparathyroidism	Depression
	Muscular weakness
	Anxiety
	Psychosis
	Coma
Hypoparathyroidism	Seizure
	Tetany
	Irritability
	Anxiety
	Depression

Diabetes

Hyperglycemia	Peripheral neuropathy
	Cranial neuropathy (pupil-sparing third nerve)
	Plexopathy
	Diabetic amyotrophy
	Thoracic radiculopathy
	Autonomic neuropathy
	Vascular complications
	Nonketotic hyperglycemic encephalopathy
	Ketotic coma
Hypoglycemia	Seizure
	Coma
	Focal deficits (e.g., hemiplegia)

■ ADRENAL DISORDERS

Hyperadrenalism (Cushing syndrome)	Pseudotumor
	Myopathy
	Psychosis
	Depression
Hypoadrenalism (Addison disease)	Memory dysfunction
	Apathy
	Confusion
	Muscle wasting
	Hyperkalemic periodic paralysis
Adrenoleukodystrophy	Peripheral neuropathy
	Myelopathy
	Posterior brain demyelination

■ GASTROINTESTINAL DISORDERS

Malabsorption	Peripheral neuropathy
	Tetany

Muscle weakness
Myedema
Myotonia
Ataxia
Subacute combined degeneration
Visual loss
Korsakoff psychosis

Liver failure   Confusion
                                       Coma
Pancreatic disease   Malabsorption
                                       Encephalopathy

■ PORPHYRIA

Syndrome of abdominal pain, followed by psychiatric dysfunction, followed by central nervous system deficits, followed by coma

Psychiatric manifestations   Insomnia
                                      Agitation
                                      Depression
                                      Hypomania
                                      Hallucinations
                                      Peripheral neuropathy

MGUS, monoclonal gammopathies of undetermined significance; POEMS, polyneuropathy, organomegaly, endocrinopathy, M protein, skin changes (syndrome).

Index

Italic pages indicate figures; pages with *t* indicate tables.